# Surgical Intervention in Corneal and External Diseases

# Surgical Intervention in Corneal and External Diseases

Edited by

## Richard L. Abbott, M.D.
Pacific Ophthalmic Consultants
Department of Ophthalmology
Pacific Presbyterian Medical Center
San Francisco, California

Illustrated by

## Steven J. Vermillion, M.D.
San Rafael, California

## Grune & Stratton, Inc.
Harcourt Brace Jovanovich, Publishers

| Orlando | New York | San Diego | London |
| San Francisco | Tokyo | Sydney | Toronto |

**Library of Congress Cataloging-in-Publication Data**

Surgical intervention in corneal and external diseases.

Includes index.
1. Cornea—Surgery.   2. Eyelids—Surgery.   3. Cornea—
Diseases—Treatment.   4. Eyelids—Diseases—Treatment.
5. Eye—Tumors—Treatment.   I. Abbott, Richard L.
[DNLM: 1. Cornea—surgery.   2. Corneal Diseases.   3. Eye—
surgery.   4. Eye Diseases.   WW 220 S961]
RE336.S87   1987        617.7'19        86-33505
ISBN 0-8089-1850-8

*Grune & Stratton, Inc.*
Orlando, Florida 32887

Distributed in the United Kingdom by
*Grune & Stratton, Ltd.*
24/28 Oval Road, London NW 1

Library of Congress Catalog Number 86-33505
International Standard Book Number 0-8089-1850-8
Printed in the United States of America
87  88  89  90   10  9  8  7  6  5  4  3  2  1

*To my wife, Chita, and our children, Galen, Alison, and Lauren,*
*for their love, understanding, and encouragement.*

# Contents

# Foreword

In managing patients with external-corneal disease problems, all too frequently the disease process does not respond to accepted methods of medical therapy. The ophthalmologist then needs to know the indications, the most appropriate techniques, and the anticipated course of surgical intervention. Hopefully, as we gain a better understanding of the pathophysiology of disease and utilize improved therapeutic modalities, the need for surgery will be reduced. In the meantime, all ophthalmologists are well served by familiarity with these surgical procedures.

Rich Abbott has selected a group of colleagues who are experienced in the surgical management of external disease. I am pleased to have worked with many of these contributors and to count them as friends, and I am honored to be able to recommend this unique text.

*Richard K. Forster, M.D.*
*Bascom Palmer Eye Institute*

# Preface

Indications for surgical intervention often are not clearly defined in disease processes affecting the cornea and external eye. Although most of these conditions are best treated medically, surgery does play a role when the pathologic process severely disrupts the integrity of the external ocular surface, when a lid or epibulbar tumor affects the function of the eye, or when an advancing melting process threatens the loss of the eye. This text provides the ophthalmologist with guidelines and recommendations for surgical intervention in both routine and complicated external ocular conditions. These conditions include eyelid malpositions and tumors, exposure keratopathy, keratoconjunctivitis sicca, recurrent and chronic epithelial defects, corneal edema, corneal perforations, tumors of the cornea and bulbar conjunctiva, pterygia, superior limbic keratoconjunctivitis, conjunctival cicatrizing disorders, scleritis, and endophthalmitis.

Each chapter presents background material on a specific condition, followed by recommendations for medical therapy. If medical treatment is not appropriate or successful, the rationale for surgical intervention is discussed along with the available surgical procedures to remedy the disease process. Surgical techniques are described and illustrated in detail, attempting to provide the clinician with a comprehensive atlas for both standard and new approaches to challenging corneal and external disease problems.

The primary goal of this project has been to produce a practical textbook and surgical atlas to be used by the clinician as a reference source in managing these difficult external ocular disorders. The contributors are respected authorities in their fields and have strived to present clear and concise information within their respective chapters. I wish to thank them for their dedication and hard work.

A major portion of this book is devoted to the many hand-drawn illustrations that appear throughout the text. Steve Vermillion worked above and beyond the "call of duty" to ensure that every detail on his drawings met the personal approval of each of the contributing authors as well as myself. He has been extremely dedicated, supportive, and diligent in his work, and I am very grateful for the privilege of working with him on this project.

I would like to extend my appreciation to my office staff, our fellows, and the residents at Pacific Presbyterian Medical Center, who frequently had to live with my excuses and delays because of my commitment to this book.

In addition, I would like to acknowledge the friendship and support of my colleagues at Pacific Ophthalmic Consultants, Wayne Fung, Bob Webster, Mike Allen, and Bill Stewart, who encouraged me in my work and stood by me throughout the entire process.

Finally, I would like to thank my father, Joseph C. Abbott, for providing me with a role model as a dedicated author and educator as well as a compassionate and sensitive human being.

# Contributors

**Richard L. Abbott, M.D.**
Pacific Ophthalmic Consultants
Department of Ophthalmology
Pacific Presbyterian Medical Center
San Francisco, California

**Walter E. Beebe, M.D.**
Cornea Associates of Texas
Dallas, Texas

**Michael W. Belin, M.D.**
Assistant Professor of Ophthalmology
Department of Ophthalmology
George Washington University Medical Center
Washington, D.C.

**J. Chandler Berg, M.D.**
Clinical Instructor
Department of Ophthalmology
Emory University
Albany, Georgia

**William W. Culbertson, M.D.**
Associate Professor
Department of Ophthalmology
Bascom Palmer Eye Institute
University of Miami School of Medicine
Miami, Florida

**David R. Demartini, M.D.**
Consultant, Corneal and External Diseases
Pacific Presbyterian Medical Center
Vice Chairman, Department of Ophthalmology
Highland General Hospital
Oakland, California

**Harry W. Flynn, Jr., M.D.**
Associate Professor
Department of Ophthalmology
Bascom Palmer Eye Institute
University of Miami School of Medicine
Miami, Florida

**Frederick T. Fraunfelder, M.D.**
Professor and Chairman
Department of Ophthalmology
Oregon Health Sciences University
Portland, Oregon

**Leslie J. Fujikawa, M.D.**
Director, Ocular Immunology/Uveitis
Department of Ophthalmology
Pacific Presbyterian Medical Center
San Francisco, California

**Ronald N. Gaster, M.D.**
Associate Adjunct Professor
Department of Ophthalmology
University of California, Irvine
Irvine, California

**Richard D. Grutzmacher, M.D.**
Assistant Professor
Department of Ophthalmology
University of Washington
Seattle, Washington

**Sadeer B. Hannush, M.D.**
Department of Ophthalmology
George Washington University
Washington, D.C.

**Alan Kozarsky, M.D.**
Assistant Professor
Department of Ophthalmology
Emory University School of Medicine
Chief of Ophthalmology
Grady Memorial Hospital
Atlanta, Georgia

**Thomas J. Liesegang, M.D.**
Associate Professor
Department of Ophthalmology
Mayo Clinic Jacksonville
Jacksonville, Florida

**Sid Mandelbaum, M.D.**
Assistant Clinical Professor
Department of Ophthalmology
Bascom Palmer Eye Institute
University of Miami School of Medicine
Miami, Florida
Assistant Attending Surgeon
Manhattan Eye, Ear, and Throat Hospital
New York, New York

**David M. Meisler, M.D.**
Department of Ophthalmology
Cleveland Clinic Foundation
Cleveland, Ohio


**Robert B. Nussenblatt, M.D.**
Chief, Laboratory of Immunology
National Eye Institute
National Institutes of Health
Bethesda, Maryland


**Edward J. Rockwood, M.D.**
Department of Ophthalmology
Cleveland Clinic Foundation
Cleveland, Ohio


**Ivan R. Schwab, M.D., F.A.C.S**
Associate Professor
Department of Ophthalmology
West Virginia University
Morgantown, West Virginia

**William B. Stewart, M.D.**
Pacific Ophthalmic Consultants
Director, Ophthalmic Plastic, Reconstructive and Orbital
    Surgery
Department of Ophthalmology
Pacific Presbyterian Medical Center
San Francisco, California


**Ira J. Udell, M.D.**
Assistant Professor
Department of Ophthalmology
State University of New York at Stony Brook
Physician-in-Charge, Division of Corneal and External
    Diseases
Long Island Jewish Medical Center
New Hyde Park, New York


**David W. Vastine, M.D.**
Consultant, Corneal and External Diseases
Pacific Presbyterian Medical Center
Chairman, Department of Ophthalmology
Highland General Hospital
Oakland, California


**Steven J. Vermillion, M.D.**
San Rafael, California

# Surgical Intervention in Corneal and External Diseases

# 1

# Trichiasis, Distichiasis, and Entropion

## William B. Stewart

The eyelids and the globe are an anatomic unit that depend on a homeostatic interrelationship to maintain normal functions. Any disruption of this relationship can result in problems.

The number and variety of lid abnormalities that may affect the cornea-conjunctiva are legion and include etiologic categories such as congenital–hereditary, dystrophic–degenerative, traumatic (including controlled trauma, i.e., surgery), infection–inflammation, neoplastic, iatrogenic, and idiopathic.

Lid and orbital abnormalities that contribute to ocular complications include not only entropion-trichiasis-distichiasis, but also ectropion, retraction-lagophthalmos, tissue loss, symblepharon, conjunctival surface abnormalities and mass lesions, proptosis-displacement, and lacrimal drainage system obstruction and infection.[19]

Entropion may be cicatricial, secondary to mucous membrane disease such as pemphigoid or Stevens-Johnson syndrome, or involutional and related to tissue laxity. Upper-lid entropion is seen more commonly in the developing countries secondary to trachoma or other infection. Surgery should be viewed as definitive, although other maneuvers may be required to maintain corneal integrity.

The in-turning of the lid margin that occurs with entropion produces direct trauma to the cornea and mechanical keratitis. A therapeutic soft contact lens, if tolerated, often is sufficient to heal the resultant keratitis. The offending lower lid can be temporarily everted to its normal anatomic position by taping the lid skin in the vertical direction to the infraorbital cheek. Mechanical epilation will also successfully remove the offending lashes, though this should be considered temporary and does not eliminate the contact of lid skin with the eye.

Trichiasis can occur without entropion in the form of misdirected or scarred aberrant follicles. Under these circumstances, mechanical epilation may be considered. A somewhat more permanent procedure, such as electrolysis of the lash follicle or cryotherapy to the offending area of the lid margin, should be considered in more extensive areas of involvement.

Distichiasis may be congenital or acquired. This condition is characterized by lashes that are more posterior on the lid margin (arising in metaplastic meibomian glands) and are directed toward the cornea. Until surgical correction, the best method for corneal protection is the application of a therapeutic soft contact lens. As with trichiasis, cryosurgery and electrolysis are effective measures for the ablation of distichiatic lashes.

## TRICHIASIS

*Trichiasis* is misalignment of the lashes where instead of being directed outward, they turn inward and come in contact with the cornea. Trichiasis is usually cicatricial, the cilia being malaligned as a result of posttraumatic, postinflammatory, degenerative, or other changes. Trichiasis frequently is associated with entropion (Fig. 1-1).

Because of the irritation it causes and probably because of its relationship to trachoma, trichiasis and its management have a long history. Complaints related to trichiasis and the recommended treatment by epilation date back to the 16th century B.C. At about 24 A.D., Celsus burned out the follicles with a red-hot needle. Ingenius operations were devised to relieve the condition. One procedure attributed by Duke-Elder to Paul of Aegina (7th century A.D.) consisted of grasping a fold of the involved eyelid skin between two pieces of reed or stick tied together so tightly that the skin underwent pressure necrosis and fell off with the stick, resulting in cicatricial ectropion and correction of the entropic lid position.[9]

Trichiasis may be localized or may involve the entire lid. The most common cause worldwide is undoubtedly trachoma. Other causes include external and internal hordeolum, blepharitis, the sequelae of chemical and thermal burns, and mechanical trauma. The initial corneal epithelial

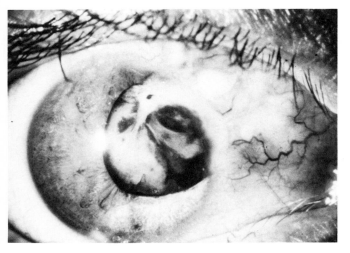

**Fig. 1-1.** Trichiasis: aberrant cilium, upper eyelid.

irritation may progress to enlarging areas of epithelial break-down, ulceration, vascularization, scarring with opacification, and resulting visual loss.

## DISTICHIASIS

*Distichiasis* is a form of polytrichia (increased number of lashes) and may be congenital or acquired. In congenital distichiasis, the cilia are usually arranged in two regular rows. The accessory lashes are present along the posterior lid lamella occupying the sites of the meibomian gland orifices. There may be only a few cilia, or a complete, well-formed row may be seen on one or more lids. The extra lashes may be small, soft, and with very little pigment, or they may be as fully developed as the normal (outer) row (Fig.1-2). Dominant inheritance has been reported.[10]

In patients with long-standing periocular inflammation, acquired distichiasis may develop. The cilia are usually stunted, fine, and nonpigmented. Magnification by use of the slit-lamp is often necessary to identify these lashes.[18]

Distichiatic cilia replace the meibomian glands, which become "modified" (metaplasia of the meibomian glands) and take on a hair-producing function. Because the meibomian glands are modified sebaceous glands and are ectodermally derived, as are hair follicles, the situation is one of heterotypical differentiation and is understandable embryologically.[10,18]

The importance of the condition, as with trichiasis, lies in the corneal irritation and damage that results. This irritation is usually less than what might be expected, because of the fineness of the lashes and the adjustment of the cornea to the chronic trauma. Many patients, although affected at birth, do not become symptomatic for many years. No treatment is necessary unless symptoms are significant and corneal changes have occurred.

## ENTROPION

*Entropion* is in-turning of the margin of the eyelid (Fig. 1-3). Unless entropion is accompanied by distichiasis or trichiasis, the lid margin itself is usually normal. In this condition, the problem lies in the malposition of the lid margin rather than in the cilia themselves.[11] Entropion may be present at birth or acquired. The cause of entropion relates to anatomic (lid laxity, cicatrix), physiologic (loss of innervation or tone of the orbicularis oculi muscle, orbicular spasm), and mechanical (presence of scar, mass) considerations. All of these possible causes must be recognized and carefully evaluated in planning treatment.[20]

## MANAGEMENT

The management of trichiasis and distichiasis depends on many factors and includes several modalities. The nature and activity of the inciting process causing the lash abnormality, which lids are involved, the number of lashes affected, the absence or presence of entropion, the severity of corneal changes, and whether the treatment is planned to achieve temporary or permanent relief must be considered

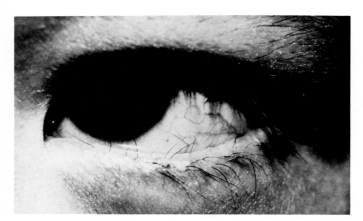

**Fig. 1-2.** Distichiasis, lower eyelid.

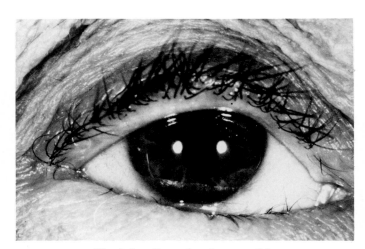

**Fig. 1-3.** Entropion, lower eyelid.

when a management protocol is being determined. In all situations, frank infection must be treated. If blepharospasm is present, causes (ocular and adnexal) should be sought and controlled.

Mechanical epilation of the lashes may be done for a few aberrant lashes and provides temporary relief. Epilating forceps, jeweler's forceps, and the Castroviejo needle holders, among many other instruments, have been employed with varied success. Mechanical epilation, however, cannot be expected to provide permanent destruction of the lash.

Electrolysis, employing galvanic or diathermy currents, when properly used, can permanently destroy follicles, but may result in significant scarring of the lid margin if too large an area is treated. Regrowth of lashes is common. A useful method used to destroy individual follicles involves the use of a battery-powered instrument. In this technique, magnification with a slit-lamp, operating microscope, or surgical loupes is useful to achieve proper placement of the electrolysis probe into the follicle shaft. Topical anesthesia may be instituted with 0.5% proparacaine, augmented by local application on the lid margin and palpebral conjunctiva of 4% lidocaine or subconjunctival or subcutaneous injection of a small volume of 0.5%–2% lidocaine with 1:200,000 epinephrine. Sufficient current should be applied to the follicle shaft base to produce bubbles in several seconds. When the follicle has been sufficiently destroyed, epilation can easily be done. This technique is useful when small segments of the lids are involved. Use of the laser for the treatment of localized trichiasis has also been described.[5]

When larger areas of the lid margin require treatment for distichiasis or trichiasis, cryosurgery is a valuable technique.[21,22] Unlike the treatment of basal cell carcinoma, which requires a liquid nitrogen system to achieve subcutaneous monitored tissue temperatures of −30°C or colder, a nitrous oxide-cooled probe may be used for the treatment of aberrant lashes. A high-flow nitrous oxide system with greater freezing capacity than the standard retina or cataract probe is recommended. Cryo-tips of various size and shape are available. Local anesthesia is instituted by injection with lidocaine/epinephrine solution. A thermocouple may be placed beneath the skin at the base of the lashes to be treated. A water-soluble lubricant or anesthetic drops are applied to enhance the probe–lid contact. The anterior or posterior lid margin is treated as indicated with a freeze-thaw-freeze technique. A tissue temperature of −20°C is considered satisfactory treatment for lash ablation. If a thermocouple is not used, a 30-second treatment application is recommended. Sullivan reported over 150 patients with trichiasis treated with cryosurgery with a recurrence rate of less than 10 percent. Retreatment is possible without undue risks and is usually successful.[22] From several lashes to an entire lid margin may be treated effectively by cryosurgery (Fig. 1-4). Surgically dividing the eyelid margin between its anterior (skin-muscle) and posterior (conjunctiva-tarsus) lamellae, as suggested by Anderson,[1] may aid in the preservation of normally positioned lashes, reduce the risk of cutaneous depigmentation, and allow more accurate placement of cryoapplications in distichiasis.

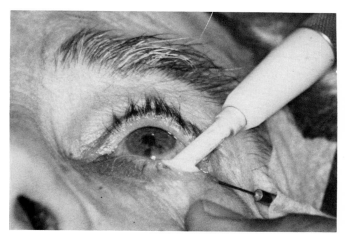

**Fig. 1-4.** Cryoablation of lashes, thermocouple needle visible laterally.

## Anatomic Considerations

The definitive management of extensive trichiasis or distichiasis and entropion causing injury to the eye will usually require surgery. In determining the proper surgical approach, careful evaluation of the anatomic disparities of the eyelids is essential. Classifying eyelid malposition usually includes categories such as cicatricial (those with scarring) and involutional (those with laxity). It is well known that a multitude of operations have been described for correcting eyelid malpositions. The "procedure of choice" can only be chosen when the anatomic abnormalities requiring correction are accurately recognized.

To this end, the eyelid can be considered to be made up of anterior (skin, orbicularis muscle) and posterior (tarsus, conjunctiva, eyelid retractors) lamellae. The status of these components of the lid structure must be determined in relationship to the lid malposition in the vertical and horizontal dimensions. Lid laxity, cicatrix, relative excesses, and inadequacies must be recognized. Because all entropion may superficially look the same, lid examination must be well directed and dynamic. The anatomic characteristics are generally readily identifiable by direct observation with or without magnification.

Evaluation of the vertical dimension of the anterior lid lamella involves assessment of skin excess or shortage. Similarly, the posterior lid lamella must be observed for scarring, inadequacy, or relative excess in comparison to the anterior lamella. The characteristic anatomic defect in cicatricial entropion is scarring, shortening of the posterior lid lamella relative to the anterior lamella. Cicatrical ectropion characteristically demonstrates shortening, scarring of the anterior lid lamella (skin).

Horizontal eyelid laxity is the anatomic abnormality commonly present in involutional entropion (and ectropion). When present, horizontal laxity should be considered as involving anterior and posterior lamellae. Its presence can be determined using several methods. Observing the presence of inferior displacement of the lower eyelid and inferior scleral show beneath the inferior limbus may provide evidence of lower eyelid laxity. Testing of springback forces reveals horizontal laxity. In this test the lower eyelid is gently drawn downward toward the cheek to distract it from the globe, and is then released. Normally the lower lid will "springback" to its normal position on the globe without the necessity of a blink. If horizontal laxity is present, however, the inferiorly retracted lid does not springback but slowly returns to its usual position, often requiring a blink to fully re-oppose to the globe. Gently pinching the lid and pulling it away from the eye can also be used to qualitatively and quantitatively assess horizontal lid laxity. Hill defined the lid as "flaccid" if it could be distracted more than 6 mm from the eye.[13]

When horizontal laxity is present as a component of eyelid malposition, a procedure designed to correct this anatomic disparity must be included in the surgical plan. Horizontal laxity can also be present in association with cicatricial changes of either the anterior and/or posterior lamellae. When significant cicatrical changes are present, the surgical procedure must reposition, rotate the abnormally positioned lid segments, and/or provide substitute tissue (grafts, flaps) to properly reconstruct the lid. The amount of lid retraction and the thickness and extent of tarsal irregularity must also be ascertained.[8]

The confusing list of procedures that have been described to manage eyelid malpositions can better be understood in light of the anatomic features contributing to the malpositions. An operation can then be selected or designed employing the proper procedures to correct the identified abnormalities (Table 1-1).

## SURGICAL APPROACH

Segmental trichiasis with entropion involving one-forth of the lid or less may be treated by a full-thickness resection of the involved segment of eyelid and primary repair of the lid margin and resultant full-thickness vertical lid defect.

Localized lid splitting and recession of the anterior lamella of skin and muscle, which is then fixed to the tarsus, is another method of displacing trichiatic lashes on a segment of the lid.[12] Infiltrative subcutaneous anesthesia is used. A gray line incision is made and extended beyond the extent of diseased lid margin. The dissection is carried along the anterior tarsal surface for up to the full vertical dimension of the tarsus. The bases of abnormal lashes are exposed, redirected, or ablated as necessary. The skin-muscle is then sutured to the anterior surface of the tarsus 3 mm from the lid margin, effecting a recession of the anterior lid lamella. The redundant skin-muscle above or below the recession is excised, and the skin is closed with running or interrupted sutures.

With extensive trichiasis of distichiasis (without entropion), not thought amenable to treatment by cryotherapy, the area of lid margin including the abnormal lash roots can be excised. Long, narrow mucous membrane grafts from the mouth (lip, cheek) or conjunctival cul-de-sac (if normal conjunctiva is available) can then be secured to the bed of the denuded lid margin with fine (7-0, 8-0) running monofilament sutures begun and completed on the cutaneous surface of the lid.[14]

The eyelid suture technique is a useful procedure for achieving lid-margin rotation in the absence of severe cicatrix or significant horizontal lid laxity (Fig. 1-5).[15] Double-armed sutures of absorbable material are passed full thickness through the lid in a horizontal mattress fashion beginning on the conjunctival surface at or below the antimarginal tarsal border. Traction is placed on the skin to rotate the lid margin as the needles are passed from conjunctiva to cutaneous surface. The sutures are tied tightly without bolsters and allowed to resorb. The procedure is effective because it creates a scar between the anterior and posterior lid lamellae, enhancing the effect of the lower eyelid retractors on the anterior portion of the lid and lid margin. Where significant horizontal lid laxity is present, full-thickness horizontal shortening must be combined with or substituted for this procedure. When a horizontal shortening procedure is

**Table 1-1**
Eyelid Malposition and Anatomic Disparity

| Lid Malposition | Vertical Abnormality | | Horizontal Abnormality |
| | Anterior Lamella | Posterior Lamella | Anterior & Posterior Lamella |
| --- | --- | --- | --- |
| Entropion | | | |
| Cicatrical | Normal or excess | Scarred or inadequate | Normal or laxity |
| Involutional | Normal or excess | Ok | Laxity |
| Ectropion | | | |
| Cicatricial | Scarred or inadequate | Ok | Normal or laxity |
| Involutional | Normal or inadequate | Ok or excessive | Laxity |

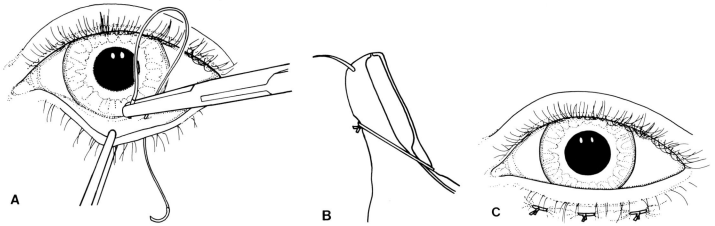

**Fig. 1-5.** Suture repair of lower eyelid entropion. (A) Transconjunctival placement of horizontal mattress sutures. (B) Cross-section of suture positioning. (C) Sutures tied on cutaneous surface of lid without bolsters effecting marginal rotation.

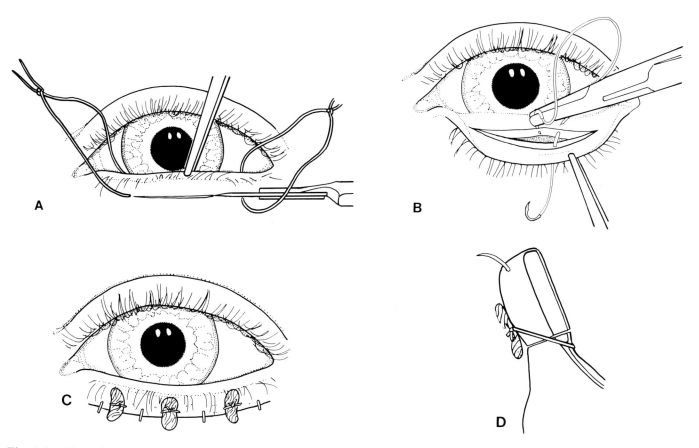

**Fig. 1-6.** Entropion repair of lower eyelid by marginal rotation (Wies procedure). (A) Full-thickness transverse blepharotomy. (B) Suture placement of horizontal mattress sutures beginning inferiorly in posterior lamella from conjunctival surface then passing through anterior lamella superiorly. (C) Sutures tied on cutaneous surface over bolsters. (D) Cross-section of suture positioning.

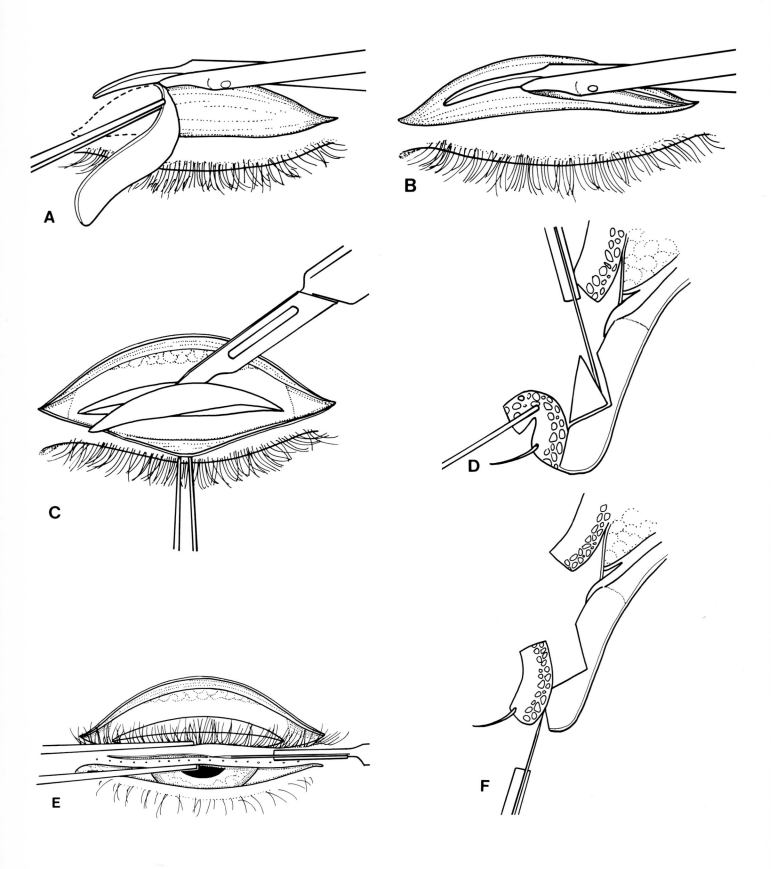

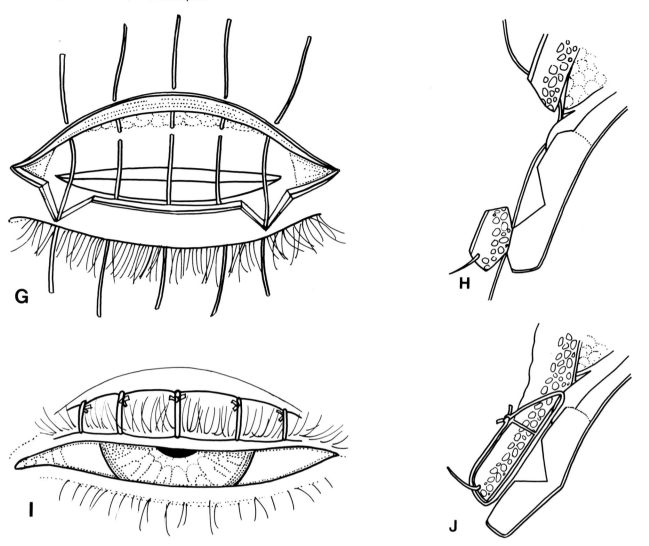

**Fig. 1-7.** Repair of upper-eyelid entropion by procedure of Cuenod-Natef. (A) Excision of skin. (B) Incision of orbicular muscle. (C) Exposure and excision of wedge of tarsus. (D) Cross-section of tarsal exposure and excision. (E) Lid-margin incision. (F) Cross-section of lid margin incision. (G) Suture placement from lid-margin incision to superior aspect of tarsus-levator to upper skin muscle edge. (H) Cross-section of suture placement. (I) Sutures tied effecting lid-margin rotation and recession of anterior lamella. (J) Cross-section of repair.

warranted, a procedure done in the lateral aspect of the lid-lateral canthal tendon complex is preferred.[2,24]

When a more pronounced cicatricial component is present in the posterior lid lamella, procedures designed to rotate the lid margin off the globe are indicated. These may involve direct marginal rotation as accomplished by the Wies procedure in the lower eyelid or tarsal fracture such as the Cuenod-Natef procedure in the upper eyelids. Or, interposition of tissue (e.g., eye bank sclera, tarsus, auricular or nasal cartilage) can be done to increase the vertical length of the posterior lid lamella and thereby allow rotation of the inturned, lash-bearing lid margin off the eye.

In circumstances in which the tarsus is adequately thick and with appropriate vertical length, tarsal rotation or fracture procedures can be elected. However, if there is significant lid retraction, or vertical tarsal shortening or thinness, a posterior lamellar graft must be done.

The Wies procedure[26] corrects entropion of the lower eyelid by effecting a marginal rotation (Fig. 1-6). A full-thickness transverse incision is made across the horizontal extent of the lateral two-thirds to three-fourths of the lid 4 mm from the margin (transverse blepharotomy). Care must be exercised to maintain the incision perpendicular to the skin and conjunctival surfaces, and to avoid angling or sloping of the incision. Double-armed nonabsorbable sutures (Wies used 5-0 silk) are then placed in horizontal mattress fashion, passing first through the inferior cut edge of the conjunctiva, which may include a portion of the tarsus and does include the lower eyelid retractors. The arms of the sutures, which are about 3 mm apart, are then brought through the superior aspect of the skin muscle incision and tied over small cotton bolsters. Three or four such sutures are placed. The skin edges are further reapproximated as necessary with interrupted sutures. The sutures are removed

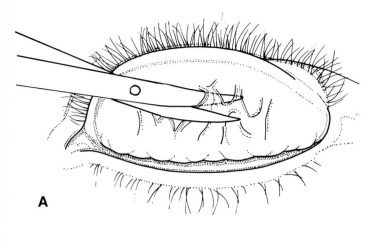

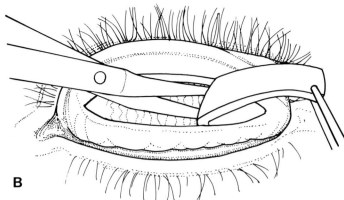

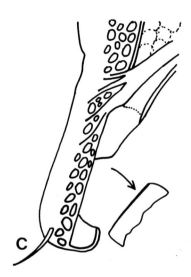

in 5–7 days. If marked overcorrection results, the bolsters can be released or the sutures removed early.

Quickert combined the principle of the Wies operation with a full-thickness horizontal lid shortening.[16] This combined procedure is indicated when significant horizontal lid laxity accompanies the entropion and trichiasis related to cicatricial factors.

Where adequate tarsus is present, rotation of the abnormal or malpositioned lid margin of the upper eyelid is effectively accomplished by the procedure of Cuenod and Natef,[23] or procedures similar in concept. This operation has been widely used in Tunisia in the surgical management of entropion and trichiasis secondary to trachoma. In this technique (Fig. 1-7), excess upper-eyelid skin is excised with the inferior aspect of the skin incision about 4 mm above and parallel to the lid margin. At this level, the dissection is carried to the anterior tarsal surface. A wedge of partial-thickness tarsus 3–4 mm wide is excised across the horizontal extent of the lid. A gray line incision is then made to a depth of 1–2 mm across the horizontal extent of the lid. The lid is divided into thirds. At each site, a 4-0 silk suture is introduced into the lid margin groove and passed superiorly on the anterior tarsal surface. The levator aponeurosis above the tarsal groove is

engaged and the suture is then passed through the upper aspect of the skin incision. The three 4-0 silk sutures are tied in their exposed position, resulting in redirection and rotation of the inferior aspect of the tarsus and recession of the anterior lid lamella at the lid margin. More deep sutures can be used if desired. The medial and lateral aspects of the incision are trimmed and closed with interrupted cutaneous sutures, as necessary.

If the tarsus is severely scarred with vertical shortening and lid retraction, lengthening of the posterior lid lamella is required. Resurfacing of the palpebral conjunctiva may also be necessary. The disparity in vertical length between the anterior lid lamella and the scarred, contracted posterior lid lamella can be corrected by release of the posterior lamella scar by a horizontal tarsal incision and interposition of graft material as tarsoconjunctival substitute. Among other donor tissues, nasal septum with mucosa,[7] eye bank sclera,[17] tarsus,[3] and auricular cartilage[4] have been employed. Tissue for mucous membrane resurfacing may be obtained from the mouth[14] or may be better accomplished using free conjunctival grafts[25] when available. Posterior lamellar grafting is particularly useful in the upper eyelid, but may also be used in the lower eyelid (Fig. 1-8).

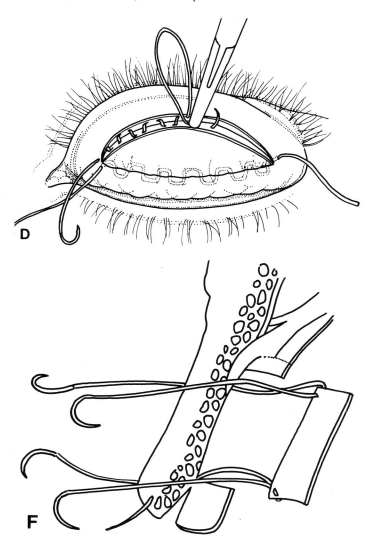

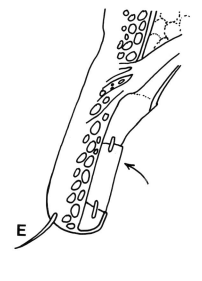

**Fig. 1-8.** Posterior lamella graft for correction of cicatricial entropion of upper eyelid. (A) & (B) Release of tarsconjunctival scarring. (C) Cross-section of posterior lamellar release. (D) Interposition of graft with intratarsal, subconjunctival closure. (E) Cross-section of graft interposition. (F) Lid-margin incision and full-thickness everting stitches between posterior lamellar graft and anterior lid lamella may be necessary.

An incision on the tarsoconjunctival surface of the lid is made several millimeters above the lid margin. The recipient bed is opened, scarred tissue is excised, and the lid is allowed to straighten and evert. This may require dissection at the level of levator aponeurosis, orbital septum, or orbicular muscle and must be complete enough to release lid retraction and malposition. Donor material is secured in the recipient bed by running sutures, mattress sutures, or both. Directing interrupted, horizontal mattress sutures from graft through the skin can aid in everting the lid margin. When these procedures need to be combined with horizontal shortening procedures to alleviate horizontal laxity, full-thickness shortening in the lateral canthal tendon complex is generally preferred. Many procedures have been described to accomplish full-thickness eyelid shortening in the lateral canthal tendon complex including those of Bick,[6] Tenzel,[24] and Anderson.[2]

The essence of these procedures includes defining a tarso-tendinous lateral strap of eyelid tissue, shortening it to proper length, and reattaching the strap/strip to the lateral periorbita (Fig. 1-9). The procedure may be done beneath a skin or skin-muscle flap if skin excision is contemplated or via an expanded lateral canthotomy. Epithelial elements

(e.g., cilia, skin and conjunctiva) must be excised from the strap. The inferior attachments of the lid (i.e., to orbital septum) should be lysed to allow upward as well as lateral release of the lid. The lid should be shortened so that apposition to the globe is secure and gentle traction on the lid margin does not distract the lid from the eye. The periosteum at the lateral orbital rim should be defined to the level of the superior limb of the lateral canthal tendon, often to the level of the inferior portion of the lacrimal gland. Intraoperatively, with the patient looking straight ahead, the reattachment should be at a height approximately even with the midpoint of the pupil. The lateral aspects of the lid should literally be directed superiorly to prevent lateral scleral show. Reattachment of the tendon strap should be made to the inner aspect of the lateral rim periosteum. The use of a double-armed, nonabsorbable suture with small full-curve needles is helpful. Skin remodeling, excision, and closure will depend on the nature and extent of the particular patient's anatomic findings.

Careful assessment of the anatomic abnormalities contributing to lid and lash malposition must be part of the evaluation of the irritated eye and will aid in the selection of the most appropriate corrective course of management.

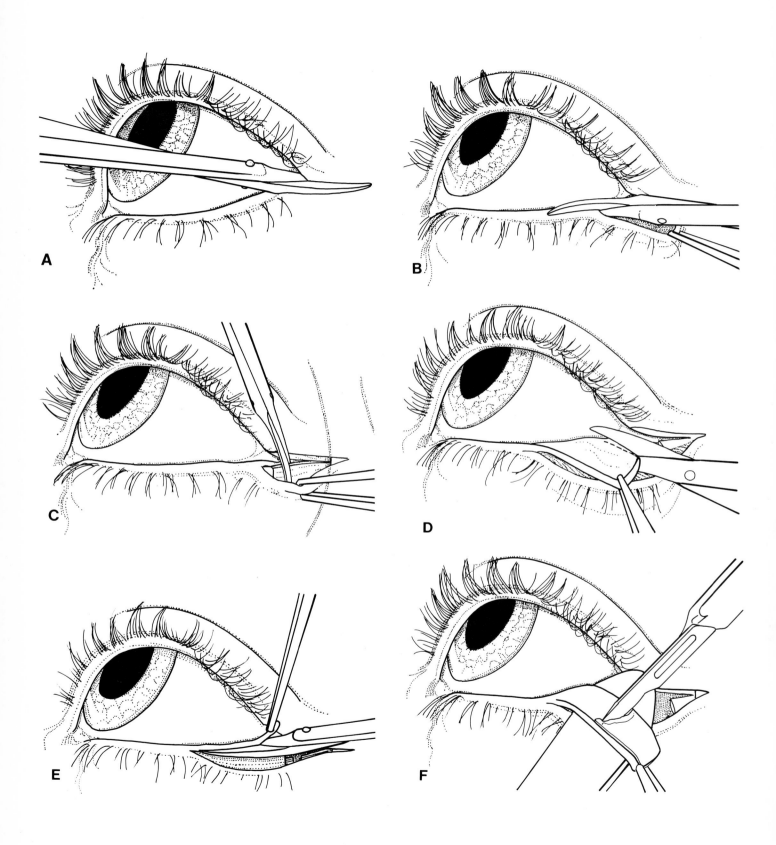

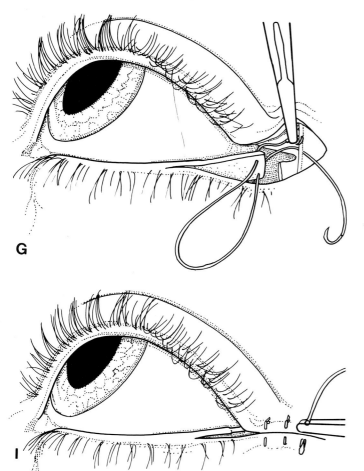

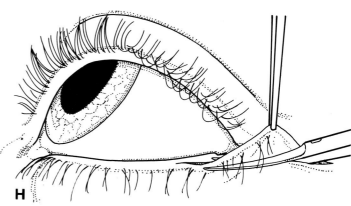

**Fig. 1-9.** Full-thickness horizontal lid shortening and refixation of lateral canthal tendon. (A) Canthotomy or lateral laugh-line incision. (B) Skin or skin-muscle mini-flap elevated. (C) Lateral cantholysis adjacent to lateral orbital rim. (D) Inferior aspect of "strap" released. (E) Marginal elements of lid excised. (F) Conjunctiva scraped from posterior aspect of "strap." (G) Strap cut to proper length and fixated to inner aspect of lateral orbital rim periosteum. (H) Excess skin resected. (I) Cutaneous closure.

## REFERENCES

1. Anderson RL Harvey, JT.: Lid splitting and posterior lamella cryosurgery for congenital and acquired distichiasis. Arch Ophthalmol 99:631–634, 1981

2. Anderson RL, Gordy DD: The tarsal strip procedure. Arch Ophthalmol 97:2192–196, 1979

3. Baylis HI, Hamako C: Tarsal grafting for correction of cicatricial entropion. Ophthalmic Surg 10:42–148, 1979

4. Baylis HI, Rosen N, Neuhaus RW: Obtaining auricular cartilage for reconstructive surgery. Am J Ophthalmol 93:709–712, 1982

5. Berry J: Recurrent trichiasis: Treatment with laser photocoagulation. Ophthalmic Surg 19:36–38, 1979

6. Bick MW: Surgical management of orbital tarsal disparity. Arch Ophthalmol 75:386–389, 1966

7. Callahan A: Correction of entropion from Stevens-Johnson syndrome. Arch Ophthalmol 94:1154–155, 1976

8. Collin JRO: Entropion and trichiasis, in Stewart WB (ed): Ophthalmic Plastic and Reconstructive Surgery. Rochester, AAO Manual, 1984, pp 131–142

9. Duke-Elder S, MacFaul PA: The ocular adnexa. Vol XIII, in Duke-Elder S (ed): System of Ophthalmology, Vol XIII. St. Louis, Mosby, 1964, pp 383–385

10. Duke-Elder S: Normal and abnormal development. Congenital deformity, in Duke-Elder S (ed): System of Ophthalmology, Vol III. St. Louis, Mosby, 1964, pp 873–876

11. Duke-Elder S, MacFaul PA: The ocular adnexa. in Duke-Elder S (ed): System of Ophthalmology, Vol XIII. St. Louis, Mosby, 1964, pp 573–580

12. Fein W: Surgical repair for distichiasis, trichiasis and entropion. Arch Ophthalmol 94:809–810, 1979

13. Hill JC: Treatment of epiphora owing to flaccid eyelids. Arch Ophthalmol 97:323, 1979

14. Leone CR: Treatment of conjunctival diseases and chalazion, in Stewart WB (ed): Ophthalmic Plastic and Reconstructive Surgery, Rochester, AAO Manual, 1984, pp 289–301

15. Quickert MH, Rathbun JE: Suture repair of entropion. Arch Ophthalmol 85:304, 1971

16. Quickert MH: The eyelids: Malposition of the lid, in Sorsby A (ed): Modern Ophthalmology (ed 2) Philadelphia, Lippincott, 1972, pp 937–954

17. Rubenzik R, Tenzel RR, Miller GR: Repair of cicatricial entropion of upper eyelid. Am J Ophthalmol 80:302–303, 1975

18. Schie HG, Albert DM: Distichiasis and trichiasis: Origin and Management. Am J Ophthalmol 61:718–720, 1966

19. Schwab LR, Abbott RL, Vastine DW, et al. Ocular complica-

tions of eyelid and orbital abnormalities. in Stewart WB (ed): Ophthalmic Platic and Reconstructive Surgery, Rochester, AAO Manual, 1984, p 63–69

20. Stewart WB: Trichiasis, distichiasis and entropion: Definition and Management. Trans Pac Coast Otoophthalmol Soc Annu Meet 61:113–123, 1980

21. Sullivan JG, Beard C, Bullock JD: Cryosurgery for the treatment of trichiasis. Am J Ophthalmol 82:117–21, 1976

22. Sullivan JH, Cryosurgery in ophthalmic practice. Ophthalmic Surg 10:37–41, 1979

23. Tenzel RR: Repair of entropion of upper lid. Arch Ophthalmol 77:675, 1969

24. Tenzel RR: Treatment of lagophthalmos of the lower eyelid. Arch Ophthalmol 81:366–368, 1969

25. Vastine DW, Stewart WB, Schwab I: Reconstruction of periocular mucous membrane by autologous conjunctival transplantation. Ophthalmol 89:1072–1081, 1981

26. Wies FA: Spastic entropion. Trans Am Acad Ophthalmol Otolaryngol 59:503, 1955

# 2

# Tumors of the Eyelids

## Thomas J. Liesegang

The majority of eyelid tumors are commonly found in other areas of the skin (e.g., squamous cell carcinoma, basal cell epithelioma, nevi, papilloma, and seborrheic keratoses). There are a number of lesions present by virtue of the unique local lid anatomy (e.g., sebaceous cell carcinoma, chalazion, and sweat gland tumors). This chapter focuses on the common tumors of the epidermis and adnexal glands of the lids. There are a variety of less common tumors of the nerves (e.g., neurofibromas, neuromas, and schwannomas), vascular system (e.g., capillary hemangiomas, varices, and arterial venous malformations), lymphoid system (e.g., lymphangiomas and lymphomas), and dermal system (e.g., dermatofibromas), which are not addressed here. The clinical characteristics of lid tumors, their biological behavior, important differentiating features, and the clinical approach to diagnosis and definitive therapy are offered. The specific histopathologic features are briefly addressed, but are presented elsewhere in detail.[2,43,75,89] The clinician must work closely with the pathologist in solving some difficult diagnostic problems.

## CLINICAL EVALUATION OF EYELID LESIONS

The history and behavior of lid lesions may offer a definitive clue as to the etiology. Benign lesions of the eyelid are much more common than malignant tumors. Eyelid lesions with a long history are generally benign; evaluation of prior photographs may allow accurate dating of the lesions. Lesions with a rapid onset or rate of growth are likely to be inflammatory or one of the benign reactive epithelial proliferations. Lesions of insidious onset or growth pattern with a history of bleeding or change in color are more characteristic of malignant lesions. Other clinical features to suggest malignancy include loss of the eyelashes, ulceration, changes in size, contour, and recurrence within a previous incision. There is a high incidence of skin tumors in patients after renal transplantation.[76] A cutaneous horn is a descriptive term with multiple clinical causes including actinic keratosis, seborrheic keratosis, squamous cell carcinoma, and others. The age of the patient, the history of prior lesions, the history of surgical or radiation therapy, or significant exposure to the sun may suggest more specific etiologies.

Evaluation of the lesion with a strong handlight, complemented by the biomicroscope, will frequently finalize the diagnosis. The soft tissues and the bony orbital rim should be palpated. Conjunctival surfaces need to be evaluated for multicentric tumors, such as sebaceous cell carcinoma or melanoma. Except for the basal cell epithelioma, the malignancies have a potential to spread by regional metastases to preauricular, submandibular, and cervical lymph nodes. Photographs, detailed drawings, and measurements of the lesion are important in documenting and then following the lesion. This is especially important if a biopsy is taken because it may be difficult to locate the lesion at a later time.

Using the history and visual clues, the clinician must decide whether the lesion in question requires a biopsy or further definitive therapy. Knowing the biological characteristics of a tumor, the surgeon can select which tissue to excise and examine.[52] In order to provide the best opportunity for diagnosis, the biopsy should be taken from a representative part of the clinical lesion, should provide adequate tissue for diagnosis, and should be submitted without excessive crush artifact. A shave biopsy is helpful for superficial epithelial lesions (Fig. 2-1). Nodular lesions are generally best evaluated with a deep incisional biopsy. An office biopsy usually allows better detail than is available with frozen section in the operating room suite, and also allows the surgeon a more leisurely period to decide on the surgical or other therapeutic course. The treatment of benign skin lesions is directed toward establishing the diagnosis and improving cosmetic appearance. Wide margins are not needed. An excisional biopsy can usually be performed on small lesions with care being taken to mark the borders if the excision turns out to be incomplete. Aspiration cytodiagnosis of lid tumors has been proposed for subepidermal lid nodules.[44]

If a malignant lesion is confirmed by biopsy, further

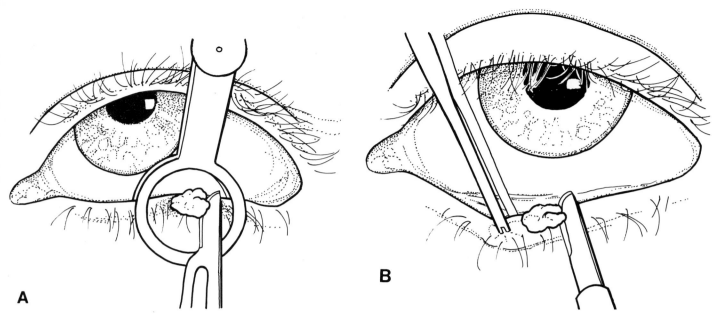

**Fig. 2-1.** Shaving technique.(A)(B) Alternative shaving techniques for removal of benign eyelid tumors and incisional biopsy of possible malignant lesions after regional anesthesia.

surgical excision with frozen section control is needed to assure complete removal (Fig. 2-2). The frozen section is valuable in evaluating for the absence or presence of tumor in the surgical margin during the definitive procedure and thus reducing recurrences.[16,58] Proper orientation and marking on a tongue blade and constant communication with the pathologist is needed. The primary aim of therapy is to remove all tumor cells; reconstructive procedures begin only after this stage.

Surgeons must be prepared for subcutaneous or bony extension with certain types of tumors and must have in their armamentarium several alternative surgical reconstructive procedures. Malignancy in the medial canthal area is especially dangerous because of the tendency to invade the orbit posteriorly. Tumors at the lid margin near the puncta pose special problems for the lacrimal drainage system. Pigmented lesions may require radical treatment.

## INFLAMMATORY EYELID LESIONS SIMULATING TUMORS

### Chalazion

The *chalazion* is a focal inflammation in the tarsal plate resulting from an obstruction to the duct or orifices of the meibomian glands or the glands of Zeis (Fig. 2-3). These holocrine lipid secretions can rupture through the tarsal plate and elicit a mixed acute inflammatory reaction and later a sterile granulomatous reaction with mononuclear cells and multinucleated histiocytes directed at phagocytosis of the lipid material. Fibrosis and scarring frequently occur. The patient may have a history of blepharitis, acne vulgaris, acne rosacea, or seborrheic dermatitis.

The chalazion usually has a rapid onset, but occasionally can enlarge slowly. It is more common in the upper lid because the sebaceous glands are more numerous there. Pain and erythema occur from stretching or irritation of the tarsal plate. The role of bacterial agents is usually negligible. The chalazion may point to the conjunctival or skin side with

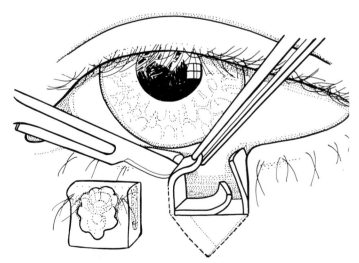

**Fig. 2-2.** Frozen section removal of a malignant tumor. The tumor margins are marked under loupes or with microscopic control. One or two millimeters of additional tissue is removed from all sides of the tumor. Slices are obtained from tumor margins, labeled, oriented on a tongue blade, and submitted for frozen section. All slices should be free of tumor before completing the pentagonal defect through the entire tarsal plate which then allows a better lid closure. (Redrawn with permission from Spaeth, G.L. (ed.): Plastic Surgery in Ophthalmic Surgery, Philadelphia, W.B. Saunders Co., 1982, p. 610.)

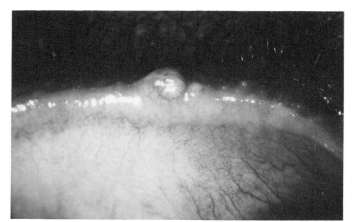

**Fig. 2-3.** A marginal chalazion of the eyelid margin arising from a localized obstruction of the gland of Zeis.

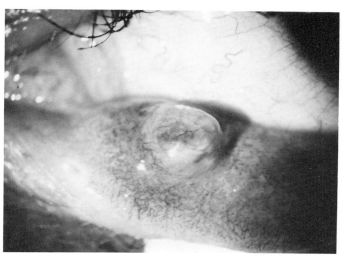

**Fig. 2-5.** Chalazion of the lower lid with a localized polypoid pyogenic granuloma on the conjunctival side.

both surfaces remaining freely mobile over the nodule. The lesions may become exuberant and stimulate a pyogenic granuloma through the rupture site on the skin or conjunctival side. (Figs. 2-4 and 2-5). A chalazion is distinguished from a hordeolum, which is an acute infection involving the meibomian glands (internal hordeolum) or the glands of Moll or Zeis on the eyelid margin (external hordeolum or stye). Compresses and topical antibiotics are indicated for these infections and only rarely is a surgical incision necessary.

The treatment of the chalazion consists of warm compresses up to four times a day. If there is no response, incision and curettage is indicated. After regional or local infiltration with 2% lidocaine with epinephrine, a chalazion clamp of the appropriate size is used to compress the surrounding tissues. A vertical incision is usually used on the conjunctival side and the fibrotic and loculated cheesy nodule is curetted. A horizontal skin incision is indicated for lesions that point toward the skin surface.

The injection of triamcinolone into the lesion and surrounding pretarsal tissue has been an effective alternative to

curettage.[61] Topical anesthesia is employed and up to 1 cc of triamcinolone is injected through a 25-gauge needle. A second injection is frequently required 1–2 weeks later to achieve complete resolution.

Recurrences are common in other areas of the lids (Fig. 2-6). If it occurs in the same location, consideration should be given to basal or sebaceous carcinoma, and the specimen should be sent for histopathologic exam with fat stain (Fig. 2-7).

## Molluscum Contagiosum

*Molluscum contagiosum* is an infection with a pox DNA virus, which leads to the formation of waxy epidermal dome-shaped nodules with a central umbilicus. The lesions are frequently multiple, are most common in children, and have

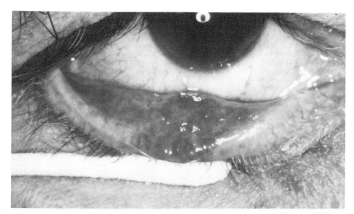

**Fig. 2-4.** A chalazion of the lower lid pointing toward the conjunctival side with exuberant tissue (pyogenic granuloma), simulating a meibomian gland carcinoma. It responded to intralesional steroid injection.

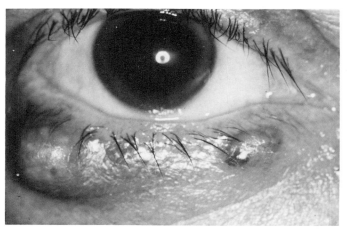

**Fig. 2-6.** Multiple confluent chalazia of the lower lid with marked thickening of the tarsus in a patient with acne rosacea. The patient was treated with an incision of the chalazion and systemic tetracycline.

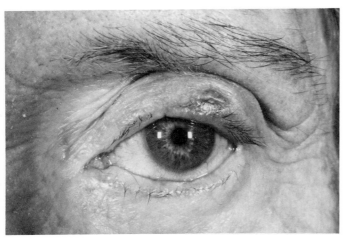

**Fig. 2-7.** A chalazion that has ruptured through the anterior tarsal plate and skin giving an ulcerated appearance, confused initially with a basal cell epithelioma.

a predilection for the skin of the lids and the eyelid margins (Fig. 2-8). An associated toxic follicular conjunctivitis is seen if the virus excreted from the surface of the nodule spills into the conjunctival sac. The lesions may wax and wane on their own.

Forms of therapy include curettage with electrodesiccation, surgical excision, or cryotherapy. The viral lesions are occasionally spread by surgical manipulation and reinfection is possible if all lesions are not eradicated. The histopathology of an excised nodule shows the intracytoplasmic inclusions, which become larger and more numerous toward the surface. Molluscum bodies are shed into the central pores as the cells desquamate.

## BENIGN TUMORS OF THE EPIDERMIS

*Keratinization* is the process of depositing several layers of relatively impermeable dead keratin. It is the end result of a

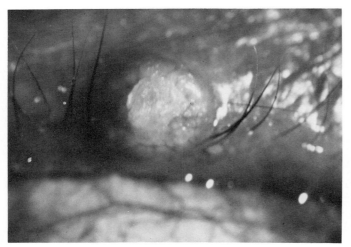

**Fig. 2-8.** A viral molluscum contagiosum infection of the eyelid margin causing a follicular conjunctival reaction and superficial punctate keratitis. It was treated successfully with cryotherapy without recurrence.

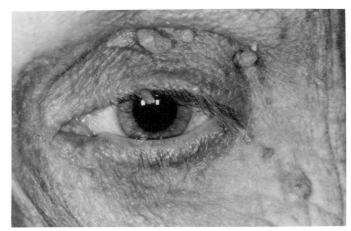

**Fig. 2-9.** Several pedunculated papillomas of the lids in an elderly man. The one on the eyelid margin was just a skin tag which was easily excised at the base without anesthesia.

number of conditions collectively called hyperkeratoses. The majority of these lesions are benign, although some malignancies may produce a keratin crust (e.g., squamous cell carcinoma). An extreme example of keratinization is typified by the cutaneous horn where there is a projected extension of solid keratin. It is necessary to obtain a sample of the underlying epidermis and dermis in order to confirm the origin of the hyperkeratoses.

## Squamous Cell Papilloma

The *papilloma* is a common proliferation of the keratinizing surface epidermis with a fibrovascular core of connective tissue. The surface may become hyperkeratotic with a superficial keratin layer. These lesions may be pedunculated (with multiple fibrovascular fingerlike processes originating from a narrow dominant stalk) or sessile (with multiple accentuations of the papillary dermis thrown into folds on a broad base) (Figs. 2-9 and 2-10). The verruca wart is a specific type

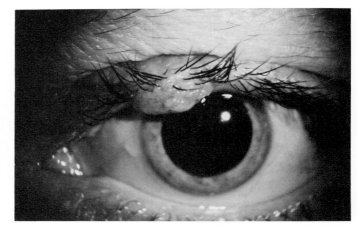

**Fig. 2-10.** A sessile papilloma of the lid margin with frondlike papillae. It was treated with a shave excision of the lid margin.

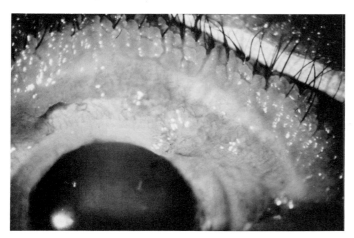

Fig. 2-11. A viral verruca papilloma of the lid and conjunctiva in an older man, which was recurrent despite multiple applications of cryotherapy.

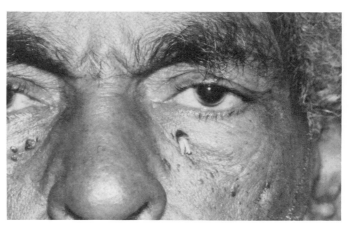

Fig. 2-13. Multiple pigmented seborrheic papules around the lids of a middle-aged black man (dermatoses papulosa nigra). One has a cutaneous horn on the surface.

of papilloma with a very rough hyperkeratotic surface caused by the papovavirus (Fig. 2-11). This virus can be seen as a small basophilic viral inclusion body within vacuolated cells.

## Seborrheic Keratosis

*Seborrheic keratosis* is a scaling or greasy lesion that develops in middle-age or older persons, especially on the face, arms, and trunk. The lesion has a soft and friable texture with a rough surface and variation in the amount of pigmentation (Fig. 2-12). In blacks, multiple pigmented hyperkeratotic papules may appear on the face and lids at the time of puberty (dermatoses papulosa nigra) (Figs. 2-13 and 2-14). The seborrheic keratosis is sharply demarcated and has a stuck-on-button appearance. The lesion has a convoluted surface and presents predominantly as an intraepidermal outward proliferation of benign basal cells with a normal dermis. There may be a hyperkeratotic surface and keratin-filled cystic spaces within a proliferating epithelium. Because

of the external proliferation it can be managed with a shave excision. It is not related to seborrheic dermatitis.

An inverted follicular keratosis is a specific type of seborrheic keratosis arising from irritation. This is usually a benign solitary nodule or papule with a predilection for the face or eyelids. The proliferation of epidermis extends into the underlying dermis with acanthosis of small basaloid cells, large squamous cells, and a squamous eddy. The lesion may clinically and histologically resemble a keratoacanthoma. This lesion would require deeper excision than a shave.

## Pseudoepitheliomatous Hyperplasia

Pseudoepitheliomatous hyperplasia is a true reactive proliferation of the nonkeratinizing squamous epithelium, with keratin production being a secondary feature. The epi-

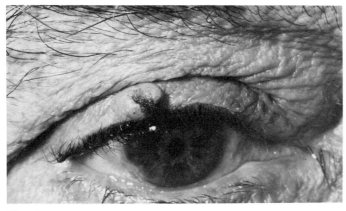

Fig. 2-12. An elevated, slightly brown, greasy button on the eyelid margin. A shave biopsy confirmed a seborrheic keratosis.

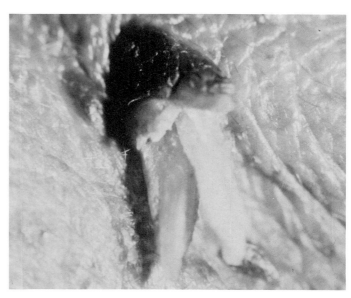

Fig. 2-14. Higher magnification of one of the pigmented seborrheic papules in Fig. 2.11, demonstrating the hyperkeratotic horn.

thelial cells invade downward into the dermis. A surface crust consists of a mixture of keratin and parakeratin with a mononuclear cell infiltration at the base.

This reactive proliferation occurs idiopathically or as a result of a variety of inflammatory stimuli, such as insect bites. It may be a reaction to an adjacent basal cell carcinoma, a fungal infection, a burn, or a histiocytic tumor. These lesions develop rapidly over weeks, in distinction to a squamous cell neoplasia which develops slowly over months or years.

## Keratoacanthoma

The *keratoacanthoma* is a rare distinctive form of pseudoepitheliomatous hyperplasia, which usually appears as a solitary large lesion developing on exposed areas of the skin in elderly people (Fig. 2-15). Occasionally there is a familial predisposition.[11] The hyperkeratotic lesion consists of a 1–2 cm dome-shaped nodule with a central keratin-filled crater, which enlarges over a few months. The tumor arises from a hyperplastic hair follicle with associated sebaceous gland metaplasia. Untreated, spontaneous regression frequently occurs in 6 months, leaving a minimal depressed scar. An immunologic process has been proposed to explain the spontaneous disappearance.[57]

The lesion must be distinguished from a squamous cell carcinoma.[71] Complete excision of the lesion allows the recognition of the specific architecture with a central keratin plug and surrounding acanthotic epithelium. Viral particles have been described within these lesions.[43]

## PRECANCEROUS TUMORS OF THE EPIDERMIS

*Precancerous tumors of the epidermis* is a term that represents a number of disease entities which could progress to malignancy. The most common lesions in the eyelid in this category include actinic keratosis, radiation dermatitis, and xeroderma pigmentosa.

*Actinic keratosis* (solar or senile keratosis) is most common in sun-exposed skin (e.g., eyelids and dorsum of the hand) of fair-skinned elderly patients. There are usually multiple lesions that may reside next to a basal or squamous cell neoplasm. The lesions are usually small, slightly elevated, scaling, and brownish or red in color. There may be a cutaneous horn on the surface. The initial histologic change with this lesion is a degenerative elastosis in the dermis with coexistent hyperkeratosis, dysplasia of the overlying epidermis, and moderately dense chronic inflammatory infiltration. Microscopically, there are various types of actinic keratosis: hypertrophic, atrophic, and Bowenoid. When actinic keratoses progresses to squamous cell carcinoma, the usual sharp demarcation between the lesion and the adjacent normal skin disappears. It may be difficult to confirm the presence of a squamous cell tumor without multiple biopsies. Fortunately, this form of squamous cell carcinoma rarely metastasizes.[4]

*Radiation dermatitis* appears in acute and chronic forms. The acute form is frequently seen within a week of radiation to the orbit or eyelids and consists of erythema, telangiectasia, and desquamation of surface epithelium with occasional scarring and pigmentation resulting (Fig. 2-16). It can occur with relatively low levels of radiation. Chronic radiation dermatitis occurs with doses of 4000 rads and is seen months after treatment. Clinically it presents an atrophic epidermis, and histopathologically an atrophic epithelium and dermis with prominant actinic elastosis and hyalinized telangiectatic vessels. A squamous cell or basal cell carcinoma may occur many years later in about 25 percent of patients.[27]

*Xeroderma pigmentosa* is a rare, autosomal-recessive inherited disease. There is a deficiency of the enzyme ultraviolet endonuclease with a subsequent defect in the repair of deoxyribonucleic acid damaged by ultraviolet light.[32,66]

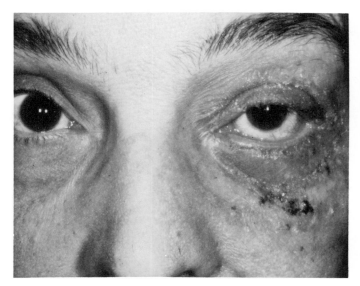

**Fig. 2-16.** Acute radiation changes to the skin with erythema, lid edema, and desquamation of the surface epithelium in a patient after radiation treatment for carcinoma of the breast metastatic to the orbit.

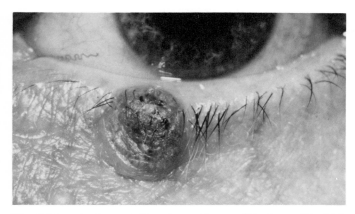

**Fig. 2-15.** A pigmented keratoacanthoma of the lower lid which demonstrated a rapid growth pattern and was developing a central umbilication.

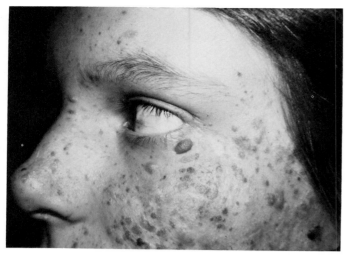

**Fig. 2-17.** Young patient with xeroderma pigmentosa demonstrating multiple pigmented lesions of the facial area, some being actinic keratosis and some being basal cell epitheliomas.

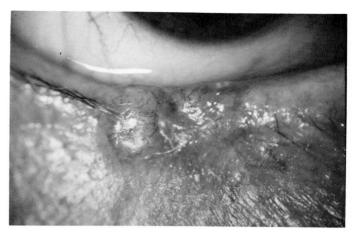

**Fig. 2-18.** Nodular and ulcerative basal cell epithelioma of the lower-lid margin demonstrating telangiectasia, loss of lashes, and slight distortion of the lid margin. The lesion was excised with frozen section control and a pentagonal wedge. It was closed primarily after a lateral cantholysis.

In this disease the skin is very sensitive to light, and becomes acutely erythematous in early childhood. Later there is increased pigmentation, telangiectasia, and solar keratosis with a high risk of basal cell carcinoma, squamous cell carcinoma, and malignant melanoma (Fig. 2-17). The eyelids additionally show atrophy, ectropion, and secondary inflammation. Most patients die of metastatic disease in their 20s.

## MALIGNANT TUMORS OF THE EPIDERMIS

### Basal Cell Epitheliomas

*Basal cell epitheliomas* are tumors of the germinal cells at the base of the epidermis and are by far the most common malignant neoplasms of the eyelids. Epitheliomas occur after prolonged exposure to light, are especially frequent on the lower lid and medial canthal area in fair-skinned adults, and may also be seen in association with benign cysts. Many patients also have other basal cell epitheliomas on the face.[83] Approximately 9 percent of the basal cell epitheliomas are pigmented as a result of benign melanocytic proliferation.[41] This feature is more common in darkly complexioned individuals. There are four clinical types of basal cell epithelioma: nodular, ulcerative, morphea, and multicentric. The types differ with regard to the completeness of excision, aggressiveness, and recurrences.[22]

The nodular form is the most common and develops insidiously as a firm nodule within the dermis, which can subsequently ulcerate the overlying epidermis and give a rolled, pearly edge with telangiectatic vessels on the surface of the thinned atrophic epidermis (ulcerative form) (Fig. 2-18). Loss of lashes is a sign of involvement of the lid margins. There is generally no hyperkeratotic surface. Histologi-

cally, small oval cells are arranged in palisading rows with dark uniform nuclei and little cytoplasm.

The morphea form clinically looks like a pale, indurated plaque and histologically has abundant fibrous connective tissue that produces cicatrization and a smooth leathery surface (Fig. 2-19). Although this tumor is less aggressive, it is dangerous because the margins are difficult to determine clinically and a high recurrence rate results.[43] The multicentric basal cell epithelioma has numerous lobules at the base of the epidermis or in the superficial corium.

A less-common histologic form of basal cell epithelioma is a netlike or pseudoglandular arrangement within loose stroma. This variant is called adenoidal basal cell carcinoma. Other basal cell epitheliomas are basosquamous with lobules of basaloid cells centrally located with an eosinophilic cyto-

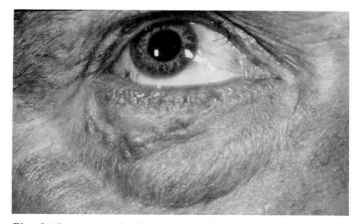

**Fig. 2-19.** A morpheaform basal cell epithelioma with an elevated, indurated, and multinodular appearance involving the whole lower lid. After frozen section control, the plastic reconstruction was completed with Mustarde skin flap supported by a periosteal posterior lamella.

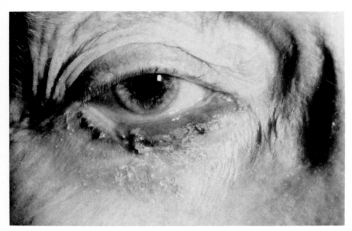

**Fig. 2-20.** Advanced ulcerative basal cell epithelioma involving the lower lid, causing an ectropion. The lesion was excised under frozen section control and was found to extend into the canalicular system nasally and up to the lateral canthal tendon temporally. The Hughes procedure and Viers rod were used for the reconstruction with good cosmetic and functional result.

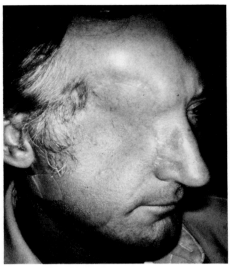

**Fig. 2-22.** Postoperative appearance of the patient in Fig. 2-19. The cosmetic defect was partially hidden by the patient's glasses.

plasm. These are aggressive and infiltrative but do not metastasize as true squamous cell carcinomas.

Multiple basal cell epitheliomas are seen in the basal cell nevus syndrome, where children present with flesh-colored nodules.[24] This may be a tumor of the basal cells outside the hair shafts. Central nervous system tumors and jaw and rib abnormalities complete the basal cell nevus syndrome.

Standardized surgery with frozen section to monitor tissue margins appears to be the best technique with 98 percent cure without recurrences.[14,21,58] All tissue margins should be examined with frozen section to assure complete removal. Nodular tumors are usually readily managed, but morphea lesions recur more often and require more complex reconstructions. When basal cell tumors involve the medial canthus, the lacrimal system may have to be removed to eradicate the tumor (Fig. 2-20). Subcutaneous extension

may be present which is not clinically obvious. Orbital, sinus, or eye invasion usually require exenteration (Figs. 2-21 and 2-22). The tumor is generally only locally invasive. Metastases are extremely rare, although the tumor can invade the skull and intracranial cavity. Close observation of an incompletely excised basal cell epithelioma is an acceptable alternative because recurrence rates are apparently less than 10 percent.[22,84]

The Mohs lamellar fresh-tissue chemosurgical technique is an alternative treatment and is especially useful because it can occasionally allow preservation of the globe.[11,53,67,68] Cryotherapy of basal cell lesions is a relatively new technique with long-term studies not yet available.[29,31,80] Early results have been encouraging, especially for small, localized central tumors. Liquid nitrogen is used and intralesional temperatures are monitored with a thermocouple probe to $-25°$ centigrade. The freeze–thaw cycle is repeated twice. Rebiopsy is necessary if recurrence is suspected.

Radiation therapy is reserved for basal cell tumors in which surgical therapy is not possible. Tumors in bone are usually resistant to this therapy. The recurrence rate of basal cell tumors is probably higher with this technique because of the inability to monitor histologic changes. If recurrence occurs, it is generally difficult to treat surgically because of the radiation damage to the tissues. Other frequent side effects are entropion, ectropion, and stenosis of the lacrimal drainage system.

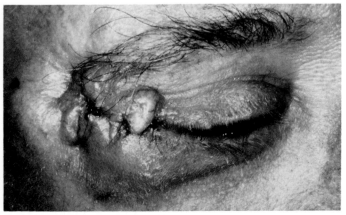

**Fig. 2-21.** A nodular basal cell epithelioma present for years which invaded the lateral orbital rim. It was treated with an exenteration, bone removal, and cranial facial reconstruction with rotation of a large skin flap.

## Squamous Cell Tumors

*Bowen's disease* is an intraepithelial squamous cell carcinoma found most commonly on nonexposed skin surfaces. The lesions are usually solitary, flat, and dark red with an indistinct outline. Growth occurs by slow, peripheral exten-

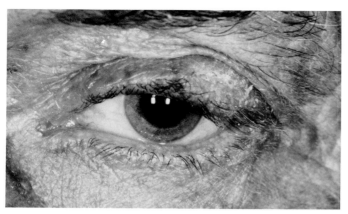

**Fig. 2-23.** A hyperkeratotic, flakey, indurated lesion of the upper lid, which showed an infiltrative squamous cell carcinoma with a surrounding actinic keratosis. After surgical excision, a Cutler-Beard flap was advanced from the lower lid and left in place for 2 months.

sion of the margins and leaves either a central ulcer or a fungating mass. Occasionally the lesion can progress to an invasive squamous cell carcinoma with metastases. Approximately 80 percent of the cases are associated with other cancers of the skin or viscera.[34] Histopathology shows very bizarre intraepithelial cells.

Squamous cell carcinomas are relatively uncommon on the lids and comprise less than 5 percent of all epithelial neoplasias.[46] They can arise from intraepithelial carcinomas, actinic keratosis, or de novo. The tumor also occurs after exposure to high-dose radiation or in multiple sites in patients with xeroderma pigmentosa. The patients are usually elderly and fair-skinned. The most common sites of involvement are the lower eyelids, followed by the upper lids, the inner canthus, and the outer canthus. Clinically there is usually an indurated thick patch, which becomes flaky white as keratin is formed (Fig. 2-23).

Invasive squamous cell carcinomas develop when the epidermis has been fully replaced and invasion of the underlying dermis has occurred. A nodule or ulceration usually signals the invasive stage and hyperkeratosis is an important feature. Histopathologically these lesions must be differentiated from similar conditions such as keratoacanthoma and pseudoepitheliomatous hyperplasia. Microscopically the lesions are usually well differentiated with evidence of pearl formation and keratinization. The cells are composed of large pale cells with abundant cytoplasm; focal keratinization is common except in the poorly differentiated lesions.

The surgical treatment of squamous cell carcinoma is the same as the approach to basal cell epithelioma. An aggressive approach is needed because of the potential to metastasize. Frozen section control with wide excision carries an excellent 5-year cure rate. The growth is usually slow and relatively benign; later occurrence, however, allows metastasizes to preauricular and submandibular lymph nodes, so lymph node removal may be appropriate.

## TUMORS OF SEBACEOUS GLANDS

### Sebaceous Adenomas

*Sebaceous adenomas* are benign overgrowths of the meibomian gland or other sebaceous glands.[62] They are usually smooth, solitary, elevated lesions approximately 5 mm in size and located on the face and scalp. Multiple sebaceous adenomas may be associated with a visceral malignancy; in most cases the skin tumors are on the trunk and the visceral malignancy is known.[66,69] The visceral malignancies are generally low grade but may metastasize. Pathologically, mature sebaceous gland cells are evident.

### Meibomian Gland Carcinoma

The eyelids contain sebaceous glands associated with the fine hair follicles of the skin (glands of Zeis) and within the tarsal plate exiting on the lid margin (meibomian glands). The lids have a definite propensity for sebaceous gland carcinoma.[64] The glands of Zeis, the caruncle, and the brow of the eyelids are unusual sites of sebaceous gland carcinomas.[6] Most sebaceous gland tumors arise from the meibomian glands, which are more numerous in the upper than in the lower lids.[56] Sebaceous gland tumors of the eyelids are rare compared to other eyelid malignancies, comprising about 2 percent of eyelid tumors.[56,62,64,85]

The tumor generally occurs in older patients but can be seen in association with prior radiation therapy. Clinically the appearance is usually of a circumscribed yellow nodule or mass within the tarsal plate (Fig. 2-24). They frequently masquerade with atypical presentations such as a unilateral chronic blepharoconjunctivitis or chalazion.[8] There may be

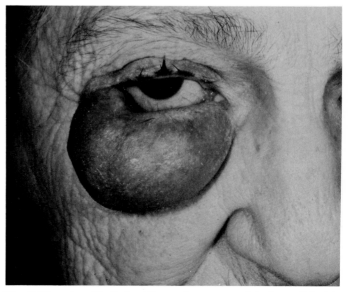

**Fig. 2-24.** A golfball-sized firm enlargement of the lower lid with enlarged preauricular and parotid lymph nodes in a patient with metastatic meibomian gland carcinoma of the lid. The patient died.

a diffuse firmness and thickening of the eyelids and an ecze-matoid reaction with loss of the eyelashes, especially when the glands of Zeis are involved. The tumor may be multicen-tric with both upper and lower lid involvement.[13,56] The con-junctival and corneal surface are frequently ulcerated or very friable. Signs indicative of a poor prognosis are the location in the upper lid; symptoms of more than 6 months; an infil-trative growth pattern; moderate or poor sebaceous pattern, multicentric origin; intraepithelial carcinoma changes in the conjunctiva, cornea, or epidermis of the skin; and invasion of vascular or lymphatic channels and the orbit.[64,65]

Sebaceous gland carcinomas are second only to malig-nant melanomas of the eyelids in lethality.[64] The mortality rate of 30 percent with a 5-year follow-up[6,43,65] may be related to the delay in recognition of the diagnosis.[77] Lym-phatic spread to unilateral preauricular, parotid, and cervical lymph nodes occurs early in up to 32 percent of patients and is more common than orbital extension. The tumor can also spread by vascular invasion to the lungs and the brain and by direct extension.

The tumor can assume a variety of histopathologic pat-terns. The most common one consists of large differentiated polyhedral acinar cells with prominent vesiculated nuclei and a frothy or foamy cytoplasm. The lipid contents on fresh tissue are confirmed with oil red O-stain. The overlying mucous membranes of the conjunctiva or cornea may con-tain cells with abundant pale cytoplasm and hyperchromatic nuclei within an unusual epithelium. This pagetoid phenom-enon may be a presenting manifestation of sebaceous carci-noma and a very poor prognostic sign.[70] Within a course of several months, the tumor may become undifferentiated with clusters of spindle-shaped cells and mitotic activity. Electron microscopy of this unusual neoplastic cell suggests an epidermoid origin because of the presence of tonofibrils and desmosomes. In this instance, the presence of fat helps to distinguish this lesion from a basal or squamous cell tumor. Sebaceous cell carcinomas of the squamoid type invade peri-neural lymphatic tissue and produce pain more commonly than other types.[56] Recognition of these different histopatho-logic features has substantially reduced the morbidity and mortality from this lesion.[20]

Tumor margins are difficult to evaluate clinically and account for a very high recurrence rate in most series, espe-cially from the less well-differentiated types of multicentric tumors.[56] If sebaceous gland carcinoma is suspected, a deep or full-thickness incision is recommended with frozen section and oil red O-stain on fresh tissue.[88] Because the lesions may mimic basal cell or squamous cell carcinoma, the pathologist must be astute. The lesion is usually larger than evident clinically because of spread within the tarsus and the page-toid spread within the conjunctiva. Wide local excision with frozen section inspection of the surgical margins is the pre-ferred definitive treatment.[37] The lesion frequently requires almost total resection of a lid. An exenteration is indicated for the extensive pagetoid spread, recurrent disease, or orbital involvement. Patients with a large diffuse tumor may do better with an initial exenteration than an exenteration after an inadequate excision. Parotid and cervical lymph

nodes are frequently involved and a radical neck dissection may be indicated. Prophylactic parotidectomy and radical neck dissection are not routinely performed. Mortality is very high with lymph node involvement and cases with dis-tant metastases are generally hopeless.[56]

Excision of the focal lid nodule coupled with cryother-apy to the intraepithelial conjunctival pagetoid spread is an alternative to exenteration in selected circumstances.[43] The radiosensitivity of the tumor is low and unpredictable, although some researchers have reported success with exter-nal beam irradiation with a short follow-up.[38]

## TUMORS OF SWEAT GLANDS

### Syringoma

The *syringoma* is a benign tumor of the intraepithelial apocrine or the eccrine sweat glands with multiple enzymes present within the cells. The lesion is more common in young or older women than in men. The tumor is character-istically white, pink, or yellow with 1–2 mm soft, waxy, or cystic papules that have a propensity for the lower eyelids (sparing the eyelid margins) as well as the axilla, abdomen, and cheek (Fig. 2-25). Histologically, the tumor is superficial with ducts lined with two rows of epithelial cells embedded in a fibrous stroma.

### Mucinous Adenocarcinoma

The *mucinous adenocarcinoma* is a very rare tumor arising from the eccrine or apocrine cells. The tumor occurs pre-dominantly in males on the lids or the inner canthus.[55,87] Clinically this aggressive tumor appears as a papillomatous lesion that may be misinterpreted clinically or histologically as squamous cell carcinoma, except for the increased amount of mucin. Regional metastases can occur. Wide excision including exenteration of orbital contents may be necessary.

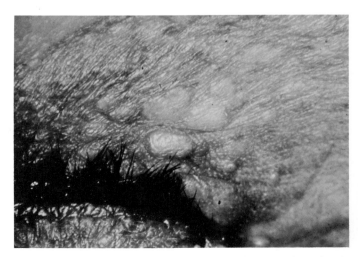

**Fig. 2-25.** Multiple benign tumors of the apocrine glands (syringoma). The soft cystic nodules spare the eyelid margin.

## TUMORS OF THE HAIR FOLLICLES

*Trichoepitheliomas* are tumors with a basaloid proliferation of the adnexal epithelium representing an attempt to produce hair. They tend to be multiple, occur on the lids and facial area, and are frequently inherited as an autosomal dominant trait (Brooke's tumor). Trichoepitheliomas resemble a basal cell epithelioma pathologically but show many horn cysts.

A *pilomatrixoma* is a tumor of the germinal cells of the hair bulb. It is more common in the brow as a cystic lesion but can occur on the eyelid skin. Histopathology reveals basaloid cells transformed into dead ghost cells with giant cells and calcification frequently present (calcifying epithelioma of Malherbe).[60]

## CYSTS OF THE EPITHELIUM

*Milia* are 1–2 mm white nodules that are retention cysts caused by occlusion of the pilosebaceous or sweat follicles of the hair (Fig. 2-26).[23] *Epidermal inclusion* cysts are larger, round, firm, nontender cysts with the wall consisting of a stratum granulosum of the epidermis with lamination of the innermost cells (Figs. 2-27 and 2-28). Horny keratin may accumulate and cause a slow enlargement of the cyst within the superficial or deep corium.[51] The cyst or multiple cysts have an epithelial wall with no intercellular bridges and the innermost cells have an increased number of filaments and fibrils which are shed into the lumen. The cystic contents contain eosinophilic material which may become calcified. There are no skin appendages in the wall as in a dermoid cyst. The lesion may be associated with significant inflammation, especially if a rupture occurs and elicits a giant cell reaction.

Comedo (blackheads) are due to intrafollicular pilosebaceous hyperkeratosis, which leads to a cystic collection of sebum and keratin (Figs. 2-27 and 2-28). The wall of the cyst may rupture causing abscesses and giant cell granulomatous reaction.

Ductal cysts (sudiforous) result from clogging of a sweat gland duct and have thin watery fluid (Fig. 2-29). They are lined by a double layer of epithelium, the outer myoepithelium and the inner layer cuboidal.

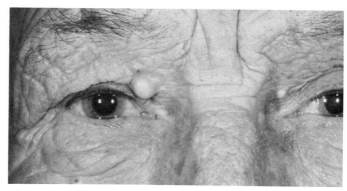

**Fig. 2-27.** An epidermal cyst of the lid containing horny keratin (not sebum) material. The wall of the cyst consists of epithelium without skin appendages.

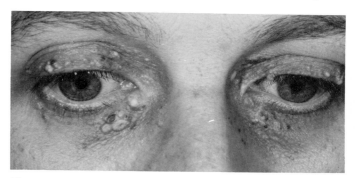

**Fig. 2-28.** Multiple epidermal cysts of both eyelids along with comedos (blackheads), which are due to intrafollicular pilosebaceous hyperokeratoses with accumulation of sebum and keratin.

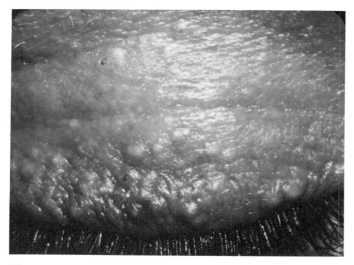

**Fig. 2-26.** Multiple retention cysts of the pilosebaceous follicles in the upper lid (milia).

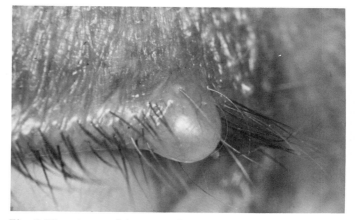

**Fig. 2-29.** A cyst of the sweat glands of the eyelid margin (sudiforous cyst) in a young patient. It is lined by a double layer of epithelium and has cloudy fluid.

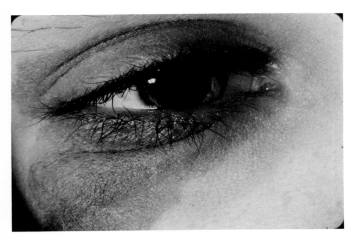

**Fig. 2-30.** A congenital intraepithelial flat brown nevus of the upper and lower lids (kissing nevi) that underwent increased pigmentation in this young boy.

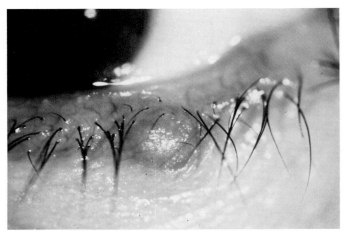

**Fig. 2-31.** A knobby, elevated, slightly pigmented, intradermal nevus at the lid margin with small telangiectatic vessels deep within the lesion and hairs on the surface. It was removed with a shave excision.

## TUMORS OF NEVUS CELLS

The nevus cell and the dermal melanocytes both originate in the neural crest and have similar melanosomes and cytoplasmic processes. Nevi of the lids are common and generally have varying shades of brown pigmentation. Very extensive kissing nevi may occur on the upper and lower lids as a congenital anomaly (Fig. 2-30). The nevus cells are generally arranged in clusters. There are four main stages of benign tumors of the nevus cells: the intraepithelial, the junctional, the compound, and the intradermal. Most nevi progress through these stages. As lesions mature, more cells drop into the dermis from the junctional nests and may adopt a verrucous brown and elevated appearance or, less commonly, become pedunulated. The clinical picture is usually sufficient to predict the histopathologic diagnosis.

The *intraepithelial* proliferation of benign nevus cells is generally flat. The nevus usually becomes pigmented in the juvenile years and generally remains stationary throughout life, although it may become nonpigmented again with older age. The *junctional* nevus has nests of cuboidal cells in the lower epidermis with a few clusters of cells in the upper dermis and is also generally flat and pigmented. The *intradermal* nevus has clusters of nevus cells confined to the dermis, with occasionally multinucleated cells and melanin confined to the superficial cells. The intradermal nevus generally has minimal pigment but tends to be dome-shaped, pedunculated, or papillomatous (Fig. 2-31). Clinically the presence of hairs on a elevated pigmented nodule indicates an intradermal nevus that has little or no malignant potential. A *compound* nevus has some features of both the junctional and intradermal nevus. The compound nevus generally is slightly elevated or papillomatous and pigmented. Both the junctional and compound nevus can become malignant, although very rarely. Malignant melanoma of the lid is extremely rare, so data on neoplastic transformation of lid nevi is not available.

A nevus on the eyelid margin is common with a distinct appearance on biomicroscopy. There is usually a knobby elevation with stretched skin over the surface and a contouring of the lesion's back surface to the globe,[43] suggesting a long presence. There may be fine blood vessels as well as pigment evident within the depth of the lesion. It has some clinical similarities to basal cell epithelioma, except the history suggests the long-standing nature. Eyelid nevi generally do not require treatment, although they might be removed for diagnosis, cosmesis, or to allow contact lens wear. Generally a shave is all that is required.

The dermal melanocytes may give rise to a benign tumor of two types: the blue nevus and the cellular blue nevus. The blue nevus is a small, blue, domeshaped tumor on the eyelids. The blue color is due to the scattering of light as it strikes the melanocytes in the deep dermis after passing through the skin. The cellular blue nevus is more darkly pigmented with a denser accumulation of nevus cells.

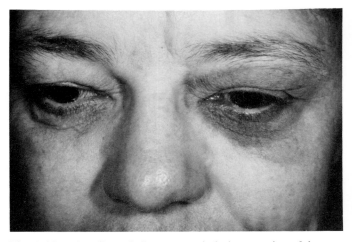

**Fig. 2-32.** A unilateral silver congenital pigmentation of the eyelid skin in a Caucasian patient with the Nevus of Ota.

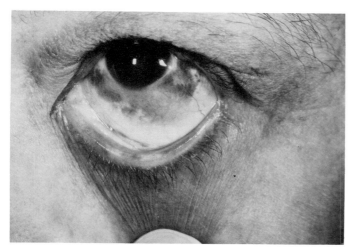

**Fig. 2-33.** A closer view of the patient in Fig. 2-32, showing the slate-blue appearance of the conjunctiva and sclera. The uveal tract is darkly pigmented on this side with no evidence of melanoma.

The *Nevus of Ota* is a congenital oculodermal melanocytosis. It is a blue nevus around the lids or brow associated with an ipsilateral blue nevus of the conjunctiva and diffuse nevus of the orbit (Figs. 2-32 and 2-33). It is quite common in blacks and orientals; when seen in whites, it has a malignant potential with rare melanoma of the skin, conjunctiva, uvea, orbit, or meninges.

## TUMORS OF THE EPIDERMAL MELANOCYTES

### Benign Tumors

The *freckle* is a flat, brown, circumscribed pigmentation which tends to increase on exposure to sunlight. The basal layer of the epidermis has large melanocytes, although the actual number of melanocytes is not increased. *Lentigo simplex* is a flat, brown or black lesion, somewhat larger in size than the freckle. This lesion has an increased number of basal melanocytes and melanophages in the upper dermis. *Lentigo meligna* (melanotic freckle of Hutchinson) occurs as an acquired brown or black, slightly raised pigmented lesion several centimeters in diameter in middle-aged patients. It occurs primarily on the face but can extend to the eyelids. This lesion has a propensity to go on to melanoma noted clinically by thickening of the lesion. Histologically it appears as a junctional nevus (but in the wrong age group).

### Malignant Melanoma

*Malignant melanomas* are extremely rare eyelid malignancies, representing only 1 percent of malignant neoplasms of the eyelid. Histologically, melanomas are composed of atypical melanocytes characterized by varying degrees of differentiation and tissue invasion. There is no good clinical evi-

dence that melanomas of the eyelids arise from preexisting nevi.

Melanomas can be divided into two main groups: intraepithelial and invading.[45] The intraepithelial (in situ) melanoma can occur as a lentigo maligna or a superficial spreading melanoma. Lentigo maligna (derived from Hutchinson's freckle) can extend or regress over periods of time and may be induced by sun exposure. When it proceeds to melanoma there are irregularly arranged melanocytes and an increased number with pigmentation. This tumor is generally less malignant than melanomas elsewhere on the skin. The superficial spreading (pagetoid) melanoma is usually small, slightly elevated, and less commonly appears in exposed areas (such as the eyelids) of middle-aged patients. Pathologically large, round melanocytes are distributed throughout the epidermis.

The invasive melanomas of the eyelids may derive from the Hutchinson's freckle, from superficial spreading melanoma, or as a nodular melanoma. The Hutchinson's freckle may invade the dermis after many decades; this change is usually heralded by the appearance of blue–black nodules. The superficial spreading melanoma is more aggressive and likely to progress to dermal invasion, as evidenced by increased pigmentation, induration, or ulceration over a 3- to 5-year period. This is the most common etiology of cutaneous melanomas elsewhere on the skin. The nodular melanoma is seen with a short history and is usually aggressive in middle-aged men (less commonly in women). It probably arises de novo or very rarely from a nevus and presents with gray or blue–black small nodules. Larger anaplastic cells are present with spindle cells and inflammatory cells. The growth may be rapid with extensive invasion.

Pigmented lesions that are stationary or present since childhood generally do not need a biopsy evaluation. In adults with acquired lesions or lesions that are increasing in size, a biopsy is needed, preferably from the center or thickest portion of the tumor. The level of skin invasion and thickness are the most important prognostic factors in predicting metastases.[15,45,54] Patients with lesions with invasive nodules less than 0.75 mm in height have almost a 100 percent survival rate, whereas those with lesions greater than 3 mm in height have an 80 percent fatality rate. The differentiation is also an important factor: the lentigo maligna rarely metastasizes and the superficial spreading melanoma frequently metastasizes. The 5-year survival rate for lentigo maligna is 89 percent, for superficial spreading is 68.5 percent, and for nodular melanoma is 60 percent. Systemic evaluation should include regional lymph node evaluation, chest x-ray, liver scan, and liver function tests.

The treatment of malignant melanoma is with a wide surgical excision for intraepithelial tumors and possible exenteration for extensive invasive or recurrent tumor once the diagnosis is firmly established. For melanoma of the skin elsewhere, a 5-cm margin is usually recommended; this is not feasible on the face. There is controversy as to whether prophylactic parotidectomy or cervical lymph node dissection should be performed for thick lesions. Adjunctive chemotherapy, immunotherapy, and hormone therapy are of unknown value in the management of eyelid malignancies without evident metastatic spread. Radiation treatment of lid melanoma has been successful in a limited reported series.[47]

## GENERAL COMMENTS ON TREATMENT OF EYELID MALIGNANCIES

There is controversy and a number of options with regard to the management of eyelid malignancies.[3] Surgery is preferred by most ophthalmologists, especially if the tumors are small and if the patients have corneal problems which might be exacerbated with radiation. Surgery with frozen section control of the tumor margin has the advantage of removing the tumor and, with the new reconstructive techniques, there are excellent cosmetic and functional results. The disadvantages of surgery are the hospitalization, expenses, inconvenience, and the cosmetic or functional blemish (e.g., trichiasis, entropion, ptosis, graft failure). The key to the surgical technique is the frozen section control of tumor removal; the functional repair and the acceptable cosmesis are secondary consideration. The surgeon must have a flexible surgical plan, and the patient should be aware that tissue may be borrowed from other areas, more than one operation may be necessary, the lids may be closed for weeks, and lacrimal reconstruction may be required.

For the best functional and cosmetic results, the reconstructed lid should have a rigid skeletal support (like the tarsus), a mucosal lining against the globe, and a skin covering. Reconstruction of the upper lid is fraught with potential functional problems related to lid instability and lid retraction. Repair of large defects in the lower lid has additional problems, including scarring of the conjunctiva, trichiasis, and ectropion of the lid. Careful attention to the vertical and horizontal dimensions of the defect, application of the appropriate tension on the lids, careful fixation of the medial and lateral canthal tendons, stripping of subcutaneous fat and connective tissue from free skin grafts, allowing stretched tissue to remain in place for the recommended times, and leaving lid margin sutures in place for an extended time are important surgical principles.

The Mohs procedure is a modification of this surgical technique in which the margin of the lid is marked with gentian violet and then excised in small lamellar tissue blocks and then examined under the microscope.[11,53,67,68] This technique can be done either with the original chemosurgical technique[53] (fixation of tissue with connected zinc chloride paste) or with a fresh tissue technique that utilizes excision guided by frozen section.[67] Originally the lesion healed by granulation. This was acceptable for the periorbital lesions but complicated because of subsequent cicatrization of the mobile eyelid. A combined team approach with a dermatologist and then plastic repair at 24–48 hours has been described.[1] This results in less operating time for the reconstructive surgeon and also allows the leisure of designing the reconstructive procedure prior to surgery. The Mohs technique is especially good for deep tumors, recurrent tumors, or extensive facial orbital tumors.[35] It may be a superior method of excising difficult lesions (e.g., morphea-type basal cell epithelioma), since it conserves as much tissue as possible. The disadvantages of this procedure relate to the time involved for the initial excision and the lack of adequately trained dermatologists to monitor the procedure.

Cryosurgery has been used to treat benign lid lesions as well as malignancy, most notably basal cell epithelioma.[30,31,80] It can also be useful as a supplementary treatment for a lesion with inadequate excision. It is ideal for elderly patients or patients with poor health where a difficult surgical repair can be avoided. The technique requires monitoring of tissue temperatures at the depth of the lesions as cells are killed by the intracellular ice crystals. There are a number of complications with this technique, including visual loss, lid notching, corneal ulceration, acceleration of symblepharon formation, cellulitis, skin depigmentation, loss of eyelashes, and a soft tissue reaction.[86] Its primary disadvantage, however, is the lack of a controlled excision.

Radiation treatment can be delivered safely be some centers where there is a good cooperation between radiologists and ophthalomogists and where there is appropriate shielding to protect the globe.[26,33,72] Basal cell epitheliomas respond well to radiation treatment (except in bone) and it is especially ideal for patients who are poor surgical risks, patients who are one-eyed and may need eyelid closure, patients with recurrence after surgical treatment, or tumors of the canalicular system. It is better for tumors of the canthal region than lesions of the central eyelid which may get ocular radiation complications. It is generally not as effective as surgical removal and tumors that persist or recur after radiation treatment are more difficult to eradicate with later surgery.[40] Radiation treatment cannot usually be repeated. The tumor limits cannot be precisely defined prior to treatment. Treatment is given with fractionated radiation so multiple visits and expense are necessary.

Complications of the procedure include stenosis of the lacrimal drainage system, loss of eyelashes, pigmentation, telangiectasis and skin atrophy, ectropion and entropion, cataract formation, and conjunctival and mucosal damage with subsequent dry eyes.

Curettage and electrocautery are the mainstay of treatment for basal cell epitheliomas by dermatologists but are useful for periorbital lesions only.[50] They are difficult to use on the mobile eyelids because they lead to subsequent contracture of tissues. Chemotherapy with flourouracil is useful for periorbital and facial lesions but should not be used near the eyelid margins. Immunotherapy has very limited potential at this time.

## RECONSTRUCTIVE TECHNIQUES OF THE EYELIDS AND CANTHAL AREA

Following total resection of the tumor with frozen section control, the choice of closure depends on the size and position of the defect, the age of the patient, the characteristics of the skin, and the preference of the surgeon. The following are guidelines, more information and detail are available elsewhere.[5,9,59,63]

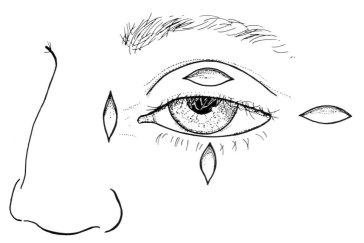

**Fig. 2-34.** Skin incisions. Elliptical skin incisions are recommended for tumors that do not involve the lid margin. Vertical incisions are recommended for the lower eyelid and medial canthus in an attempt to avoid ectropion. Regional anesthesia is preferred to infiltration which may distort the tumor.

## Closure of Defects Without Lid Margin Involvement

Direct closure is preferred, although care must be taken to avoid any tension on the eyelid which might create an ectropion. Direct closure is generally possible for smaller lesions but slightly larger lesions can be closed by transfer flaps, including sliding flaps, 0-to-Z plasties, and rotational flaps. Generally, elliptical incisions are made in the horizontal direction in the supper lid and lateral canthus area. Elliptical incisions in the vertical direction are generally performed on the lower lid (to avoid ectropion) and in the medial canthal area (Fig. 2-34).[63] Large defects can be closed with a full-thickness skin graft. Sites for obtaining this tissue, in order of preference, are from the same or opposite upper lid, retroauricular skin, or the supraclavicular area. Split-thickness skin grafts are less desirable around the eyelids because of the cosmetic match of tissue and the 25–50 percent contracture that takes place.

## Closure of Small Defects Involving the Eyelid Margin

Direct closure of an eyelid defect is usually employed when up to one-fourth to one-third of the horizontal lid margin is involved (Fig. 2-35). This varies depending on the age of the patient and the tension on the wound. The creation of a pentagonal defect with parallel cuts through the margin will help to minimize the amount of redundant skin at the extremity of the wound. The most important aspect of direct closure is reapproximation of the tarsal plate.[18]

If more than one-third of the upper or lower lid margin is removed and at least 2 mm of the lateral lid margin is preserved, then transfer of tissue can be employed. The horns of the lateral canthal tendon on the same lid is cut, allowing for medial mobilization of the eyelid. The direct

layered closure of the lid margin is accomplished and the skin is closed in the lateral canthal area (Fig. 2-36).

Larger defects of the upper or lower eyelids (approximately 40 percent) can be repaired with an advancement of the lateral segment of the lid. The lateral canthal tendon is incised and a semicircular skin flap is made below the lateral portion of the brow to allow further mobilization of the lateral segment of the eyelid (Fig. 2-37).[79]

## Large Defects of the Upper Lid

With large (50 percent or more) defects of the upper lid, tissue is usually borrowed from the lower lid (the Cutler-Beard technique).[17] The full-thickness flap of skin, muscle, and conjunctiva is advanced from the lower lid, brought underneath a bridge of the lower eyelid margin, and placed into the defect in the upper lid (Fig. 2-38). Depending on the tightness of the tissue, the flap is opened in approximately 8 weeks. This lid-sharing technique produces a dynamic movable lid with good cosmetic appearance. Its main disadvantages are that it is a two-stage procedure necessitating a closed lid for 2 months, and it has some subsequent functional complications.[12] Other reconstructive techniques include a sliding tarsal flap with a full-thickness skin graft or a tarsal conjunctival advancement flap.[49]

## Large Defects of the Lower Lid

Large (50 percent or more) defects of the lower eyelid may be repaired by transfer of a tarsal-conjunctival flap (Hughes procedure) from the upper lid into the defect in the lower lid (Fig. 2-39).[39] The skin layer is obtained from adjacent skin or from a free skin graft from the opposite upper lid, postauricular tissue, or beneath the upper arm. Alternatively, repair of large or total defects of the upper or lower lid involve the creation of a mucosal graft, a mucosal cartilage graft, or a mucosal tarsal flap from the opposite lid to create the posterior lamella of the lid. Alternative sites for mucosa and the skeletal framework for stability are the nasal septum or retroauricular cartilage. The anterior lamella is created by a rotational cheek flap,[10] the rotation of a medial forehead pedicle flap, or from a free skin muscle donor site. The Mustardé flap is a full-thickness rotational cheek flap that allows lower-lid reconstruction in one operation[10] (Fig. 2-40). It is especially useful in patients with vertically deep defects or nasal defects. Disadvantages of the technique are the necessity to remove a large triangle of tissue, a long facial scar, and the atonicity of the new lid leading to lower-lid sagging and ectropion.

## Medial Canthal Defects

Defects of the medial canthus are technically more difficult to repair because primary closure is usually not possible. One of the primary techniques employed is a spontaneous natural granulation or laissez-faire.[25,28,36,48] Disadvantages of this technique are the length of the healing process and the cicatricial scarring that may occur if the eyelids are

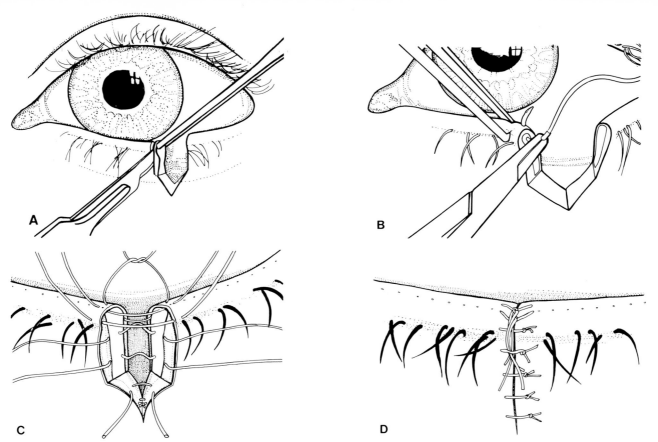

**Fig. 2-35.** Primary lid-margin closure. (A) The defect is sharpened, made perpendicular to the eyelid margin, and extended into a pentagonal defect to include the whole tarsal plate (which avoids buckling of the tarsus and lid notching). (B) A 6-0 silk suture is placed in the posterior lid margin in an oblique fashion, tied, and then placed on a stretch. (C) The tarsal plate is closed with several 7-0 or 6-0 absorbable sutures, as is the orbicularis muscle. There are no sutures in the conjunctiva. A 6-0 silk suture is placed at the meibomian gland orifices and the anterior lid margin and tied. (D) A 6-0 silk suture is placed just anterior to the lashes and the three posterior 6-0 silk sutures are brought anteriorly and tied. The skin is closed with interrupted 7-0 silk sutures, which are lubricated frequently with the antibiotic ointment and removed at 5 days; the lid margin sutures are removed at 10 days.

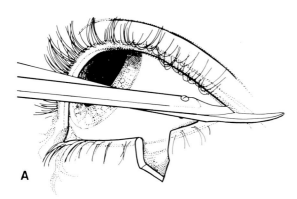

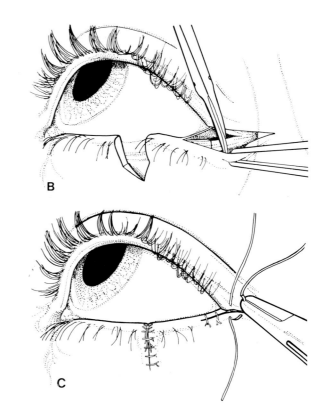

**Fig. 2-36.** Lateral cantholysis for primary closure of eyelid defects. (A) If direct closure is not possible, a lateral cantholysis is performed by making a scissors incision horizontally (canthotomy) at the lateral canthus through skin down to the orbital rim. (B) Scissor or blade can be used to isolate and then detach the limb of the lateral canthus tendon from the bony orbital rim (cantholysis) between the conjunctiva and the skin. The amount of detachment can be graded. (C) The central defect is then closed with a primary repair as described in Fig. 2-35. The skin in the lateral canthus area is closed with interrupted 7-0 silk sutures. The skin sutures are lubricated frequently with the antibiotic ointment and are removed at 5 days; lid margin sutures are removed at 10 days.

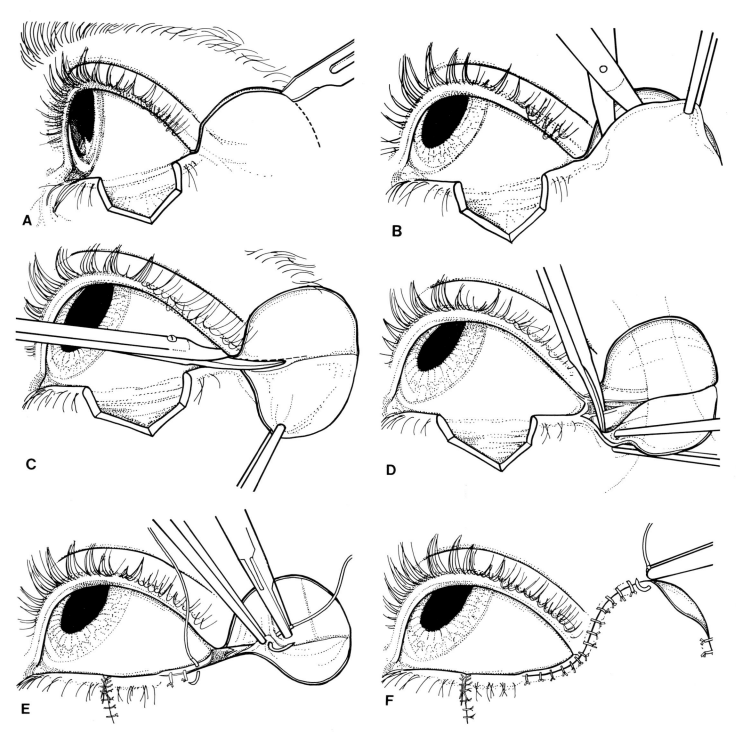

**Fig. 2-37.** Tenzel lateral rotational flap for closure of moderate eyelid defects. Variation of this same technique can be used for defects of the upper or lower lid. (A) A superior arching line is drawn with methylene blue beginning at the lateral canthus with a diameter of 20 mm. The skin and muscle are incised with a blade. (B) The tissue is undermined. (C) Additional dissection is performed down the lateral orbital rim. (D) The inferior ramus of the lateral canthal tendon is cut to mobilize the lateral aspect of the lid. (E) With the lid mobile, the central defect is approximated with the primary closure technique. The inferior ramus of the lateral canthal tendon is recreated by suturing the dermis of the flap to the periosteum of the lateral orbital rim. The conjunctiva is undermined, advanced to the skin edges of the lid margin, and sutured with 7-0 silk. (F) The lateral incision is closed with subcutaneous sutures and then mattress 7-0 silk sutures, depending on the tension present. Antibiotic ointment is applied frequently to the sutures which generally are removed after 10 days.

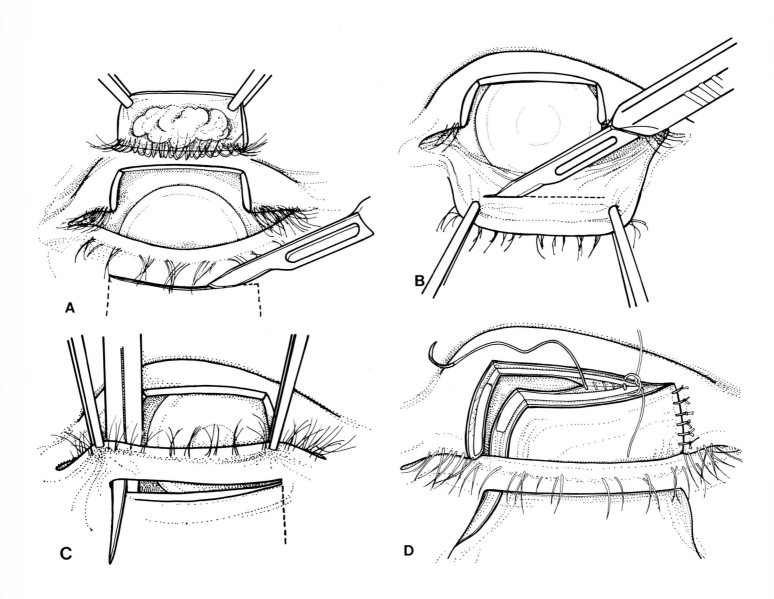

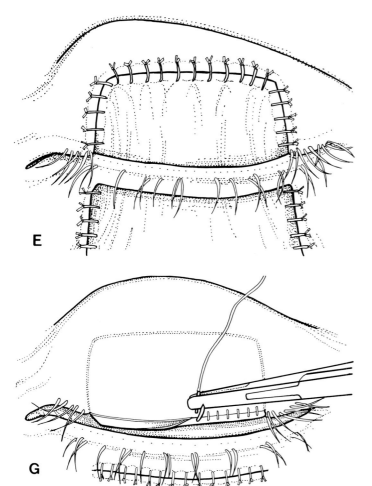

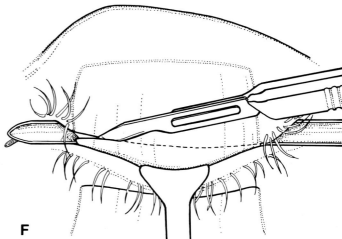

**Fig. 2-38.** Cutler-Beard full-thickness flap for large upper eyelid defects. (A) The upper eyelid defect is cut into a rectangular shape. There may be total excision of the tarsal plate with only the lateral and medial canthal tendons remaining. The flap of tissue marked on the lower lid should be approximately the same width as the defect in the upper lid (after checking the amount of stretch possible). A full-thickness horizontal incision is made in the lower eyelid 3–4 mm below the lid margin with a corneal protector in place. (B) Separate incisions on the skin and conjunctival side are preferred to insure the corrected viability of the marginal artery. (C) At the extremes of the horizontal incision, a full-thickness incision is made vertically down to the inferior fornix and the tissue undermined and loosened as necessary. (D) The tissue is pulled up through the skin tunnel; the conjunctival layer of the flap is sutured to the conjunctiva of the upper lid defect with running 6-0 plain gut. The tarsal plate from the lower lid is sutured laterally to the remnants of the tarsal plate (or the medial and lateral canthal tendons) and to the cut edge of the levator and Mullers muscles above with 6-0 absorbable sutures. Alternatively, the use of donor eyebank sclera in conjunction with the tarsal plate may add more stability to the new upper lid. (E) The skin from the lower lid is sutured to the skin of the upper and lower lid with interrupted 7-0 silk sutures. (F) Separation of the flap is carried out about 2 months later. A groove director is placed under the flap and a knife and/or scissor used to make the incision which should be beveled to leave a longer posterior edge on the upper lid. (G) The skin can be trimmed and the extra conjunctiva pulled over the new upper lid and sutured with 7-0 silk to create a mucous membrane edge to the upper lid. These sutures are removed at one week. The lower lid is sutured back in position after smoothing out any irregular surfaces. A ptosis or swelling of the upper lid generally resolves in a few weeks. The absence of lashes on the upper lid is generally cosmetically acceptable.

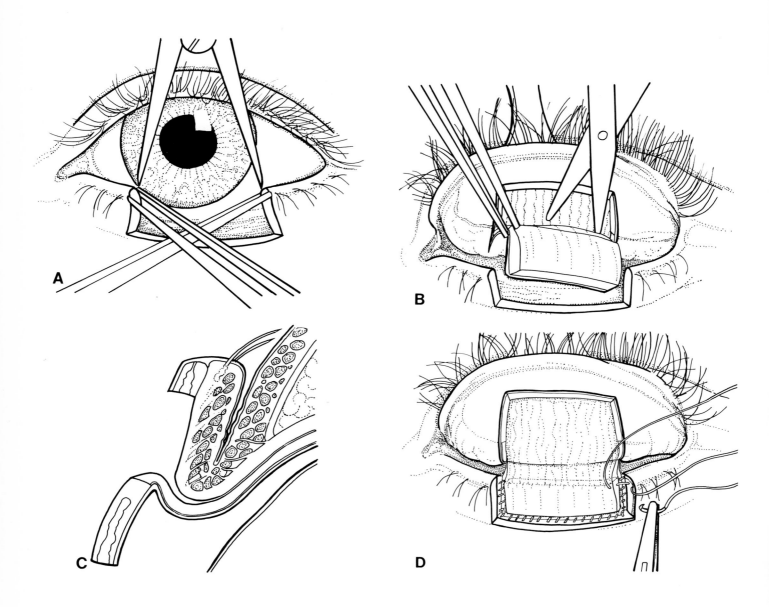

A

B

C

D

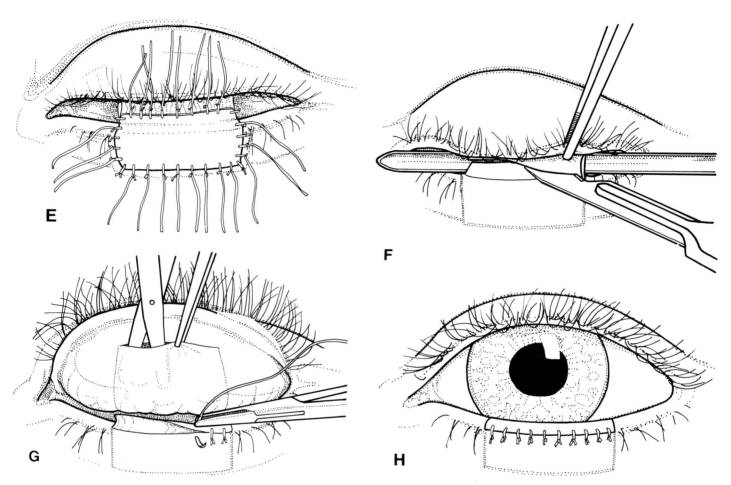

**Fig. 2-39.** Hughes procedure for closure of large lower eyelid defects. (A) Perpendicular margins are fashioned in the lower lid defect; the lid edges are stretched and calipers are used to measure the horizontal length of the defect to be filled by the upper lid tissue. (B) A Desmarres retractor everts the upper lid. A horizontal incision, the appropriate length needed, is marked and created through the conjunctiva and tarsus 4 mm from the lid margins until the plane is found between the tarsus and levator aponeurosis. The blunt dissection is carefully continued superiorly between Muller's muscle and levator aponeurosis until the tissue is sufficiently mobilized. (C) This cross-section of the upper lid indicates the correct plane of dissection. (D) The flap of conjunctiva, tarsus, and Mullers muscle is placed into the lower lid defect. Some surgeons remove Mullers muscle from the dissection to avoid distortion of the upper lid. The conjunctiva is closed with a running 6-0 gut suture and the tarsal plate is sutured to the tarsal plate of the lower lid with 6-0 gut. If the tarsus is absent in the lower lid, the medial canthal and lateral canthus can be recreated with permanent fixation sutures. A periosteal flap can be created temporally. (E) Skin to cover the tarsal plate is usually obtained from a free skin graft from the upper lid or postauricular skin. If the skin of the lower lid is lax, this can be undermined and slid up to fill in the defect. The skin is sutured with 7-0 silk to the tarsus approximately 2 mm higher than the existing lower lid margin. The wound is covered with a moderate pressure dressing and the skin sutures are removed in about 5 days. (F) After 8 weeks of stretch, the wound can usually be opened using a sharp knife with a groove director placed under the bridge. The cut is beveled to leave a longer posterior edge of conjunctiva on the lower lid. (G) The conjunctiva is draped over the lower lid and sutured with 7-0 silk to the anterior lid margin. The conjunctiva should cover the whole lower lid margin in order to prevent entropion or corneal irritation. The under surface of the upper lid is everted with a Desmarres retractor and the released tarsal conjunctival flap is undermined to allow retraction of Muellers muscle to the level of the superior fornix. (H) The appearance of the lids after the second stage has been completed. The silk sutures can be removed after 5 days.

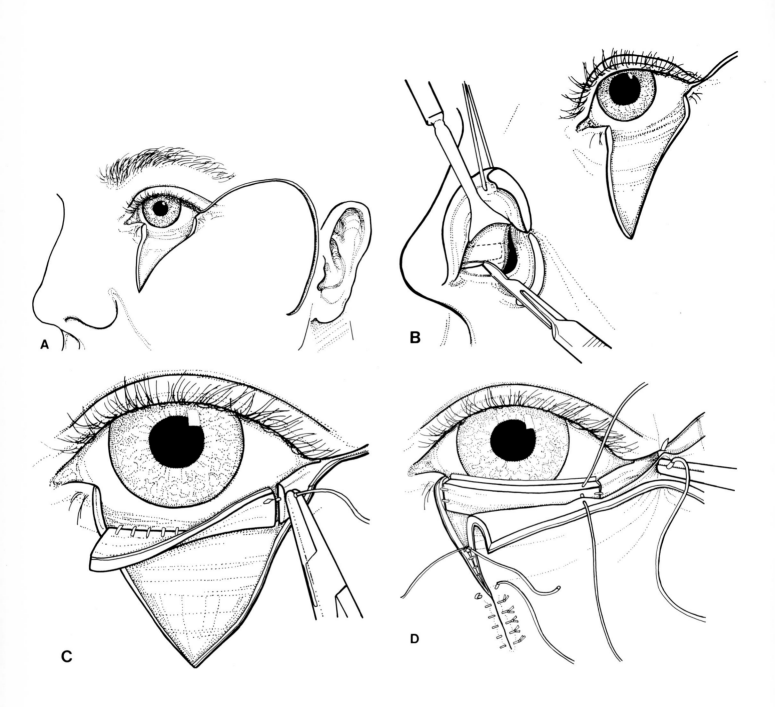

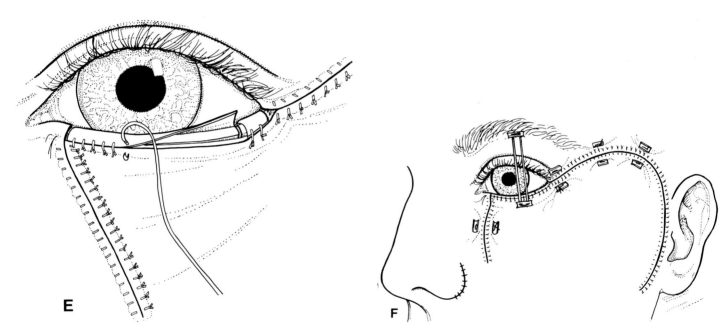

**E**

**F**

**Fig. 2-40.** Mustardé rotational cheek flap for large lower lid defects. (A) This flap is preferred with nasal defects up to the nasolabial fold. A large triangular defect based superiorly is created. A semicircle flap is begun at the lateral canthus and extending to the auricular tragus. The flap should extend at least to the level of the brow in order to avoid potential sagging of the lower lid. Undermining is performed, avoiding vessels and the facial nerve. (B) The supporting posterior lamella of the newly created lid is obtained by a chondromucosal graft from the nasal septum and mucosa. This can be obtained by making a relaxing incision through the ala nasal in the plane of the facial skin. The nasal septum is then exposed and a 10 × 5 mm strip of nasal mucosa and cartilage is removed. The nasal ala is resutured with 4-0 silk and the naris is packed with petroleum-jelly impregnated gauze. An alternative technique is to simply expose the inside of the nose with a speculum and fashion the graft. (C) The chondromucosal graft is sutured to the conjunctiva in the inferior fornix with 5-0 plain gut and to the remaining tarsus laterally and medially, or it can also be sutured directly to the periosteum or to a periosteal flap. (D) The chondromucosal graft is sutured to the posterior margin of the cheek flap with 5-0 gut to create a new lid margin. The dermis of the rotational flap is sutured to the periosteum of the inner aspect of the lateral orbital rim with a 4-0 mersiline suture to recreate a new lateral canthus. (E) The dermis and skin flap is then closed with 5-0 catgut subcuticular and 7-0 silk vertical mattress skin sutures. The (nasal) mucosa and the remaining conjunctiva can be rotated over the lid margins and sutured to the advanced skin flap. (F) Frost sutures are used to put tension on the new flap for the first few days.

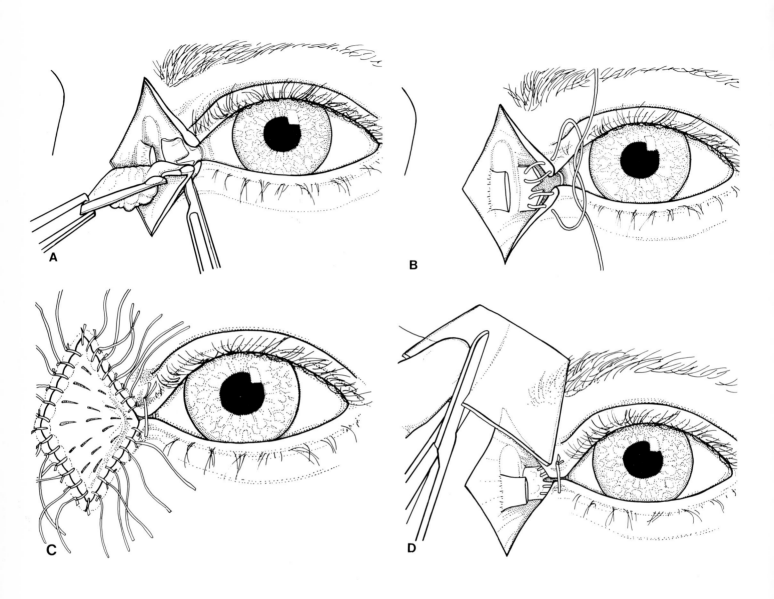

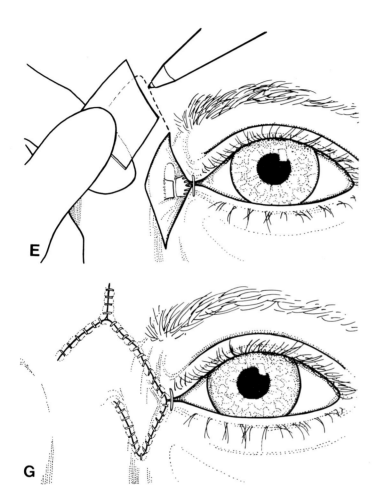

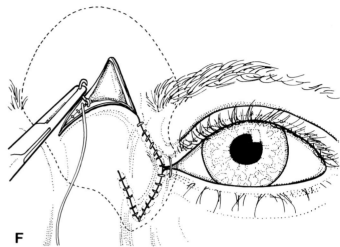

**Fig. 2-41.** Repair of medial canthal defects. (A) A diamond-shaped defect is easier to close either primarily, with natural granulation, or with the use of skin grafts. If granulation is chosen, frequent dressing changes are necessary. This method is preferred if free tumor margins have not been assured. (B) The edge of the lid remanant is attached to the posterior reflection of the medial canthal tendon with permanent sutures (such as mersiline) to obtain the desired posteriorly directed pull to the medial canthal angle. If the lacrimal canaliculus cannot be preserved, a Quickert tube stint may suffice but in all likelihood a Jones tube will be needed and can be placed primarily or in the future. (C) If a skin graft is chosen, the full-thickness tissue can be obtained from the upper eyelid or retroauricular skin. It is sutured in place with multiple 7-0 silk sutures. A telfa pad is placed and firm pressure is applied. The sutures are removed at 1 week. Free grafts are especially useful in the medial canthus and a bolus may not be necessary if the graft is "pie crusted" to allow for seepage of secretions or if it is sutured to the underlying tissue. (D) A glabellar forehead flap can be rotated into place using the surgical principles involved in movable pedicle flaps. X-ray film can be used to fashion a template of the correct size. (E) After appropriate measurement of the defect, a flap of vertical skin is outlined, incised, and elevated. (F) The surrounding tissue is undermined and rotated into the donor site. The donor site and the primary site are closed with subcutaneous 5-0 catgut and the skin with 4-0 silk mattress sutures. If the undersurface of the flap covers the globe, it should be lined with a mucosa from a free buccal graft, from a nasal chondromucosal graft, or from a flap from the lower conjunctiva. (G) The appearance of the lids at the completion. After 8 weeks, the tissue can be thinned and/or the base of the pedicle flap replaced back into the glabellar area to reduce the bulk. (Redrawn with permission from McCord CD: Oculoplastic Surgery. New York, Raven Press, 1981.)

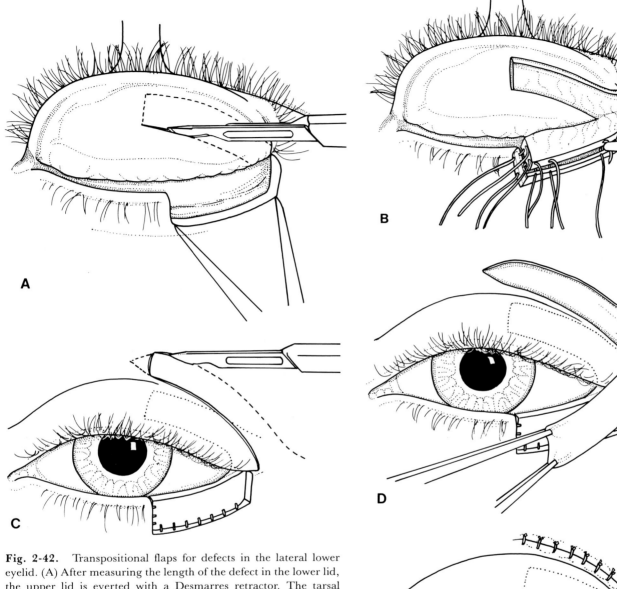

**Fig. 2-42.** Transpositional flaps for defects in the lateral lower eyelid. (A) After measuring the length of the defect in the lower lid, the upper lid is everted with a Desmarres retractor. The tarsal conjunctival graft is prepared by making parallel incisions 4-mm wide into the lateral canthus and 3 mm from the lid margin. (B) The tarsal conjunctival flap is rotated into the defect and sutured to the inferior conjunctiva with 6-0 catgut and to the tarsus of the lower lid with 6-0 catgut. (C) The anterior lamella (skin muscle flap) can be obtained from the upper lid along a crease line extending to the lateral canthus and with a line parallel to this. This flap should be taken from an area superior to the previous tarsal conjunctival flap. (D) The skin muscle flap is rotated into position and sutured with interrupted 6-0 silk sutures. Another alternative for obtaining this anterior lamellar tissue is a free skin graft from the upper lid or retroauricular tissue. (E) The skin donor site can be closed with 6-0 silk. A cotton bolster can be used as a stent over the transpositional flap. The tarsal conjunctival donor flap site does not need to be sutured.

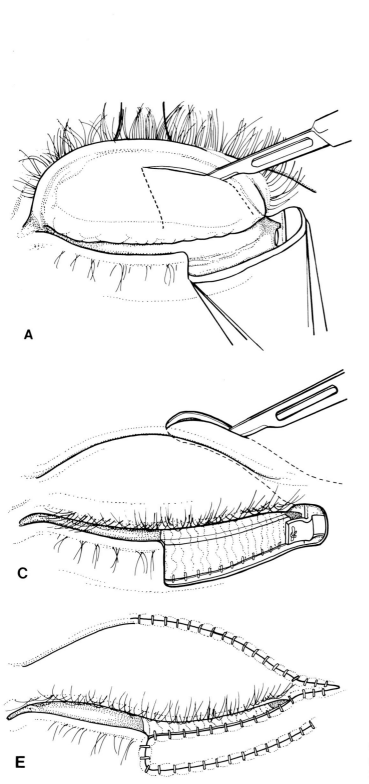

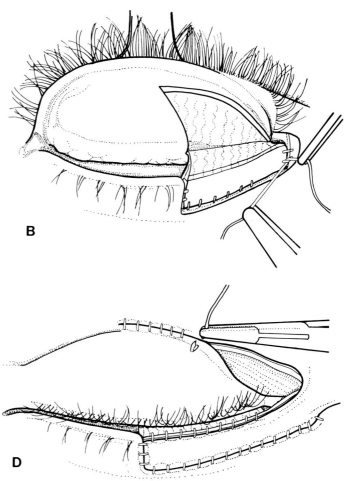

**Fig. 2-43.** Closure of large lateral canthal defects. (A) The support framework for the lower lid defect can be provided by the residual upper lid. A tarsal conjunctival flap is constructed similar to the Hughes procedure with a careful dissection between the levator aponeurosis and Mullers muscle up to the superior fornix and then rotated obliquely to fill the defect. (B) The lateral edge of the newly created tarsal flap is sutured to the periosteum of the lateral canthus. The medial edge of the tarsal flap is sutured to the remaining lateral tarsal plate of the lower lid with absorbable sutures. (C) An alternative here and for other lateral canthal defects is to create a periosteal flap to supply support and a firm structure for suturing. The skin of the lateral upper lid can be advanced with a transpositional flap (as shown) or the residual covered with a full-thickness free skin graft from the upper lid or retroauricular tissue. (D) The transpositional skin flap can be sutured in place with interrupted 7-0 silk sutures and the donor site sutured with 7-0 silk sutures. (E) The appearance of the lid at the completion of this stage with the advanced tarsal plate and the overlying transposed skin flap. The lid should remain on a stretch for about 2 months and can then be opened in a similar manner as illustrated in Figs. 2-39F–2-39H.

not in proper position at the time of granulation. Advantages of this technique are that it is usually cosmetically satisfactory and recurrences of the tumor are more easily detected.

It is important to sacrifice and later repair the lacrimal system if it is involved with tumor; recurrences here are difficult to detect and treat. If the puncta or lacrimal system is removed, a Viers rod or Quickert tube can be placed or a marsupialization of the canalicular system can be done. Occasionally the use of a Jones pryex lacrimal drainage tube is necessary. All surgical repairs should make an effort to maintain or create the anatomy and physiology of the medial and lateral canthal tendon. Procedures necessary to employ in medial canthal reconstruction are transnasal wiring and plication of the medical canthal tendon.

Free full-thickness skin flaps from the upper eyelid or retroauricular area may be used to close defects, or a medial forehead flap (glabellar) can be rotated into position. (Fig. 2-41). This is a good versatile alternative to reconstruct the medial canthus or eyelids, especially when the recipient site has a poor blood supply, standard procedures have failed, or extensive tissue loss is present.[19] Another alternative is a rhomboid flap.[73]

## Lateral Canthal Defects

Large defects that cannot be closed by direct approximation are best corrected with a tarsal conjunctival graft for the posterior lamella and an advancement or free skin flap for the anterior lamella (Fig. 2-42).[5,50,78] Because lateral canthal defects often are large and involve the upper as well as the lower lids, ingenuity in closing the defects may be necessary (Fig. 2-43). Periosteal strips[82] can be used to close extensive lateral canthal and temporal eyelid defects. Strips are reflected nasally and are sutured to residual tarsal stumps and covered anteriorly with myocutaneous flaps. The periosteal tissue is strong, readily available, and allows a free skin graft to survive on the surface. Other options for the posterior lamella are the nasal cartilage or tarsal conjunctival grafts from uninvolved eyelids.

## REFERENCES

1. Anderson RL, Ceilly RI: A multispecialty approach to the excision and reconstruction of eyelid tumors. Ophthalmology 85:1150–1162, 1978
2. Apple DJ, Rabb MF: Ocular Pathology. Clinical Applications and Self-assessment. St. Louis, Mosby, 1985, pp 465–486
3. Beard C: Management of malignancy of the eyelids. Am J Ophthalmol 91:1–6, 1981
4. Bendl BJ, Graham JH: New concepts of the origin of squamous cell carcinomas of the skin: solar (senile) keratosis with squamous cell carcinoma. A clinicopathologic and histochemical study, in Proceedings of the Sixth National Cancer Conference, Philadelphia, Lippincott, 1970, pp 471–488
5. Boniuk M: Surgical management of eyelid tumors, with emphasis on a new reconstructive technique: advancing tarsoconjunctival flap from the adjacent lid, in Transactions of the New Orleans Academy of Ophthalmology, St. Louis, Mosby, 1982, pp 410–440
6. Boniuk M, Zimmerman LE: Sebaceous gland carcinoma of the eyelid, eyebrow, caruncle, and orbit. Trans Am Acad Ophthalmol Otolaryngol 72:619–642, 1968
7. Brooks NA: Curettage and shave excision. J Am Acad Dermatol 10:279–284, 1984
8. Brownstein S, Codere F, Jackson WB: Masquerade syndrome. Ophthalmology 87:259–262, 1980
9. Callahan M: Techniques of eyelid reconstruction after malignancy, in Jakobiec FA (ed): Ocular and Adnexal Tumors. Birmingham, AL, Aesculapius, 1978, pp 484–507
10. Callahan MA, Callahan A: Mustarde flap lower lid reconstruction after malignancy. Ophthalmology 87:279–286, 1980
11. Callahan A, Monheit GD, Callahan MA: The Mohs' technique in ophthalmic plastic surgery, in Transactions of the New Orleans Academy of Ophthalmology, St. Louis, Mosby, 1982, pp 364–379
12. Carroll RP: Entropion following the Cutler-Beard procedure. Ophthalmology 90:1052–1055, 1983
13. Cavanagh HD, Green WR, Goldberg HK: Multicentric sebaceous adenocarcinoma of the meibomian gland. Am J Ophthalmol 77:326–332, 1974
14. Chalfin J, Putterman, AM: Frozen section control in the surgery of basal cell carcinoma of the eyelid. Am J Ophthalmol 817:802–809, 1979
15. Clark WH Jr, From L, Bernadino EA, et al.: The histogenesis and biological behavior of primary human malignant melanomas of the skin. Cancer Res 29:706–727, 1969
16. Cole JG: Histologically controlled excision of eyelid tumors. Am J Ophthalmol 70:240–244, 1970
17. Cutler NL, Beard C: A method for partial and total upper lid reconstruction. Am J Ophthalmol 39:1–7, 1955
18. Divine RD, Anderson RL: Techniques in eyelid wound closure. Ophthalmic Surg 13:283–287, 1982
19. Dortzbach RK, Hawes MJ: Midline forehead flap in reconstructive procedures of the eyelids and exenterated socket. Ophthalmic Surg 12:257–268, 1981
20. Doxanas MT, Green WR: Sebaceous gland carcinoma. Review of 40 cases. Arch Ophthalmol 102:245–249, 1984
21. Doxanas MT, Green WR, Iliff CE: Basal cell carcinoma. Am J Ophthalmol 91:726–736, 1981
22. Doxanas MT, Green WR, Iliff CE: Factors in the successful surgical management of basal cell carcinoma of the eyelids. Am J Ophthalmol 91:726–736, 1981
23. Epstein W, Kligman AM: The pathogenesis of milia and benign tumors of the skin. J Invest Dermatol 26:1–11, 1956
24. Feman S, Apt L, Roth A: The basal cell nevus syndrome. Am J Ophthalmol 78:222–228, 1974
25. Fier RH, Older JJ: Spontaneous repair of the medial canthus after removal of basal cell carcinoma. Ophthalmic Surg 13:737–740, 1982
26. Fitzpatrick PJ, Thompson GA, Easterbrook WM, et al.: Basal and squamous cell carcinoma of the eyelids and their treatment by radiotherapy. Int J Radiat Onchol Biol Phys 10:449–454, 1984
27. Forrest AW: Tumors following radiation about the eye. Trans Am Acad Ophthalmol Otolaryngol 65:694–717, 1961
28. Fox SA, Beard C: Spontaneous lid repair. Am J Ophthalmol 58:947–952, 1964
29. Fraunfelder, FT, Wallace TR, Farris HE, et al.: The Role of cryosurgery in external ocular and periocular disease. Trans Am Acad Ophthalmol Otolaryngol 83:713–724, 1977

30. Fraunfelder FT, Zacarian SA, Limmer BL, et al.: Cryosurgery for malignancies of the eyelid. Ophthalmology 87:461–465, 1980

31. Fraunfelder FT, Zacarian SA, Wingfield DL, et al.: Results of cryotherapy for eyelid malignancies. Am J Ophthalmol 97:184–188, 1984

32. Gaasterland DE, Rodrigues MM, Moshell AN: Ocular involvement in Xeroderma Pigmentosum. Ophthalmology 89:980–986, 1982

33. Gladstein AH: Radiotherapy of eyelid tumors, in Jakobiec F (ed): Ocular and Adnexal Tumors. Birmingham, AL, Aesculapius, 1978, pp 508–516

34. Graham JH, Helwig EB: Bowen's disease and its relationships to systemic cancer. Arch Dermatol 83:738–758, 1961

35. Grove AS Jr: Staged excision and reconstruction of extensive facial-orbital tumors. Ophthalmic Surg 8:91–109, 1977

36. Harrington JN: Reconstruction of the medial canthus by spontaneous granulation (laissez-faire): a review. Ann Ophthalmol 14:956–960, 1982

37. Harvey JT, Anderson RL: The management of meibomian gland carcinoma. Ophthalmic Surg 13:56–61, 1982

38. Hendley RL, Rieser JC, Cavanagh HD, et al.: Primary radiation of meibomian gland carcinoma. Am J Ophthalmol 87:206–209, 1979

39. Hews EH, Sullivan JH, Beard C: Lower eyelid reconstruction by transportation. Am J Ophthalmol 81:512–514, 1976

40. Hirshowitz B, Mahler D: Incurable recurrences of basal cell carcinoma of the mid-face following radiation therapy. Br J Plast Surg 24:205–211, 1971

41. Hornblass A, Stefano JA: Pigmented basal cell carcinoma of the eyelids. Am J Ophthalmol 92:193–197, 1981

42. Jakobiec FA: Sebaceous adenoma of the eyelid and visceral malignancy. Am J Ophthalmol 78:952–960, 1974

43. Jakobiec FA: Tumors of the lids, in Symposium of disease and surgery of the lids, lacrimal apparatus and orbit. Transactions of the New Orleans Academy of Ophthalmology. St. Louis, Mosby, 1982, pp 264–307

44. Jakobiec FA, Chattock A: Aspiration cytodiagnosis of lid tumors. Arch Ophthalmol 97:1907–1910, 1979

45. Kopf AW, Bart RS, Rodriquez-Sains RS: Malignant melanoma: a review. J Dermatol Surg Oncol 3:41–125, 1977

46. Kwitko ML, Bonuik M. Zimmerman LE: Eyelid tumors with reference to lesions confused with squamous cell carcinoma. I. Incidence and errors in diagnosis. Arch Ophthalmol 69:693–697, 1963

47. Lederman M, Wybar K, Busby E: Malignant epibulbar melanoma: natural history and treatment by radiotherapy. Br J Ophthalmol 68:605–617, 1984

48. Leone CR Jr, Hand Si Jr: Reconstruction of the medial eyelid. Am J Ophthalmol 87:797–801, 1979

49. Leone CR: Tarsal-conjunctival advancement flaps for upper eyelid reconstruction. Arch Ophthalmol 101:945–948, 1983

50. Leone CR, Van Gemert JV: Lower eyelid reconstruction with upper eyelid transpositional graft. Ophthalmic Surg 11:315–318, 1980

51. Lever WF, Schaumberg-Lever G: Histopathology of the Skin, (ed 5), Philadelphia, Lippincott, 1975

52. McCord CD Jr, Cavanagh HD: Microscope features and biological behavior of eyelid tumors. Ophthalmic Surg 11:671–681, 1980

53. Mohs FE: Chemosurgical treatment of cancer of the eyelids. A microsurgical controlled method of excision. Arch Ophthalmol 39:43–59, 1948

54. Naidoff M, Bernardino V, Clark W: Melanocytic lesions of the eyelid skin. Am J Ophthalmol 82:371–382, 1976

55. Ni C, Dryja TP, Albert DM: Sweat gland tumors in the eyelids: a clinicopathological analysis of 55 cases. Int Ophthalmol Clinics 22:1–23, 1982

56. Ni C, Searl SS, Kuo Pk, et al.: Sebaceous cell carcinomas of the ocular adnexa. Int Ophthalmol Clin 22:23–61, 1982

57. Nicolau SG, Bandanoiu A, Balus L: Untersuchungen über spezifische antitumorale. Reaktinonen bei an Keratoakanthom leidenden Kranken. Arch Klin Exp Dermatol 217:308–320, 1963

58. Older JJ, Quickert MH, Beard C: Surgical removal of basal cell carcinoma of the eyelids utilizing frozen section control. Trans Am Acad Ophthalmol Otolaryngol 79:658–663, 1975

59. Stewart WB (ed): Ophthalmic Plastic and Reconstructive Surgery. San Francisco, American Academy of Ophthalmology, 1984

60. Perez RC, Nicholson DH: Malherbe's calcifying epithelioma (pilomatrixoma) of the eyelid: clinical features. Arch Ophthalmol 97:314–315, 1979

61. Pizzarello L, Jakobiec FA, Hofeldt A: Intralesional corticosteroid therapy of chalazia. Am J Ophthalmol 85:818–821, 1978

62. Prioleau PG, Santa Cruz DJ: Sebaceous gland neoplasia. J Cutan Pathol 11:396–414, 1984

63. Putterman AM: Eyelid tumor surgery. Int Ophthalmol Clin 18:1–18, 1978

64. Rao NA, Hidayat AA, McLean IW, et al. Sebaceous carcinoma of the ocular adnexa: a clinicopathologic study of 104 cases with 5-year followup data. Hum Pathol 13:113–122, 1982

65. Rao NA, McLean IW, Zimmerman LE: Sebaceous carcinoma of the eyelids and caruncle: Correlation of clinicopathologic features with prognosis in FA Jakobiec (ed): Ocular and Adnexal Tumors, Aesculapius, Birmingham, AL, 1978, pp 461–476

66. Robbins HH, Kraemer KH, Andrews AD: Inherited DNA repair defects in *H. sapiens:* their relationships to UV-associated processes in xeroderma pigmentosum, in JH Yuhas, RW Tennant, Regan RD (eds): Biology of Radiation Carcinogenesis. New York, Raven Press, 1976, p 115

67. Robins P. Mohs FE: Chemosurgery for tumors in the periorbital area, in Jakobiec FA (ed): Ocular and Adnexal Tumors. Aesculapius, Birmingham, AL, 1978, pp 525–531

68. Robins P, Rodriquez-Sains R: Recurrent basal cell carcinoma of the eyelids managed by Mohs' surgery, in Jakobiec FA, Sigelman J (eds): *Advanced Techniques in Ocular Surgery,* Philadelphia, Saunders, 1984, pp 563–571

69. Rulon D, Helwig E: Multiple sebaceous neoplasms of the skin: an association with multiple visceral carcinomas, especially of the colon. Am J Clin Pathol 60:745–752, 1973

70. Russell WE, Page DL, Hough AJ, et al.: Sebaceous carcinoma of meibomian gland origin. The diagnostic importance of pagetoid spread of neoplastic cells. Am J Clin Pathol 73:504–511, 1980

71. Schnur PL, Bozzo P: Metastasizing keratocanthomas. The difficulties in differentiating keratoacanthomas from squamous cell carcinomas. Plast Reconstr Surg 62:258–262, 1978

72. Sealy R, Baret E, Cleminshaw H, et al.: Progress in the use of iodine therapy for tumors in the eye. Br J Radiol 53:1052–1060, 1980

73. Shotton FT: Optimal closure of medial canthal surgical defects with rhomboid flaps: ''rules of thumb'' for flap and

rhomboid defect orientations. Ophthalmic Surg 14:46–52, 1983

74. Sommerville J, Milne JA: Familial primary self-healing squamous epithelioma of the skin (Ferguson Smith type). Br J Dermatol 62:485–490, 1950

75. Spencer WH: Ophthalmic Pathology. An Atlas and Textbook (ed 3) vol. 3. Philadelphia, W.B. Saunders Co., 1985

76. Stewart WB, Nicholson DH, Hamilton G, et al.: Eyelid tumors and renal transplantation. Arch Ophthalmol 98:1771–1772, 1980

77. Straatsma BR: Meibomian gland tumors. Arch Ophthalmol 56:71–93, 1956

78. Tenzel RR: Lower lid and laternal canthal reconstruction. Trans New Orleans Acad Ophthalmol. St. Louis, C.V. Mosby Co., pp 308–320, 1982

79. Tenzel RR, Stewart WB: Eyelid reconstruction by the semi-circle flap technique. Ophthalmology 85:1164–1169, 1978

80. Torre D: Cryosurgical treatment of eyelid tumors, in Jakobiec FA (ed): Ocular and Adnexal Tumors. Aesculapius, Birmingham, AL, 1978, pp 517–531

81. Weigent CE, Staley NA: Meibomian gland carcinoma: report of a case with electron microscopic findings. Hum Pathol 7:231–234, 1976

82. Weinstein GS, Anderson RL, Tse DT, et al.: The use of a periosteal strip for eyelid reconstruction. Arch Ophthalmol 103:357–359, 1985

83. Wesley RE, Collins JW: Basal cell carcinoma of the eyelids as an indicator of multifocal malignancy. Am J Ophthalmol 94:591–593, 1982

84. Wiggs EO: Incompletely excised basal cell carcinoma of the ocular adnexa. Ophthalmic Surg 12:891–896, 1981

85. Wolfe JT, Yeatts RP, Wick MR, et al. Sebaceous carcinoma of the eyelid: errors in clinical and pathologic diagnosis. Am J Surg Pathol 8:597–606, 1984

86. Wood JR, Anderson RL: Complications of cryosurgery. Arch Ophthalmol 99:460–463, 1981

87. Wright JD, Font RL: Mucinous sweat gland adenocarcinoma of eyelid. Cancer 44:1757–1768, 1979

88. Wright P, Collin RJO, Garner A: The masquerade syndrome. Trans Ophthalmol Soc UK 101:224–250, 1981

89. Yanoff M, Fine BS: Ocular Pathology (ed 2). New York, Harper and Row, 1982, pp 209–263

90. Zelickson AS, Lynch FW: Electron microscopy of viral-like particles in keratoacanthoma. Invest Dermatol 37:79–83, 1961

# 3

# Exposure Keratopathy

## J. Chandler Berg    Alan Kozarsky

Exposure keratitis results from prolonged exposure of the corneal surface with secondary dessication. Symptoms include blurred vision and discomfort with the potential for visual loss. Corneal thinning, opacification, and perforation may occur in any patient with exposure keratitis regardless of etiology. Medical therapy with lubricants is essential; however, the best management in many cases is surgical treatment of the underlying condition. This chapter discusses the etiology, medical, and surgical management of exposure keratitis with emphasis on specific surgical techniques useful for the general ophthalmic practitioner.

## ETIOLOGY

Exposure keratitis may be precipitated by local or systemic disorders that affect eyelid function, position, and shape. Common causes of exposure keratitis are as follows.

1.  Ectropion
       Lower eyelid
          Involutional-senile
          Paralytic-seventh nerve
          Trauma
          Postoperative-blepharoplasty
          Inflammatory-chronic skin disorders
          Tarsal kink
          Congenital
       Upper eyelid
          Floppy eyelid syndrome
          Posttraumatic
          Postoperative
          Inflammatory
          Congenital
2.  Lagophthalmos
       Peripheral seventh nerve paresis
       Supranuclear seventh nerve paresis
       Nocturnal
       Restrictive-Graves disease, cicatricial

Post surgical-ptosis, superior rectus recession
Inflammatory-chronic skin disorders with cicatricial changes
Coma-absent closure reflex
Psychiatric disorder-inadequate blink
3.  Proptosis
       Orbital disease-dysthyroid states, tumor

Conditions such as Bell's palsy may be temporary, requiring only medical therapy or a temporizing surgical procedure. Unfortunately, many causes of exposure keratitis do not undergo spontaneous resolution and require definitive surgery. Table 3-1 lists common surgical procedures used to treat exposure keratitis.

## Ectropion

*Ectropion* is the outward rotation or eversion of the eyelid margin away from the globe. Regardless of etiology, the conjunctiva and cornea may become dry leading to keratitis, conjunctivitis, and their subsequent complications. In most patients, surgical correction of the ectropion provides a cure for the exposure keratitis.

The most common type of ectropion is due to relaxation and lengthening of the canthal tendons of the lower eyelid. This is known as involutional or senile laxity ectropion. A variety of eyelid-shortening techniques have been utilized successfully to treat involutional ectropion. The most popular procedures are discussed later in this chapter under "Surgical Techniques."

Upper-lid laxity with eversion and secondary corneal exposure is described by Culbertson and Ostler[4] and named the floppy eyelid syndrome. Dutton[6] achieved complete resolution of the condition in five of five cases by surgically tightening the upper eyelid. When ectropion of the upper or lower lid is due to cicatricial changes, reconstructive surgery including skin grafting with the release of adhesions is required.

SURGICAL INTERVENTION IN CORNEAL AND EXTERNAL DISEASES
ISBN 0-8089-1850-8

**Table 3-1.**
Surgical Procedures for Exposure Keratitis

| Procedure | Disorder |
|---|---|
| Tarsorrhaphy | |
|    Temporary | Bell's Palsy with keratopathy |
| | Metabolic coma |
|    Permanent | Seventh nerve paresis |
| | Proptosis with keratopathy |
| Canthoplasty | Seventh nerve paresis |
| Horizontal lower-lid shortening | Involutional ectropion |
| | Paralytic ectropion |
| Horizontal upper-lid | |
|    shortening | Floppy eyelid syndrome |
| Conjunctival flap | Seventh nerve paresis or |
| | combined seventh and fifth |
| | nerve paresis |

## Seventh Nerve Paresis

Lesions of the seventh nerve may be supranuclear, nuclear, or peripheral. All lesions result in weakness of the lower facial muscles, lagophthalmos, and laxity ectropion. Patients with supranuclear lesions may have partial retention of orbicularis oculi and upper facial muscle movement. A typical lesion of the peripheral seventh nerve includes drooping of the corner of the mouth, lower-lid laxity (with ectropion), inability to close the lids, and depending upon location, hyperacusis and loss of taste. The diagnosis is generally not difficult; however, management of the improper lid closure while maintaining useful vision is a challenge.

The most common cause of seventh nerve paresis is Bell's palsy. This condition usually develops acutely and lasts 1–4 months. Fortunately, about 80 percent of patients will have partial or complete recovery of their seventh nerve function[8] and will only require temporary procedures. For the patients that have permanent paresis and significant keratopathy, a more aggressive surgical approach is needed.

A common surgical treatment for patients with permanent seventh nerve paresis and exposure keratopathy is the tarsorrhaphy. The tarsorrhaphy can be lateral, medial, both lateral and medial, or central. Central closure gives the most corneal protection but is restrictive visually. Other effective procedures include lower-lid tightening, and the Arion sling.[1] The lid-tightening procedures are often combined with a tarsorrhaphy for greater effect. Patients with complete seventh nerve paresis have continued stretching of the orbicularis postoperatively and may require periodic surgical revision. Ocular lubricants should be continued after surgery and the patient followed closely.

## Lagophthalmos

*Lagophthalmos* is failure of the eyelids to close properly. If the cornea remains exposed, it becomes susceptible to drying and infection. Lagophthalmos has multiple etiologies including lid retraction and exophthalmos due to dysthyroid states,

lid paralysis due to seventh nerve lesions, tissue shortage following eyelid surgery or burns, and loss of muscle tone during coma or sleep.

Nocturnal lagophthalmos occurs whenever the eyelids fail to adequately cover the globe during sleep. This condition is usually transient and is best treated conservatively with lid taping and/or lubricants. Only in the rare patient for whom medical therapy fails is surgery indicated. The best procedure for these patients is a simple tarsorrhaphy that can be reversed at a later date if desired.

Patients in metabolic coma should also be treated conservatively with lid taping and lubricants. A temporary tarsorrhaphy is useful in patients for whom the coma is expected to be transient. For patients with prolonged coma a more permanent procedure is indicated. The tarsorrhaphy should be central for maximum protection, unless the pupil or cornea needs to be examined.

Patients with dysthyroid eye disease, eyelid tissue shortage, and cicatricial deformities require complex reconstruction procedures beyond the scope of this text. The reader should consult comprehensive oculoplastic texts for the treatment of these disorders.

## MEDICAL MANAGEMENT

Medical therapy for exposure keratitis includes ocular lubricants, lid taping, moist chamber dressings, and therapeutic contact lenses. All patients with exposure keratopathy should be treated medically. Many of the patients undergoing surgery continue to benefit from medical treatment postoperatively.

### Lubricants

Useful ocular lubricants include nonpreserved artificial tears, nonpreserved saline, and ophthalmic ointments. Patients generally prefer drops to visually disturbing ointments; however, the clinical situation should dictate the lubricant selected. As with keratitis sicca, the corneal epithelium becomes devitalized and may not tolerate the preservatives used in most tear preparations. Nonpreserved tears (Refresh, Allergan, Irvine, CA) or nonpreserved saline (Unisol, CooperVision, San German, PR; BSS, Alcon, Fort Worth, TX) are preservative-free and avoid this potential toxicity. Useful ointments include Duolube (Muro, Tewksbury, MA) or Hypotears (CooperVision, San German, PR), which do not contain lanolin or chlorbutanol.

### Lid Taping

Eyelid taping at bedtime is an effective therapy for nocturnal lagophthalmos. Lid taping is also helpful in patients with atony of the orbicularis as seen with seventh nerve paresis. The tape should be applied directly to the eyelids without the use of a patch. Care should be exercised to insure that the eyelids are clean and do not have ointment present that would weaken the adhesion and allow the lid to open. Foster

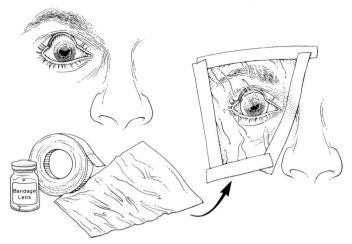

**Fig. 3-1.** Moist chamber for corneal protection with extensive eyelid defects. A moist chamber to prevent corneal desiccation can be purchased commercially or made with readily available materials. A bandage contact lens may be used underneath the moist chamber. A piece of plastic wrap is cut to the shape indicated. One-half inch surgical tape is then used to seal the edges of the plastic wrap to the skin of the brow and cheek. Complete occlusion is indicated by fogging up the moist chamber. Careful attention is indicated to assure that the edges of the moist chamber remain sealed to the skin.

recommends that ointment be avoided for several hours before tape application to lessen adhesion problems.[13]

## Moist Chamber Dressings

The creation of a moist chamber environment helps decrease surface evaporation in patients with corneal exposure. Moist chambers are a useful alternative for patients who need lid closure but desire visual function (Fig. 3-1). For example, the patient may undergo a lateral or medial tarsorrhaphy and use the moist chamber for additional protection in dry or windy environments. The moist chamber is also useful when eyelid tissue is absent after trauma or during staged reconstructive surgery. Useful devices for providing a moist environment include swimmer's goggles, the Guibor shield (Concept Inc., Clearwater, Florida), and cellophane wrap.

## Therapeutic Contact Lenses

Therapeutic bandage lenses can be used effectively in selected cases of exposure keratopathy. An important example of their good use is a large eyelid defect with grossly inadequate corneal coverage. In such a case, the combination of a moist chamber and therapeutic bandage lens is a good temporizing measure to protect the ocular surface prior to definitive surgical repair of the eyelid. The use of any high water content, 14- to 16-mm diameter lens is appropriate in this setting. This may either be a specially designated therapeutic bandage lens or a low-power myopic extended wear contact lens adapted for this purpose.

## SURGICAL TECHNIQUES

The goal of surgery in patients with exposure keratitis is to improve corneal coverage and wetting. This goal is usually achieved by repositioning the eyelids, improving lid motility, or reducing palpebral fissure size. Although the best management of exposure keratitis is elimination of the underlying etiology, this is not always possible. Surgery on patients with chronic cicatricial diseases and seventh nerve paresis may only be palliative and require periodic revisions. All of the following techniques except for the conjunctivial flap are intended to provide improved eyelid protection of the diseased cornea. A list of techniques described in this chapter follows.

1. Tarsorrhaphy
   Temporary
     Mattress suture over bolsters
     Running intermarginal
   Permanent
     Simple intermarginal adhesions
     Sliding tarsal flap
2. Horizontal lower-lid shortening
   Wedge resection
     Full-thickness pentagonal wedge
     Kuhnt-Szymanowski, Smith modification
   Lateral canthal tightening
3. Horizontal upper-lid shortening
4. Conjunctival flap

For more advanced techniques such as the Arion sling[1] for seventh nerve paresis, full-thickness skin grafting, and correction of a tarsal kink[3,10,15,17], the reader is referred to specialized oculoplastic texts.

## Tarsorrhaphy

Tarsorrhaphy is an effective technique for reduction of palpebral fissure size, decreasing surface evaporation, and improving closure of paretic lids. The procedure can be rapidly performed at the patient's bedside or in the office. Positioning of the adhesions must be determined according to the clinical situation. Factors include the severity of keratitis, underlying etiology, and need for visualization of the cornea and pupil. Patients with a tear deficiency and poor blinking benefit from a small lateral tarsorrhaphy, however, patients with metabolic coma should have a temporary closure of the entire eyelid. The marginal excision technique is effective in patients with Bell's Palsy when multiple temporary tarsorrhaphies have been performed and a more permanent but reversible closure is needed. As the condition resolves the intermarginal adhesions can be easily severed restoring fissure size. The tarsal flap technique is more appropriate for patients with irreversible seventh nerve palsies to decrease stretching of the adhesions.

### Temporary Tarsorrhaphy

The following technique is commonly used for temporary lid closure (Fig.3-2). It gives excellent results for 2–3 weeks and can be repeated if needed.

Temporary                    Permanent

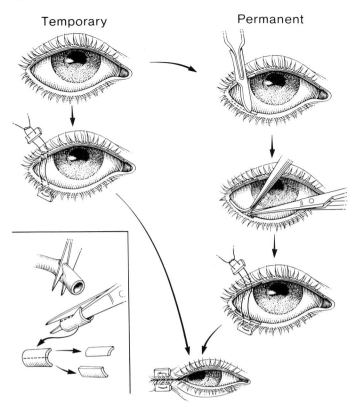

**Fig. 3-2.** Lateral tarsorrhaphy. Lateral tarsorrhaphy can be performed with or without preparation of the eyelid margin depending on whether a permanent intermarginal adhesion is desired. When performing a permanent tarsorrhaphy, a shallow incision is made along the lateral mucocutaneous border on the upper and lower lid. This is elevated with a fine forcep and a thin sliver of posterior lid margin is removed with scissors dissection. Rubber bolsters can be made from a sterile urinary catheter as shown. A double-armed 4-0 prolene suture is then inserted in a mattress fashion using the bolsters and is tied snugly with special care to externalize the eye lashes and to ensure that the prepared eyelid margins are approximated. The suture can be removed in 2–3 weeks. If total tarsorrhaphy is indicated, an identical procedure can be performed in the medial aspect of the eyelids with special care to avoid the lacrimal punta.

Lid anesthesia is obtained with local infiltration of lidocaine with epinephrine. One arm of a double-armed 4-0 prolene suture is inserted into the upper eyelid 4–5 mm from the lid margin. The needle is passed anterior to the tarsal plate and emerges from the lid margin anterior to the gray line. The needle is then passed through the adjacent lower eyelid margin and emerges from the skin 4–5 mm away. The second arm of the prolene is passed in an identical fashion. Small cotton or rubber bolsters are positioned to support the horizontal suture loops and the prolene is tied securely.

### Permanent Tarsorrhaphy

Two techniques are described for forming a permanent tarsorrhaphy. The marginal excision technique is easy to perform and can be easily reversed, but it may stretch, decreasing its effectiveness.

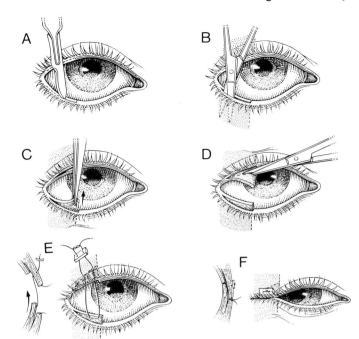

**Fig. 3-3.** Lateral tarsorrhaphy with use of a sliding tarsal conjunctival flap. (A) A shallow incision is made in the lateral mucocutaneous border of the upper and lower lid. (B) Wescott-type scissors can be used to extend this dissection into the lid and provide a freely mobile tarsal conjunctival flap. (C) The flap is further mobilized by a perpendicular cut along the medial border of the tarsal conjunctival flap. (D) A small triangle of tarsus and conjunctiva is removed from the superior tarsal conjunctival flap. (E) Using a double-armed 4-0 prolene suture and a rubber bolster, a mattress stitch is placed through the inferior tarsal conjunctival flap and used to approximate it to the defect created by the excision of the triangle of tissue superiorly. (F) The suture is tied snugly over the bolster and left in place for 2–3 weeks.

*Technique 1: simple tarsorrhaphy with intermarginal adhesion.* Lidocaine with epinephrine is used to infiltrate the upper and lower eyelids in their lateral aspect. The mucocutaneous border of the lateral upper and lower eyelid is marked with a shallow incision using a #15 blade. The posterior aspect of the eyelid margin is then excised. A double-armed 4-0 prolene suture is then passed through bolsters, and through the upper eyelid and tarsus emerging from the lid margin. The needle is then passed through the lower-lid margin with a symmetrical path through the lower lid emerging from the skin 4–5 mm inferior to the lid margin. The suture is tied over a bolster and remains in place for 3–4 weeks to allow optimal formation of intermarginal adhesions (Fig. 3-2).

*Technique 2: tarsorrhaphy with sliding flap.* Following infiltration anesthesia with lidocaine and epinephrine, an incision is made along the mucocutaneous border of the lateral upper and lower eyelids using a #15 blade. Blunt dissection is used to separate the anterior and posterior lamellae of the lateral upper and lower eyelid. The upper and lower tarsal flaps are created by a vertical incision of the tarsus. The vertical cut should begin at the medial aspect of the lid margin incision (Fig. 3-3). The lateral aspect of the upper and lower tarsal plates should be sufficiently loose to allow sliding. The superior tarsal flap is pulled downward and a small triangle is excised. The lower tarsal flap is advanced and sutured to the upper lid in the space created by excision of the upper tarsal triangle using a double-armed 4-0 prolene suture. A partial-thickness bite is taken through the superior aspect of the lower tarsal flap, then passed from the exposed undersurface of the upper lid externally through the skin and tied over a bolster. The suture and the bolster are removed in 3–4 weeks.

## HORIZONTAL LOWER-LID SHORTENING

Shortening of the lower eyelid is an effective treatment for many cases of ectropion due to eyelid laxity. By tightening the lower lid, the margin is repositioned against the eye and elevated to improve tear dynamics. The lower eyelid can be tightened by a mid-lid resection, lateral canthal shortening or medial canthal shortening. The wedge resection is familiar to almost all ophthalmic surgeons, is easily performed and effectively tightens the lower eyelid. A disadvantage of this technique is that healthy tarsus is removed.[11] The lateral lid-tightening techniques remove tissue where the laxity occurs and allow more tightening than mid-lid resections.[11]

### Pentagonal Wedge Resection

Infiltration anesthesia is obtained using lidocaine with epinephrine. Starting 3–4 mm from the lateral canthus a perpendicular incision is made through full-thickness eyelid. The incision should extend approximately 3.8 mm (to the end of the lower tarsus)[16] and is redirected nasally for 3–4 mm to form the lateral half of the pentagon. The medial edge of incised eyelid is pulled laterally overlapping the incision to determine the amount of lid to be resected. The second perpendicular incision is then made to the lower edge of the tarsus and redirected to join the lateral incision. A pentagon of full-thickness lid is removed and hemostasis obtained.

A 6-0 silk suture is placed through the lid margin but not tied. The suture is used for alignment and control of the lid margin during tarsal closure. Three or four interrupted 6-0 vicryl or 7-0 silk sutures on a spatula needle are used to close the tarsus. The tarsal sutures should remain anterior to the conjunctiva to prevent corneal irritation. Next, the lower-lid retractors inferior to the tarsus are reapproximated with additional interrupted vicryl or silk sutures. The 6-0 retention suture is removed and the lid margin is reapproximated with two 6-0 silk sutures: one through the gray line and one through the lash line. The ends are left long to be secured to the skin sutures. A horizontal mattress suture of 4-0 prolene is used to decrease wound tension and the skin is closed using interrupted or running 6-0 silk.

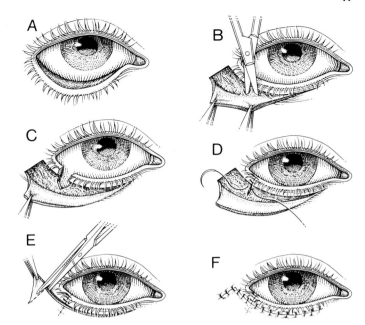

**Fig. 3-4.** Repair of lower lid ectropion by Smith modification of the Kunht-Szymanowski procedure. (A) A senile-type lower lid ectropion. (B) A blepharoplasty-type subciliary incision is made with dissection of a skin flap. (C) A pentagonal wedge of tarsus and conjunctiva is removed from the lower lid. (D) The tarsus and conjunctiva is then approximated with a 4-0 silk suture at the mucocutaneous border and 6-0 chromic sutures at the tarsus inferiorly. (E) A triangular piece of redundant skin is excised laterally. (F) Interrupted or continuous 6-0 silk or nylon sutures are used to approximate the skin incision completing this procedure. The skin sutures are removed in 4–7 days and the 4-0 silk suture approximating the tarsal conjunctival border is removed in approximately 2 weeks.

### Kuhnt-Szymanowski Procedure, Smith Modification

The Kuhnt[9]-Szymanowski[14] procedure is no longer used since this technique is associated with a high incidence of trichiasis and scarring of the eyelid margin.[5] Smith modified the procedure combining a skin flap anteriorly with a block resection of the eyelid posteriorly resulting in a safer more effective procedure.[12]

#### The Technique

A marking pen is used to define the skin incision (Fig. 3-4). The infraciliary incision begins 2–3 mm temporal to the punctum and extends to the lateral canthal angle. The incision is redirected in an oblique fashion along the skin lines. A skin-muscle flap is elevated and hemostasis obtained. The skin is retracted and a pentagonal wedge resection is performed as described previously. If there is redundant skin, it may be excised using the following triangulation technique of McCord.[11] The skin-muscle flap is stretched toward the ear until the appropriate tension is obtained, the lateral triangle for excision is marked and excised. Next, the skin-muscle flap is fixed to the lateral canthus with 4-0 silk and the superior triangle is conservatively removed. A small strip of muscle is removed from the edge of the flap to create a smoother closure. The skin is closed with interrupted or running 6-0 silk suture.

## Lateral Canthal Approach for Horizontal Lid Shortening

Lateral canthal tightening is a popular technique for repair of laxity ectropion. The lateral canthal approach avoids lid notching and allows more tightening of the eyelid than mid-lid procedures. There are many effective techniques described for lateral canthal tightening.[2] The procedure by McCord[11] has proven to be a very simple and effective treatment for most cases of laxity ectropion.

### The Technique

The skin is marked and a horizontal canthotomy is performed along the natural skin lines (Fig. 3-5). The lateral canthal tendon is then released by cutting infratemporally along the orbital rim with scissors. The lateral lower lid should become freely mobile and easy to rotate away from the globe. Next, the lid is stretched temporally and a triangle of tissues marked for excision. The lid incision should be perpendicular to the lid margin for the length of the lower tarsus (3.9 mm) and then directed toward the initial cantholysis incision. A double-armed 4-0 polydek with ME-2 needle is placed through the edge of the tarsal plate as illustrated and attached to the inner aspect of the lateral orbital rim. The suture tension is adjusted and the suture tied. The skin is closed with 6-0 silk or prolene. Sometimes a dog ear will form at the distal portion of the incision and this is removed using a standard oblique extension.

## Horizontal Upper-Lid Shortening

The upper eyelid can be effectively shortened with a pentagonal wedge resection. This technique was used by Dutton[6] to treat five eyes of four patients with the floppy eyelid syndrome. In all five eyes the shortening and resultant tightening of the upper lid resulted in complete resolution of symptoms. The amount of lid excised varied from 7 to 15 mm. As with the lower-lid pentagonal wedge resection, care must be taken to incise the eyelid perpendicular to the lid margin for the entire length of the tarsus. After parallel incisions are made for the length of the tarsus, they are connected to create a pentagonal shaped defect.

### The Technique

The area for excision is defined with a marking pen. Vertical incisions should be perpendicular to the lid margin and extend for the full length of the tarsus (10–11 mm). The incisions are redirected at a 45° angle to join in a pentagonal shape. Full-thickness eyelid is resected using tissue scissors and hemostasis is obtained. A 6-0 silk retention suture is placed through the lid margin but not tied. This suture is used for control of the lid margin during tarsal closure. The tarsal closure is the most important aspect of the lid repair and should be performed meticulously. The tarsus can be reapproximated with 6-0 absorbable sutures or 7-0 silk on a spatula needle. Three to five sutures are placed through the tarsus in a vertical line. The sutures should be placed anterior to the tarsus to prevent corneal irritation. The 6-0 retention suture is removed and the lid margin is closed with two 6-0 silk sutures: one through the lash line and one through the gray line. The ends of the lid margin sutures are left long to be secured to the skin sutures. A 4-0 prolene horizontal mattress suture is placed to decrease wound tension. The skin is closed with interrupted or running 6-0 silk.

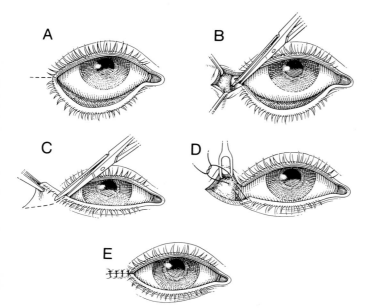

**Fig. 3-5.** Repair of lower lid ectropion using lateral lid-shortening procedure. (A) A senile-type lower lid ectropion. (B) A skin incision is made perpendicular to the eyelid margin at its most lateral aspect exposing lateral canthal tendon. Inferior arm of lateral canthal tendon is visualized and cut with scissors. (C) Triangular wedge of full-thickness skin and tarsus is excised. (D) A double-armed a 4-0 or 5-0 absorbable suture is used to approximate cut edge of lateral eyelid to periosteum. (E) The skin incision is closed with interrupted 6-0 silk or nylon sutures.

## Conjunctival Flaps

In 1958 Gundersen described an effective technique for using conjunctival flaps in the treatment of corneal ulceration and recalcitrant keratitis.[7] Although improved therapeutic capabilities such as surgical Adhesive and bandage lenses have lessened the need for conjunctival flaps, they remain an effective alternative for severe exposure keratitis. This technique should only be used when other therapies have failed to stabilize the cornea. The most likely clinical condition in which a flap is useful is in patients with combined fifth and seventh nerve paresis. These patients have a combined exposure and neurotropic keratitis and are at high risk for melting and perforation.

*The Technique*

The quantity of conjunctiva elevated and the area covered should be according to the individual case. The procedure has the following steps: (1) preparation of the corneal bed, (2) elevation of the flap, and (3) suturing of the flap in position. The corneal epithelium should be removed only in the area to be covered by the graft because uncovered cornea remains at risk for ulceration. The epithelium being removed is unhealthy and can usually be removed by wiping gently with a cellulose sponge. Chemical agents should be avoided because they may damage the adjacent epithelium and underlying basement membrane.

A subconjunctival injection of 1% lidocaine with epinephrine is used to balloon the conjunctiva superiorly. A horizontal incision is made parallel to the tarsal fold and the flap is dissected to the superior limbus for 180°. A peritomy is performed for 360° and the limbus is bared of remaining epithelium in the areas to be covered by the conjunctival flap. The flap is positioned and sutured in place. The suture should be nonreactive if bites are taken in clear cornea, preferably 9-0 or 10-0 nylon in a running or interrupted fashion.

## REFERENCES

1. Arion HG: Dynamic closure of the lids and paralysis of the orbicularis muscle. Int Surg 57:48, 1972
2. Bick MW: Surgical management of orbital tarsal disparity, Arch Ophthalmol 80:494, 1966
3. Biglan AW, Burger GE: Congenital horizontal tarsal kink. AM J Ophthalmol 91:552, 1980
4. Culberson WM, Ostler HB: The floppy eyelid syndrome. AM J Ophthalmol 92:568–575, 1981
5. Dryden RM, Doxanas MT: Eyelid Malpositions, Part II: Ectropion and entropion, in McCord CW (ed): Oculoplastic Surgery. New York, Raven Press, 1981, p 128
6. Dutton JJ: Surgical management of the floppy eyelid syndrome. Am J Ophthalmol 99:557–560, 1985
7. Gundersen T: Conjunctival flaps in the treatment of corneal disease with reference to a new technique of application. Arch Ophthalmol 60:880, 1958
8. Jonghees LBW: On peripheral facial nerve paralysis. Arch Otolaryngol 95:313–317, 1972
9. Kuhnt, H: Beitrage zur Operationen Augenheilkunder. Jena, G. Fischer, 1883, pp 44–55
10. McCarthy RW; Lamellar tarsoplasty-A new technique for correction of horizontal tarsal kink. Ophthalmic Surg 15:859–860, 1984
11. McCord CD: Surgery of the eyelids, in Duane T (ed): Clinical Ophthalmology, vol 5. Philadelphia, Harper and Row, 1985, pp 18–29
12. Smith B, Cherubini TD: Oculoplastic Surgery: A Compendium of Principles and Techniques. St. Louis, C.V. Mosby, 1970, pp 92–94
13. Smolin G, Thoft RA: The Cornea: Scientific Foundations and Clinical Practice. Boston/Toronto, Little, Brown, 1983, p 319
14. Szymanoski J, Hindbuch D: Operation Chirurgie. Berlin, Brauschweig, 1870 p 243
15. Wesley RE: Tarsal ectropion form detachment of the lower eyelid retractors. Am J Ophthalmol 93:491, 1982
16. Wesley RE, McCord CD, Jones JA: The height of the tarsis on the lower eyelid. AM J Ophthalmol 90:102, 1980
17. White JH: Method of correction of tarsal ectropion, Am J Ophthalmol 72:615–617, 1971

# 4

# Keratoconjunctivitis Sicca

## Ivan R. Schwab

*Keratoconjunctivitis sicca* is a protean disease with many diverse causes; yet the physical findings remain remarkably constant regardless of cause. Simply stated, keratoconjunctivitis sicca exists when the production of tears is inadequate in quantity or quality to maintain the health and normal physiology of the corneal and conjunctival epithelium.

Holly and Lemp have suggested a five-part classification of dry eye, which includes (1) aqueous deficiency, (2) mucin deficiency, (3) lipid abnormality, (4) lid abnormality, and (5) epitheliopathy (anesthetic cornea, epithelial irregularity of any cause).[21]

Primary keratoconjunctivitis sicca includes aqueous deficiencies, mucin deficiencies, and in some cases lipid abnormalities. Aqueous deficiencies are a diverse group of diseases best represented by Sjogren's syndrome, an autoimmune disease usually associated with rheumatologic problems. Mucin deficiencies result from conjunctival diseases such as Stevens-Johnson syndrome, ocular pemphigoid, and trachoma. Although pure mucin deficiencies are less common than pure aqueous deficiencies, the mucin and aqueous deficiency states often coexist in the same patient.

Lipid composition is controlled by the meibomian glands, and any disruption or change in the function of these glands may result in a decrease in the stability of the lipid layer. For example, the infectious agents in chronic blepharitis may produce lipase, which often hydrolyzes lipids, thus liberating free fatty acids. These short-chain fatty acids decrease stability, leading to dry spots in the tear film and eventually to keratopathy. Occasionally, one of the lipid disorders is severe enough to be considered a primary dry eye, but many of these diseases are managed as primary lipid disorders with little regard to the dry eye.

Though the secondary dry eye conditions such as lid abnormalities and the epitheliopathy group are not emphasized in this chapter, it is important to distinguish them from the primary dry eye because their medical and surgical management are entirely different. Lid abnormalities such as lagophthalmios, lid notches, entropion, ectropion, and related problems may cause disruption of the tear film resulting in chronic (often localized) drying. The epitheliopathy group, like the lid abnormalities, is not primarily a dry eye, but rather is secondary to another condition. An epitheliopathy such as an anesthetic cornea may result from an acoustic neuroma. Tear quality and quantity are both relatively unaffected. Still, the anesthetic cornea may have permanent dry spot formation or even corneal ulceration. Neuronal stimulation may be required for the corneal epithelium to participate in the integrity of tear film. As these examples illustrate, secondary dry eyes may require a very different treatment than the primary dry eyes. Thus, their treatment is beyond the scope of this chapter.

## DIAGNOSIS OF KERATOCONJUNCTIVITIS SICCA

### History

A careful history is quite helpful in establishing the diagnosis of dry eye. Patients with dry eye will often complain of a sensation of dryness, irritation, or burning, especially with various stimuli such as bright lights, air conditioning, wind, fumes, or even reading. Patients should be queried regarding medications, because many preparations and drugs such as antihistamines, anticholinergics, birth control pills, and marijuana can temporarily decrease aqueous tear production.

Dermatologic and rheumatologic diseases should be considered because many of these systemic diseases have dry eye as one of their components. Ichthyosis, psoriasis, pemphigoid, and eczema are examples of dermatologic problems that may have dry eye as an associated finding. Rheumatoid arthritis, scleroderma, and systemic lupus erythematosus often have keratoconjunctivitis sicca as an associated finding.[12] Furthermore, these autoimmune and rheumatologic diseases are frequently part of Sjogren's syndrome, which includes keratoconjunctivitis sicca, xerostomia, and arthritis.

SURGICAL INTERVENTION IN CORNEAL AND EXTERNAL DISEASES
ISBN 0-8089-1850-8

## Examination

Examination must begin with a general inspection of each patient. Any physical findings such as rheumatoid nodules or skin rashes should be palpated or inspected. A facial examination should focus on the periocular and ocular tissues but should not ignore the remainder of the facial skin in the search for such things as telangiectases, seborrhea, pustules, or other rashes. It is important to perform an inspection of both globes and lids in natural light that will reflect the pattern of conjunctival injection, subconjunctival or scleral inflammation, or changes in lid coloration or configuration.

Biomicroscopic examination should reveal many, if not all, of the common, important findings, including debris in the tear film, decreased tear film meniscus, meibomian oversecretion, mucus strands, filaments, conjunctival injection (especially in the palpebral aperture), and punctate epithelial keratopathy.

Staining is another important diagnostic tool. Fluorescein will stain the punctate epithelial keratopathy but is even more valuable in assessing the tear meniscus height which is normally 0.5- to 1-mm in width.[2,24] Fluorescein is also important in assessing tear break-up time. Although somewhat controversial and subject to many potential sources of error, tear break-up time is an important assessment of quantity and quality, or stability, of tears, especially in ocular diseases with a primary mucus[5,32] or aqueous deficiency.[10,27] Rose bengal stain is also useful because it stains devitalized, injured epithelial cells, mucus threads, and filaments.[10,42] Also, rose bengal staining of the keratopathy is prominent, especially in the palpebral aperture, since drying injures epithelial cells, allowing for the uptake of stain.[42] Rose bengal staining is one of the most sensitive and specific tests for keratoconjunctivitis sicca.

Tear volume can be assessed by using Schirmer's tear strips, an objective measure of aqueous production. Schirmer's tear-strip testing depends upon the amount of wetting of a standardized strip, and is sometimes difficult to interpret in marginal cases.[42,44] Although there is some debate as to whether Schirmer's test is best performed with or without anesthesia, we prefer to perform it without anesthesia. Abnormal Schirmer's test result without anesthesia is less than 5 mm of wetting, although 5–15 mm is still not a normal value.[10] An abnormal Schirmer's test result with anesthesia is less than 3 mm.[26]

Tear lysozyme can also be measured with the tear-wetted Schirmer's strips. Lysozyme level is an accurate measure of the antibacterial quality of a patient's tears and is probably a good indicator of aqueous tear production.[7,42] Unfortunately, this test is time-consuming and somewhat difficult to perform, especially if only a few specimens are encountered each month.

Measurement of tear osmolarity and tear lactoferrin levels are newer diagnostic methods to assess keratoconjunctivitis.[13,19] Tear osmolarity rises with the concentration of tears in cases of dry eye. Lactoferrin levels also rise with keratoconjunctivitis sicca. Both measurements seem to be

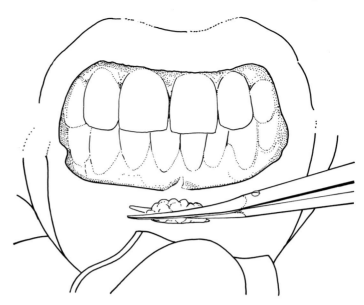

**Fig. 4-1.**   Labial salivary gland biopsy of lower lip. The gland has prolapsed through a horizontal incision in the oral mucosa.

quite effective as diagnostic tests, but each is time-consuming and requires rather expensive equipment.

The diagnosis of Sjogren's syndrome can be documented by labial gland biopsy, which will show focal lymphocytic and plasma cell infiltrates with ductal aberrations suggesting an autoimmune disease.[6,8] Lacrimal gland biopsy would show similar findings but is not advocated, since any loss of lacrimal tissue could potentially inhibit the tear production.

Labial salivary gland biopsy can be performed as follows. The minor salivary glands of the lower lip are chosen because they are accessible and lie above the muscle layer. The lower lip is everted and 2% Xylocaine (Astra, Worcester, MA) with epinephrine is injected beneath the mucosa in the midline. A 2-cm horizontal incision is made through just the epithelium. Blunt dissection is used to remove surrounding fascia and avoid sensory nerves. The gland will prolapse readily. Several (5 to 10) of these small glands must be excised to obtain an adequate histologic sample (Fig. 4-1). Repair of the incision is performed using three interrupted sutures of 4-0 or 5-0 plain gut.[6,8]

## MEDICAL TREATMENT OF KERATOCONJUNCTIVITIS SICCA

Artificial tears are the principal treatment for keratoconjunctivitis sicca, and mild or moderate cases of dry eye respond well to this therapy. There are several different commercial brands of tear substitutes, each with a different theoretical objective. These can be given to patients as frequently as every hour, though medicamentosa or toxic keratopathy may be a problem for patients using any of these solutions frequently. Toxic keratopathy, probably due to preservatives such as benzalkonium chloride and thimerosal, can lead to conjunctivitis, keratopathy, frank epithelial cell loss, uveitis, and infection. If toxic keratopathy develops, nonpreserved tears may be substituted. Any patient using nonpreserved solutions should be cautioned to take care not to contaminate solutions.

Large molecular weight polymers such as methyl cellulose will prolong the time of evaporation but are somewhat viscous.[30,38] Patients may complain of lid crusting or visual symptoms with these polymers. Polyvinyl alcohol, another polymer, is much less viscous and better tolerated.[25] Newer polymers seem to have an increased surface affinity, but still suffer from short duration. Recently, hypotonic tear solutions have been shown to have better penetration and some advantages.[18,19] It is probably best to try several agents with each patient, seeking the best regimen. A combination of a large molecular weight polymer four or five times a day with frequent supplement of a newer, less-viscous polymer might be an attractive form of therapy. Ointments and emollients may be used at bedtime as an adjunct to tear substitutes or may be added as a diurnal therapy. Unfortunately, these ointments blur vision and make the skin oily to touch, which can be disagreeable for some patients.

Long-term release pellets of hydroxypropyl cellulose have been used in the last few years with varying degrees of success.[22,23,43] Although blurring of vision, foreign body sensation, and loss of the pellet can be disturbing side effects, these pellets greatly help some patients. In patients with moderate or severe dry eye, tear substitutes may have to be instilled to dissolve these pellets. The combination of body temperature and moisture work to dissolve the cellulose in a time-release fashion over 8–12 hours. This is an excellent concept, although the problems of practical application have yet to be overcome. Because some authors believe there is little difference clinically between one tear substitute and the next,[29] perhaps the best approach is to try several different tear substitutes to find the ones that give the most subjective improvement.

In the most severe cases of dry eye, or in cases of toxicity from the tear substitutes themselves, specially prepared solutions deserve some consideration. Healon (Pharmacia, Piscataway, NJ) has been tried with success either undiluted or diluted 1:10.[35,37] This solution of sodium hyaluronate is highly viscous, biologically inert, and has been successfully used intraocularly.[33] Although there are enthusiastic reports as to its efficiency without appreciable toxicity, this medication should be carefully investigated before it can be assumed both useful and safe.

Commercially available albumin prepared in small (5–10 cc) aliquots may be provided to patients at relatively little expense. This unpreserved solution must be constituted in a sterile fashion, and patients warned of the increased risk of infections. Although data have not yet been published, there have been enthusiastic reports as to albumin's success (JD Lanier, personal communication). This modality has not, however, been officially approved in the United States.

Similarly, artificial tears made with autologous serum have been used successfully to treat patients with severe keratoconjunctivitis sicca.[15] This serum has several theoretical advantages, but relatively few patients have been treated. Also, it is unpreserved, so bacterial contamination is a potential complication. Autologous serum, like albumin, is not an officially approved treatment. Some patients may benefit from a 10% solution of N-acetylcysteine. This collagenase inhibitor is thought to be helpful in breaking the disulfide cross-linkage in mucus, producing a less-viscous tear solution.[28] This solution must, however, be carefully prepared to a neutral or slightly alkaline pH with the use of sodium bicarbonate and it requires refrigeration because it is unpreserved and therefore subject to breakdown. If this treatment is too difficult and inconvenient, mucus removal with irrigation, a warm wet cloth, or a moistened applicator may be quite effective and symptomatically useful to patients.

Tseng et al. have recently documented improvement in keratoconjunctivitis sicca with topical vitamin A.[39] This exciting work has been suggested in previous studies.[20,36,41] However, confirmation of clinical success by other investigators is important before this medication can be generally accepted. Still, it is theoretically promising, and clinically exciting in the medical management of dry eye.

Other solutions that have yet to gain wide clinical acceptance include bromhexine hydrochloride and pilocarpine. Bromhexine hydrochloride seems to improve tear production and prolongs tear break-up time but has not had great acceptance clinically. Pilocarpine may increase tearing in patients with relatively normal lacrimal glands, but it has not been shown to be effective in keratoconjunctivitis sicca.[11]

A note of caution should be raised regarding medicamentosa. Patients with keratoconjunctivitis sicca have a compromised ocular surface that is more susceptible to injury from active topical compounds such as preservatives. To add to this problem, these patients may have an increased risk of topical sensitization leading to an increased prevalence of allergic syndromes. Hence, patients taking topical medications should be supported and followed closely for worsening of their signs or symptoms.

In addition to topical medications, simple mechanisms of tear preservation also should be mentioned and discussed with each patient. For example, permanent humidity units for the home (especially during winter when the average humidity is much lower) and a portable unit for the work place are often a great help. Patients should be told to avoid sources of hot, dry air such as hair dryers, hot air vents, and arid environments. Patients should be advised to stop or limit administration of medication or drugs that contribute to dry eye, such as antihistamines, diuretics, birth control pills, anticholinergics, and marijuana. Also, all dry eye patients should wear at least glasses, and if possible goggles, when in a dusty windy environment.

For severe cases of keratoconjunctivitis sicca, swimmers' goggles, buller shields, or side shields attached to glasses are often helpful in retaining the tear volume present. These work by decreasing or preventing evaporation. The goggles, however, are inconvenient for patients to wear and maintain, and are helpful to only a small percentage of cases.

Therapeutic soft contact lenses have been advocated by

some practitioners because theoretically they would limit evaporation of tears from the ocular surface. The lenses, however, increase surface area and probably do not decrease evaporation. In fact, infections (and probably toxicity) are more common with soft contact lenses in dry eye patients. Increased risk of corneal ulcer, a potentially devastating complication of soft contact lenses, serves to prohibit widespread use of these devices in dry eye patients. Still, soft contact lenses are effective in relieving the pain and problems with filamentary keratoconjunctivitis and exposure keratitis. Perhaps the best use of these therapeutic lenses is in the treatment of mucus deficiency with sufficient lacrimal outflow. Caution should, however, be exercised because of the added risk of infection. Generally, soft contact lenses are probably of little help and may cause significant problems.

## SURGICAL TREATMENT OF KERATOCONJUNCTIVITIS SICCA

### Punctal Occlusion

If medical therapy has been unsuccessful, punctal occlusion should be considered. Punctal occlusion is safe and effective, with a low prevalence of complications.[9,10,40]

#### Temporary Punctal Occlusion

Because the major complication is epiphora, temporary punctal occlusion should be tried first, particularly in the mild and moderate cases. Some authors feel that the eye should have 2 mm or less of wetting before punctal occlusion is considered, but this test does not predict the therapeutic effect of the procedure or the likelihood of complications. Certainly, irreversible punctal occlusion should be reserved for patients with severe keratoconjunctivitis sicca. If doubt remains, temporary occlusion should be performed first.

Temporary occlusion can be obtained with 2-0 plain suture, collagen implants, tissue adhesive,[31] punctal plugs,[16] gelatin implants,[14] or temporary closure by suturing. Although there is virtually no literature to support (or contradict) the use of plain suture as a canalicular plug, it has been used anecdotally for years with no known significant side effects. (Allergy to the suture material is possible but must be rare).

Canalicular occlusion with suture plugs is performed as follows. Upper and lower puncta are anesthetized with proparacaine and then with 4% Xylocaine®. Punctal dilation is performed (Fig. 4-2). Approximately 4–5 mm of 2-0 plain suture is inserted into the lower punctum (Fig. 4-3). The suture is cut at the punctum and pushed slightly beyond the orifice with the punctal dilator (Figs. 4-4 and 4-5). The upper punctum is treated in a similar fashion. The suture material will swell in the canaliculus, occlude the passage, and then dissolve in 2–6 weeks. This will allow for a satisfactory clinical trial of occlusion.

Commercially available collagen implants have been tested and approved by the FDA. These implants are similar

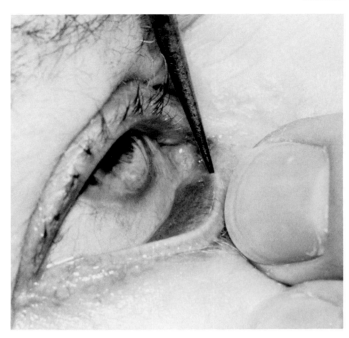

**Fig. 4-2.** Temporary punctal occlusion can be achieved with 2-0 plain suture. After topical anesthesia, the upper and lower puncta are dilated with a punctal dilator.

to the suture material although the collagen implants are designed to be the correct punctal diameter (0.2 mm). These will also resorb in the canaliculus.

Tissue adhesive (N-butyl cyanoacrylate) occlusion is also effective[34] and may be performed as follows. The upper and lower puncta are anesthetized with proparacaine and then with 4% Xylocaine®. Both puncta are dilated with a punctal dilator. The epithelium of each dilated punctum is removed mechanically with a corneal burr bit used for rust rings. The orifice and surrounding area must be dried care-

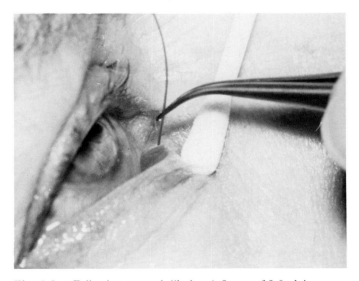

**Fig. 4-3.** Following punctal dilation 4–5 mm of 2-0 plain suture is directed into each punctum.

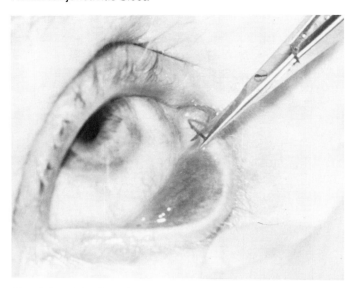

**Fig. 4-4.** After insertion of 2-0 plain suture into the lower punctum, the suture is cut flush with the orifice.

fully and the lid everted. A small drop of tissue adhesive is applied to each punctum. The lid should remain everted until the tissue adhesive dries. This adhesive can be removed with a small pair of forceps, or it will drop off within 1–3 weeks. This procedure is relatively free of complications although the medical-grade tissue adhesive is difficult to obtain. Also, it can be hard to place a small drop of adhesive that occludes the punctum without creating a large plaque that might abrade the cornea.

Punctal plugs (Freeman Punctum Plug, Eagle Vision, Memphis, TN) have also been used for temporary occlusion.[16] Following application of topical anesthesia, gentle punctal dilation is performed with care taken to preserve the punctum connective tissue ring. These silicon plugs are then inserted into each punctum. Migration is discouraged by a small flange. Occasionally, these can be accidentally dislodged by rubbing or during sleep.[16] Keratitis has been reported as another potential complication. Migration of the plug would be possible, and certainly retrieval from the canaliculus or lacrimal sac could be difficult. Silicone foreign bodies can produce a chronic granulomatous inflammation within the lacrimal sac, resulting in occlusion.

### Permanent Punctal Occlusion

Permanent punctal occlusion can be effectively achieved by diathermy or cautery.[9,40] First, the skin around the upper and lower puncta is infiltrated with 2% Xylocaine® with epinephrine (Fig. 4-6). The disposable (battery-operated) ophthalmic cautery tip is inserted into the lower punctum and the tissue is burned until a 1- to 2-mm area of cauterization is achieved.[40] Alternatively, a diathermy unit (e.g., HyFrecater, Birtcher, Elmonte, CA) with a thin needle is inserted approximately 10 mm into the lower canaliculus (Fig. 4-7). The current is turned on and increased until a whitening effect is achieved. The needle is removed and the punctum is then cauterized.[9]

Both puncta should be occluded with the chosen technique. Antibiotic drops should be prescribed for 2–5 days following either procedure. Cautery with a disposable unit is

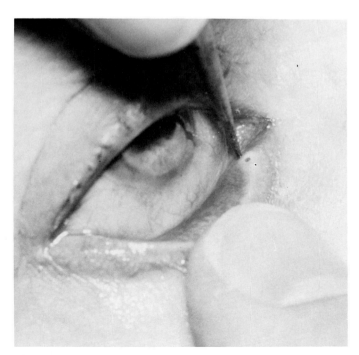

**Fig. 4-5.** The punctal dilator is used to push the distal end of the suture material beyond the orifice to "countersink" the suture. The 2-0 plain suture can be seen in the punctum, and the dilator is being held beside the orifice.

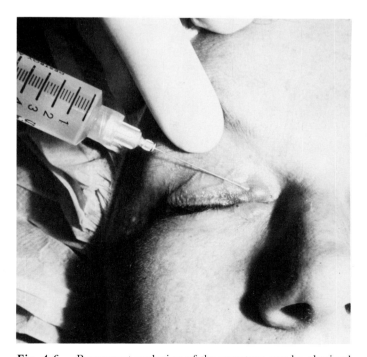

**Fig. 4-6.** Permanent occlusion of the punctum can be obtained by cautery or diathermy. First, local infiltration with 2% xylocaine with epinephrine is performed in the skin surrounding each punctum. Topical anesthesia may also be of assistance.

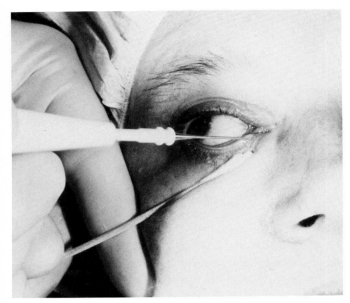

**Fig. 4-7.** After appropriate anesthesia, the thin diathermy needle is inserted approximately 5 mm into the punctum. Because of local factors, it is difficult to predict the setting of the instrument. Hence, the lower settings should be used, and the settings gradually increased until a whitening effect is achieved. Once the needle is removed, the punctum itself is cauterized, although the settings required for the superficial punctum are much lower than those for the internal canaliculus.

more likely to produce failure than cautery of the full length of the canaliculus by diathermy. Both procedures are effective and safe, with perhaps as much as a 30 percent failure rate. That is, as many as one-third may reopen after several weeks. This procedure can be repeated if necessary. It should, however, be regarded as permanent because repair of cicatricial canalicular obstruction is very difficult.

Recent ophthalmic tabloid reports of greater success with laser occlusion of the punctum offer no data to support their claims, and no literature report has substantiated these results. Excessive costs of laser treatment, and the use of inappropriate technology seem unjustifiable with such a high rate of success with simple cautery. Until scientific reports document a higher success rate, fewer complications, or lower cost, laser punctal occlusion appears to be a costly treatment awaiting an indication.

## Parotid Duct Transposition

Parotid duct transposition is a surgical procedure that has been largely abandoned because of poor long-term success. It was and remains a desperate procedure, suitable for only one eye per patient, with a poor prognosis for success. The limited indications for this procedure are often contradictory. The patient must have total xerophthalmia, yet a relatively normal production of saliva from both parotids. The patient's disease process must be stable, yet severe, including keratinization, ankyloblepharon, and corneal opacifications. Potential complications are not insignificant. Only

one parotid duct may be transplanted because of the potential for dry mouth if both were transplanted. Dry mouth may result even if only one duct is transplanted, because the remaining parotid duct may not be producing a normal quantity or quality of saliva. There can be no guarantee that, if successful, the parotid duct transposition will halt any progression of the ocular surface complications, because saliva does not contain the proper constituents for the trilaminer structure of tears. Consequently, even if successful, the operation may provide 30–40 mm of Schirmer's wetting and overflow "epiphora," yet still provide incomplete and inadequate wetting. It is unlikely that any keratinization of symblepharon will be reversed by the saliva even if the newly transplanted duct remains patent.

The procedure requires that a horizontal incision be made over the anterior border of the masseter where the parotid duct turns to enter the mouth. A large cuff of buccal mucosa surrounding the parotid duct orifice is necessary to create a funnel of mucosal tissue since the duct is frequently too short to reach the inferior cul-de-sac. This pericanalicular oral mucosa is then sewn into the inferiorlateral fornix.[3,4] Potential complications of the surgery include overflow "epiphora," especially with meals,[31] and facial paralysis from inadvertent section of the seventh nerve during surgery. Overall, this procedure has few if any indications.

## Lid Procedures

Inadequate tear production will not be improved by lid surgery, but oculoplastic procedures may reduce ocular exposure, improve the blink, and conserve tears. Also, any coexistent lid malposition worsens the keratoconjunctivitis sicca; thus repair of this condition will benefit the patient.

### Cyrotherapy

Trichiasis may cause keratitis as well as disrupt the tear film. Also, trichiasis is commonly caused by diseases of conjunctival shrinkage that typically produce keratoconjunctivitis sicca. If associated lid repair is not required, however, isolated trichiasis can be well managed by cryotherapy.[28] Indications for this procedure in dry eye patients include normal or nearly normal lid position and a limited number of misdirected lashes with an associated keratitis. Cryotherapy is not a substitute for appropriate lid repair if there is lid malposition responsible for the trichiasis. Relative contraindications for cryotherapy include such diseases as ocular pemphigoid that may be activated by cryotherapy.

Following skin preparation, the lid is infiltrated locally using xylocaine with epinephrine. A thermocouple needle can be placed beneath the skin near the follicles of the lashes to be treated. The oculoplastic cryoprobe is placed on the lid margin and activated until −25°C is measured by the thermocouple. The usual retinal or cataract cryoprobe will not freeze the tissue rapidly enough to produce reliable treatment, even if the final temperature reaches −25°C. Therefore, the lid is allowed to thaw and the cryotherapy spot is repeated in the identical manner to complete a second cycle of treatment. The lashes will spontaneously drop out in 3–6 weeks.[28] Complications include depigmentation of the overlying skin and, in certain cases, reactivation of the disease.

### Lid-Tightening Procedures

Keratoconjunctivitis sicca is occasionally accompanied by senile lower-lid laxity, ectropion, or paralytic lower-lid laxity, with or without the element of lagophthalmus. While this may be classified as exposure in many cases, these conditions may accompany dry eye. Repair of these eyelid malpositions with the technique described by Anderson and Gordy is important to the treatment of these cases.[1] This discussion is limited to the repair of the lower lid because this defect is more commonly associated with keratoconjunctivitis sicca, or siccalike symptoms. However, the lateral tarsal strip procedure is applicable to either upper- or lower-lid laxity.[1]

When lower-lid ectropion or laxity has been identified, the lateral tarsal strip procedure is performed as follows (see Fig. 1-9). The lateral canthus, including skin and muscle overlying the superior lateral orbital rim and the tissues just inside the rim, are infiltrated with xylocaine containing epinephrine. A lateral canthotomy is performed to the orbital rim, and the inferior crus of the lateral canthal tendon is lysed. The lateral 1–2 cm of the lower eyelid is then split into anterior and posterior lamellae, slightly anterior to the gray line. The length of the tarsal strip required is determined by the amount of the laxity present. The conjunctiva is then cut from the lower tarsal edge for the length of the lid splitting and the conjunctiva is scraped from the inner surface of the tarsal strip. The mucocutaneous margin is excised from the tarsal strip. The tarsal strip is then sutured to the periosteum on the inner surface (orbital) of the lateral orbital rim. The vertical and posterior placement determines the effect achieved. The proper placement of these sutures is greatly facilitated by using a small, stout, half-circle needle (G-2) on a 4-0 polygalactin (or similar material) suture. It is important to place these sutures on the inner aspect of the orbital rim to prevent anterior displacement of the new canthus. The anterior lamelae (skin surface) is then excised to allow for interrupted closure of the lateral canthotomy with 6-0 or 7-0 silk or nylon sutures in a vertical mattress suture fashion. Skin sutures should be removed in 5–6 days.

Intermittent entropion may accompany keratoconjunctivitis sicca. Patients may have marginal tear production but do well until they are stressed by their environment. Once dry eye symptoms begin, frequent blinking and blepharospasm may initiate the entropion in a spastic fashion, which will only worsen the keratitis and symptoms. Control of the entropion may be enough to alleviate the symptoms but will not help the tear production. The variety of entropion procedures and indications for each procedure are beyond the intended scope of this chapter.

## ACKNOWLEDGMENTS

Supported in part by an unrestricted grant from Research to Prevent Blindness Inc.

The authors gratefully acknowledge the assistance of Patricia Tyrpak, editor, and Amy Clark, secretary.

## REFERENCES

1. Anderson RL, Gordy DD: The tarsal strip procedure. Arch Ophthalmol 97:2192–2196, 1979
2. Baum JL: Systemic disease associated with tear deficiencies. Int Ophthalmol Clin 13(1):157–184, 1973
3. Bennett JE, Bailey AL: A surgical approach to total xerophthalmia. Arch Ophthalmol 58:367–371, 1957
4. Bennett JE: The management of total xerophthalmia. Arch Ophthalmol 81:667–682, 1969
5. Brown SI: Further studies on the pathophysiology of keratitis sicca of Rollet. Arch Ophthalmol 83:542–547, 1970
6. Chisholm DM, Mason DK: Labial salivary gland biopsy in Sjogren's disease. J Clin Pathol 21:656–660, 1968
7. Copeland JR, Lamberts DW, Holly FJ: Investigation of the accuracy of tear lysozyme determination by the quantiplate method. Invest Ophthalmol Vis Sci 22:103–110, 1982
8. Daniels TE: Labial salivary gland biopsy in Sjogren's syndrome. Arthritis Rheum 27:147–156, 1984
9. Dohlman CH: Punctal occlusion in keratoconjunctivitis sicca. Ophthalmology 85:1277–1281, 1978
10. Dohlman CH, Lemp MA, English FP: Dry eye syndromes. Int Ophthalmol Clin 10(2):215–251, 1970
11. Dresner SC, Codere F, Brownstein S, et al.: Lacrimal drainage system inflammatory masses from retained silicone tubing. Am J Ophthalmol 98:609–613, 1984
12. Ehlers N: The precorneal film. Acta Ophthalmol 43:(suppl 81), 1965
13. Farris RL, Gilbard JP, Stuchell RN, et al.: Diagnostic tests in keratoconjunctivitis sicca. CLAO J 9:23–28, 1983
14. Foulds WS: Intra-canalicular gelatin implants in the treatment of kerato-conjunctivitis sicca. Br J Ophthalmol 45:625–627, 1961
15. Fox RI, Chan R, Michelson JB, et al.: Beneficial effect of artificial tears made with autologous serum in patients with keratoconjunctivitis sicca. Arthritis Rheum 27:459–461, 1984
16. Freeman JM: The punctum plug: Evaluation of a new treatment for the dry eye. Trans Am Acad Ophthalmol Otolaryngol 79:874–879, 1975
17. Gifford SR, Puntenney I, Bellows J: Keratoconjunctivitis sicca. Arch Ophthalmol 30:207–216, 1943
18. Gilbard JP, Farris RL: Tear osmolarity and ocular surface disease in keratoconjunctivitis sicca. Arch Ophthalmol 97:1642–1646, 1979
19. Gilbard JP, Farris RL, Santamaria II J: Osmolarity of tear microvolumes in keratoconjunctivitis sicca. Arch Ophthalmol 96:677–681, 1978
20. Hatchell DL, Faculjak M, Kubicek D: Treatment of xerophthalmia with retinol, tretinoin, and etretinate. Arch Ophthalmol 102:926–927, 1984
21. Holly FJ, Lemp MA: Tear physiology and dry eyes. Surv Ophthalmol 22:69–87, 1977
22. Katz IM, Blackman WM: A soluble sustained-release ophthalmic delivery unit. Am J Ophthalmol 83:728–734, 1977
23. Katz JI, Kaufman HE, Breslin C, et al.: Slow-release artificial tears and the treatment of keratitis sicca. Ophthalmology 85:787–793, 1978
24. Klein M: The lacrimal strip and the precorneal film in cases of Sjogren's syndrome. Br J Ophthalmol 33:387–388, 1949
25. Krishna N, Brow F: Polyvinyl alcohol as an ophthalmic vehicle. Am J Ophthalmol 57:99–106, 1964
26. Lamberts DW, Foster CS, Perry HD: Schirmer test after topical anesthesia and the tear meniscus height in normal eyes. Arch Ophthalmol 97:1082–1085, 1979

27. Lemp MA, Dohlman CH, Holly F: Corneal desiccation despite normal tear volume. Ann Ophthalmol 2:258–261, 1970

28. Levine MR: Medical and surgical treatment of the dry eye. Int Ophthalmol Clin 18(3):101–119, 1978

29. Marner K, Prause JU: A comparative clinical study of tear substitutes in normal subjects and in patients with keratoconjunctivitis sicca. Acta Ophthalmol 62:91–95, 1984

30. Mims JL: Methyl cellulose solution for ophthalmic use. Arch Ophthalmol 46:664–665, 1951

31. Nicholas JP, Brown FA: Management of epiphora following parotid duct transposition for xerophthalmia. Arch Ophthalmol 68:529–53l, 1962

32. Norn MS: Desiccation of the precorneal film: 1. Corneal wetting-time. Acta Ophthalmol 47:865–880, 1969

33. Pape LG, Balazs EA: The use of sodium hyaluronate (Healon) in human anterior segment surgery. Ophthalmology 87:699–705, 1980

34. Patten JT: Punctal occlusion with N-butyl cyanoacrylate tissue adhesive. Ophthalmic Surg 7(2):24–26, 1976

35. Polack FM, McNiece MT: The treatment of dry eyes with Na hyaluronate (Healon). Cornea 1:133–136, 1982

36. Sommer A: Treatment of corneal xerophthalmia with topical retinoic acid. Am J Ophthalmol 95:349–352, 1983

37. Stuart JC, Linn JG: Dilute sodium hyaluronate (Healon) in the treatment of ocular surface disorders. Ann Ophthalmol 17:190–192, 1985

38. Swan KC: Use of methyl cellulose in ophthalmology. Arch Ophthalmol 33:378–380, 1945

39. Tseng SCG, Maumenee AE, Stark WJ, et al.: Topical retinoid treatment for various dry-eye disorders. Ophthalmology 92:717–727, 1985

40. Tuberville AW, Frederick WR, Wood TO: Punctal occlusion in tear deficiency syndromes. Ophthalmology 89:1170–1172, 1982

41. Ubels JL, Edelhauser HF, Austin KH: Healing of experimental corneal wounds treated with topically applied retinoids. Am J Ophthalmol 95:353–358, 1983

42. van Bijsterveld OP: Diagnostic tests in the sicca syndrome. Arch Ophthalmol 82:10–14, 1969

43. Werblin TP, Rheinstrom SD, Kaufman HE. The use of slow-release artificial tears in the long-term management of keratitis sicca. Ophthalmology 88:78–81, 1981

44. Wright JC, Meger GE: A review of the Schirmer test for tear production. Arch Ophthalmol 67:564–565, 1962

# 5

# Recurrent and Chronic Corneal Epithelial Defects

Leslie S. Fujikawa          Robert B. Nussenblatt

The corneal epithelium is essential for corneal integrity. It not only provides a smooth outer surface in conjunction with tears for good visual acuity, but it is the protective barrier against invading microorganisms and against degradation of the corneal stroma by proteolytic enzymes.[23]

Under normal circumstances, damage to the corneal epithelium is followed by rapid healing with migration of the epithelium to cover the denuded area. In certain pathologic states, however, recurrent or chronic epithelial defects may occur, leading to prolonged pain, photophobia, corneal infection, and melting of the stroma with possible perforation of the cornea.[5,22] Loss of the corneal epithelium may, therefore, lead to significant ocular morbidity and potential blindness.

This chapter reviews the current state of knowledge regarding the etiology and medical and surgical therapy of recurrent and chronic corneal epithelial defects.

## DEFINITION

Recurrent and chronic corneal epithelial defects are clinical entities in which the corneal epithelium is unable to maintain an intact layer and breaks down in recurrent episodes or is broken down chronically.[5,22]

*Recurrent corneal erosion* is characterized by episodes of spontaneous breakdown of the epithelial layer.[22] An acute episode may begin with the sensation of a foreign body when the eye is first opened upon awakening in the morning. This progresses to photophobia with pain and tearing. Ocular examination reveals an epithelial defect, and the damaged epithelial sheet may float on the tear film as a gray filament. The epithelium that surrounds the defect may be edematous and loosely adherent to the underlying stroma. The epithelial defect usually heals within 1–2 days depending upon the size, and the eye becomes quiet and comfortable. The entire process, however, recurs at irregular intervals from several

days to weeks or months later. Between attacks, the cornea may appear normal or there may be small gray–white cystic or linear areas in the epithelium at the site of the erosions. Less commonly, there may be subepithelial scarring, depending upon the length of time the erosions take to heal.

*Chronic corneal epithelial defects,* also termed persistent corneal epithelial defects, usually occur in more severely damaged corneas and often are associated with abnormal corneal sensation.[5] There is varying degree of discomfort depending upon the level of corneal sensation. Ocular examination reveals an epithelial defect with rolled, raised edges of piled up epithelial cells. The epithelium that surrounds the defect may be edematous and loosely adherent to the stroma. The stroma underlying the defect is edematous and ulcerates at differing rates depending upon the underlying corneal disease. Usually there is corneal opacity due to stromal damage and scarring. The epithelial defect may change in size and in configuration with time, or it may remain relatively static in one location. These chronic corneal epithelial defects have a predilection for the central cornea.

The complications associated with epithelial defects include incapacitation from discomfort, infection, stromal ulceration (especially with chronic corneal defects), and loss of vision from corneal scarring or perforation.[5,22]

## BASIC PATHOGENESIS OF RECURRENT AND CHRONIC EPITHELIAL DEFECTS

Corneal epithelial defects may be caused by a variety of conditions and insults to the cornea. The following list summarizes the conditions associated with both recurrent and chronic corneal epithelial defects; in all of these conditions the basic underlying mechanism is the inability of the epithelium to effectively adhere to its stromal substrate:

SURGICAL INTERVENTION IN CORNEAL AND EXTERNAL DISEASES
ISBN 0-8089-1850-8

1. Dystrophies
   Cogan's microcystic, map/dot/fingerprint dystrophy
   Meesman/Stocker-Holt
   Reis-Bücklers
   Lattice
   Granular
   Fuch's endothelial
   Posterior polymorphous dystrophy
2. Degenerations
   Salzmann's nodular degeneration
   Band keratopathy
3. Traumatic
   Mechanical
   Chemical
   Thermal
4. Postsurgical
   Diabetes—postvitrectomy
   Postpenetrating keratoplasty
   Postradial keratotomy
   Postepikeratophakia
5. Associated with infectious agents
   Bacterial
   Viral, e.g., metaherpetic
   Fungal
6. Other
   Tear deficiency
   Lid abnormality
   Corneal edema—postoperative or postinflammatory
   Neurotrophic/neuroparalytic

The epithelial basement membrane (EBM) is the structure that forms the connection between the epithelium and the stroma, and it is crucial in maintaining tight adhesions between the epithelium and stroma.[37] Figure 5-1 summarizes its ultrastructure as seen by the electron microscope. Two of these structures, hemidesmosomes and anchoring fibrils, play important roles in epithelial attachment.[24]

In addition to the ultrastructural components, recent work has characterized the components of the basement membrane from a biochemical standpoint.[37] Figure 5-2 indicates these basement membrane components, which include fibronectin (FN), the bullous pemphigoid antigen (BPA), laminin, type IV collagen, and herapan-sulfate proteoglycan

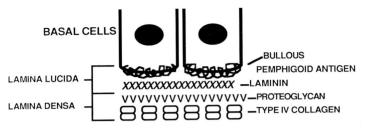

**Fig. 5-2.** Schematic diagram of the basement membrane glycoproteins that are important in corneal epithelial adhesion.

(HSPG), all of which are basement membrane glycoproteins that play important roles in epithelial adhesion. FN is deposited on the surface of corneas with epithelial defects where it may provide a scaffold for the migration of epithelial cells.[16,17,39] BPA is a component of hemidesmosomes, which may connect to the lamina lucida of the basement membrane.[28] Laminin and type IV collagen are also part of the basement membrane, located more closely to the lamina densa where they play important roles in epithelial adhesion.[14,48] HSPG is also part of this complex.[25] It may bind to FN, laminin, and type IV collagen forming a supramolecular structure for epithelial adhesion. These components are also found in the basement membrane of skin epidermis where they play a similar role in adhesion.[37]

The normal sequence of events during epithelial healing may be outlined as follows.[17,37] FN is initially deposited onto the wounded area where it plays a role in the initial attachment of the epithelium to the substrate. Laminin, HSPG, and BPA help to bind the basal epithelial cells to the substrate when hemidesmosomes are synthesized. Type IV collagen is secreted in segments until a new lamina densa is deposited. Any dystrophic or traumatic abnormality of the basement membrane may compromise the bond between epithelium and stroma and could lead to recurrent or chronic corneal epithelial defects. In recurrent corneal erosion, the epithelium is able to migrate across the wound, but it is unable to establish tight adhesion. In chronic corneal epithelial defects, the stromal substrate is very abnormal and is unable to support either epithelial migration or adhesion.

## CLINICAL CONDITIONS ASSOCIATED WITH EPITHELIAL DEFECTS

Minor trauma is the most common cause of recurrent corneal erosion.[22] If the condition is bilateral and without a history of trauma, there may be an underlying dystrophic process.[22] Other causes all have an underlying abnormality of the basement membrane with associated periodic breakdown of the corneal epithelium.

Chronic corneal epithelial defects are usually associated with more severe damage to the basement membrane and stromal substrate.[5] Often there may be no basement membrane remaining with bare stroma exposed at the site of the corneal epithelial defect. Metaherpetic keratitis is the most frequent cause of chronic corneal epithelial defects.[5]

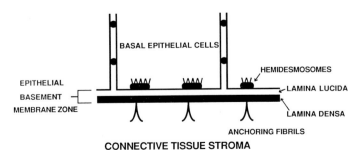

**Fig. 5-1.** Schematic diagram of the ultrastructure of the epithelial basement membrane of the cornea which is analogous to that of skin. Structures important for epithelial adhesion include the hemidesmosomes and anchoring fibrils.

The list on page 60 summarizes the causes of recurrent corneal erosion and chronic corneal epithelial defects, and several of these clinical conditions are discussed below.

Anterior corneal dystrophies may lead to recurrent corneal erosion. These include Cogan's microcystic, map-dot-fingerprint dystrophy, Meesmann/Stocker-Holt dystrophy, and Reis-Bücklers dystrophy,[3,6,34] and Grayson-Wilbrandt[18] and honeycomb dystrophy (Thiel and Behnke),[40] which are possible variants of Reis-Bücklers. In these conditions, there is abnormality of the EBM that allows the loosely adherent epithelium to shift, leads to formation of abnormal epithelial configurations, and causes a predisposition to symptomatic corneal erosions.

Stromal dystrophies of the cornea may be manifest on the surface, such as in patients with lattice or granular dystrophies.[13] In lattice, the amyloid deposits may be seen in a subepithelial location, and likewise, in granular dystrophy, the hyaline material may be seen in a similar location. The abnormal material leads to irregularity of the basement membrane and poor epithelial adhesion.

Elevated surface irregularities overlying nodules in Salzmann degeneration and band keratopathy may be prone to epithelial breakdown, slow healing, and increased scarring.[23,32,45]

Traumatic damage to the basement membrane may occur from a variety of insults, such as physical trauma, and chemical or thermal damage.[12,15,36]

Alkali-burned cornea is the classic chemical injury that frequently leads to chronic corneal epithelial defects with associated stromal melting, vascularization, and defective wound healing.[36] This injury is quite severe, damaging the substrate to the point that the epithelium cannot migrate to cover the defect. In addition to injury to the stromal substrate, the epithelium is usually compromised, making it virtually impossible for the defect to heal.

Thermal damage may result from thermal cautery for keratoconus, and complications of poor epithelial healing have been seen in patients who have received thermal cautery.[12]

Diabetes mellitus patients may have problems with epithelial wound healing.[15] They do not usually experience spontaneous corneal epithelial breakdown, but do have difficulty in healing after operative procedures such as vitrectomy, in which the corneal epithelium is traumatized during surgery.[15] The corneal epithelium after surgery is slow to heal and may result in a chronic corneal epithelial defect.

Postoperative corneal epithelial defects may be devastating in radial keratotomy and epikeratophakia patients.[1,8,21] After radial keratotomy, the epithelium usually heals over the incisions rapidly, although stromal healing may be prolonged.[8] Occasionally, however, recurrent corneal erosion may result, and there have been reports of chronic corneal epithelial defects resulting in severe keratitis, delayed wound healing, and neovascularization and perforation requiring corneal transplantation.[21] After epikeratophakia, nonhealing corneal epithelial defects may lead to loss of the lenticle.[1]

Herpes simplex keratitis usually heals without difficulty when the process is acutely infective. However, epithelial healing difficulties may be encountered when metaherpetic keratitis is present due to a damaged basement membrane.[4] This may be the result of multiple recurrences of viral infection, overly vigorous debridement using chemical cauterization, toxic effects of antiviral drugs, or collagenolytic enzymes. A chronic corneal epithelial defect very resistant to therapy results.

Keratoconjunctivitis sicca may result in corneal wound healing problems.[33] Conditions such as rheumatoid arthritis, sarcoidosis, erythema multiforme, cicatricial pemphigoid, vitamin A deficiency, and trachoma may all lead to sicca with epithelial abnormalities and chronic corneal epithelial defects. Filamentary keratitis is commonly encountered in keratoconjunctivitis sicca or superior limbic keratoconjunctivitis.[20] It produces erosive symptoms with strands of desiccated epithelial cells detached from the corneal surface.

If an epithelial defect is allowed to persist, the cornea is prone to infection due to loss of the protective epithelium. In addition, the corneal stroma is at risk of melting from the action of enzymes secreted by the damaged corneal epithelium, stromal keratocytes, and by inflammatory cells, especially neutrophils.[2] This process of corneal melting may occur rapidly or very slowly depending upon the condition, and it leads to corneal scarring with loss of vision and may ultimately lead to corneal perforation. Thus, it is important to attempt to heal an epithelial defect as rapidly as possible.

## MEDICAL APPROACH TO THERAPY

The objective in medical therapy of both recurrent and chronic corneal epithelial defects is to promote epithelial regeneration and maintain an intact epithelial surface for a sufficient period of time to allow reformation of the normal basement membrane complexes for tight adhesion.[5,22]

Mild erosive symptoms may be treated with 5% sodium chloride ointment at night. This dehydrates the epithelium and leads to closer apposition of the epithelium and Bowman's layer. In addition, it lubricates the cornea leading to decreased friction between the lids and cornea.

If the symptoms are more extensive, gentle debridement of the loose epithelium with a moist cotton-tipped applicator may be performed followed by a pressure patch for several days. It is important not to scrape too vigorously or cauterize with chemicals, as these may lead to a damaged basement membrane and more problems with healing. Erythromycin or sulfacetamide ointment may be used once daily while the pressure patch is maintained. An intermediate-acting cycloplegic may be used once daily for patient comfort. After healing has been achieved, 5% sodium chloride ointment and/or antibiotic ointment may be used for at least 2 months to prevent a recurrent erosion.

Patching time is 24–48 hours for small epithelial defects and longer for larger defects. If there are neurotrophic influences, an associated keratitis, or metabolic problems, the epithelial defect may require longer periods of patching as well.

If there is any suspicion of infection with evidence of cellular infiltration into the stroma, appropriate scrapings and cultures should be performed to rule out active bacterial, viral, or fungal infection.

The use of topical corticosteroids must be judicious because healing may be inhibited and steroids do predispose the cornea to infection. Thus, the anti-inflamatory effects of steroids must be balanced with the side effects.

Therapeutic soft contact lenses have been used with increasing frequency in the treatment of recurrent corneal erosion and for the therapy of chronic corneal epithelial defects.[27] The lenses reduce pain, provide mechanical protection for the ocular surface, as well as facilitate corneal epithelial healing and maintain proper surface hydration. They may also improve vision by smoothing the corneal surface, although visual improvement is not the purpose of therapeutic lenses.

In recurrent erosion, the decision as to when to use a therapeutic soft contact lens depends upon the severity, frequency, and duration of attacks. If attacks lasting hours to days occur more frequently than once a month, a soft lens may be useful. If attacks are only a few minutes to hours and occur very frequently, a soft lens may not be necessary.

Usually thin lenses of medium water content may be used for erosive disorders. If there is a component of dry eyes, a lens with high water content may be more useful, and sterile saline or artificial tears should be used copiously to prevent drying and to promote epithelial healing. If mechanical protection is the major goal, a less-fragile lens with water may be used (e.g., in patients who have abnormal lids or lashes contributing to the corneal epithelial defect). When any of these lenses are used, antibiotic drops should be prescribed to prevent infection. Gentamicin drops or chloramphenicol drops may be used twice daily.

After fitting a therapeutic lens, follow-up should be done in 24 hours to ensure a good fit. If the lens is too tight, hypoxia with lens intolerence may result. The patient may complain of pain, photophobia, and there may be conjunctival chemosis, corneal edema, and possibly a worsening of the epithelial erosion beneath the lens. A mild anterior chamber reaction may also result. If a therapeutic lens must be left in place for some time, superficial stromal neovascularization may result.[9]

If the lens is tolerated well initially, then follow-up may be in 1 week, then 1 month, and finally at monthly intervals. The lens should be left in place for at least 2 months after healing to encourage tight adhesion of the epithelium to its basement membrane. After lens removal, 5% sodium chloride ointment or lubricants should be used at night for several more months.

In certain conditions, which have a predisposition to corneal scarring, a prophylactic soft contact lens should be considered on a chronic basis. For example, in Reis-Bücklers' and lattice corneal dystrophy, this may be useful not only in preventing symptoms from recurrent corneal erosion, but also in preventing subsequent corneal scarring. Success with a soft contact lens thus may prevent or delay the need for corneal transplantation in these patients.

Therapeutic contact lenses are also very useful in the treatment of chronic corneal epithelial defects of many causes, including metaherpetic disease, keratitis sicca, and postsurgical and posttraumatic (chemical and thermal) chronic corneal defects.

Special considerations for the treatment of chronic corneal epithelial defects include avoiding preservatives in topical medications if possible, avoiding any other toxic drugs that may delay healing (e.g., antiviral, antibiotic, or antifungal agents, and using topical steroids only with great caution (discontinuing them if melting occurs). N-acetylcysteine 20% every 2 hours may help to slow stromal melting.

Possible complications of the use of therapeutic contact lenses are discussed here.[9] Minor complications include epithelial edema, stromal edema, vascularization, and lens deposits. Major complications include sterile infiltrates, sterile hypopyons, and bacterial ulcers, which are serious problems that may lead to permanent corneal scarring. It is not possible in most cases to distinguish between a sterile process and an infective process. Therefore, in all cases, the lens must be removed and cultured for bacteria and fungi. Appropriate scraping and cultures should be performed from the corneal defect, and therapy initiated if scrapings are positive. Although most of the inflammatory reactions associated with these lenses are not infective, it is important to view all of them as infective until proven otherwise. A hypopyon without an infiltrate does not necessitate an anterior chamber tap because these represent lens intolerance without infection.

Other medical therapies that may assist in the healing of certain epithelial defects include epidermal growth factor, retinoic acid, and fibronectin (FN).[7,29,30,31,35,44] These topical therapies are experimental and require further study before they are proven for use clinically.

Epidermal growth factor is a polypeptide hormone that may shorten the time of corneal reepithelialization by stimulating a marked cell proliferation of the corneal epithelium.[35] It has been tested clinically in limited trials where it appeared to promote epithelial healing in certain conditions but not in others.[7]

Retinoic acid is a form of vitamin A that has been advocated for the treatment of various dry eye disorders in which it may facilitate the healing of chronic corneal epithelial defects.[44] It may act by reversing the squamous metaplasia often associated with dry eye disorders. Vitamin A is necessary for proper epithelial growth and differentiation, and retinoic acid may work by reversing a local vitamin A deficiency. It is currently under clinical investigation.

FN is a glycoprotein that circulates in the blood and has been shown to be an essential component of corneal wound healing.[16,17,39] It is deposited at sites of corneal wounds, and it may help to form the necessary substrate for corneal epithelial wound healing. Preliminary studies have shown that fibronectin given in topical drop therapy may help to heal epithelial defects that previously were recalcitrant to therapy.[29,31] FN is purified from a patient's blood and given back to that patient in the form of an eyedrop. Its efficacy is currently being tested.

These substances may be proven to be useful alone or in concert with one another. There is some experimental evidence to suggest that EGF may increase FN synthesis in the cornea.[30] In addition, it is possible that retinoic acid may allow for a more normal epithelium, and fibronectin might help to provide a more favorable substrate upon which the epithelium may migrate and firmly attach.

## SURGICAL THERAPY

When conventional medical therapy, as discussed above, fails and the corneal epithelial defect persists with resultant corneal stromal thinning and scarring, surgical therapies should be considered. These include superficial keratectomy, tarsorrhaphy, conjunctival transplantation, conjunctival flap, and correction of any other contributing factors, such as lid malposition.

Superficial keratectomy may be of great benefit to patients who have failed medical therapy, including hyperosmotic agents, lubricants, patching, or bandage lenses.[38] Removal of the abnormal stroma may allow the epithelium to migrate over more normal stroma and reconstruct a normal basement membrane upon this stroma. The technique includes the removal of only the most superficial layers of the stroma to remove the diseased scarred tissue. Conditions for which this is useful include, among others, Salzmann's nodular degeneration, band keratopathy, and superficial corneal dystrophies.

Careful attention should be directed toward dissection within a horizontal plane in the corneal stroma. Vertical nicks or cuts in the stroma may lead to increased corneal scarring and opacity and poor epithelial healing. Following the surgical procedure, a therapeutic soft contact lens should be instituted as discussed in this chapter under "Medical Approach to Therapy." It is important to note that the adhesion of the corneal epithelium to the stroma requires resynthesis of the epithelial basement membrane and therefore may take weeks to months to completely re-form. Precautions must be taken to protect the intact epithelial surface during this healing period.

Tarsorrhaphy is a simple, safe, effective treatment for corneal epithelial defects that are unsuccessfully treated with medical therapy.[10] It may be partial or total, temporary or permanent. Tarsorrhahpy serves as a more complete form of patching, and in many cases will allow an epithelial defect to heal when patching and soft contact lenses have failed. It is especially useful in severe dry eye syndromes, especially if combined with abnormal lids. In addition, it may greatly help exposure keratitis and neurotrophic keratitis in which it may save the cornea from perforation.

Conjunctival transplantation is used in corneas with recalcitrant epithelial defects to provide a source of normal surface epithelial cells. This stabilizes the ocular surface and allows the cornea to provide better vision.[41,42] It is used in cases in which there has been unilateral damage to the cornea and conjunctiva, allowing the conjunctiva from the opposite eye to be used as a donor source. This autologous graft is therefore not associated with problems of HLA incompatibility, and there is no chance of immunologic rejection as in homologous transplants such as corneal transplantation. Some experimental work has suggested that homologous conjunctival transplants may be beneficial in providing a source of normal epithelium. The underlying stromal substrate, however, undergoes more fibrosis and inflammation than the autologous graft.[46] There is some experimentation in which epithelial cells are transplanted, but this is preliminary and requires further experimental work.

Prognosis for good vision is best when the scarring and vascularization is located in the superficial cornea since this may be removed by superficial keratectomy. Conditions for which conjunctival transplantation are useful include unilateral chemical or thermal burn, chronic persistent defects after herpes simplex keratitis, after penetrating keratoplasty, or in association with toxicity from medications, (e.g., pseudopemphigoid).[43]

The following technique as advised by R.A. Thoft is illustrated in Figure 5-3. Local or general anesthesia is used. The conjunctiva is resected 5 mm posterior to the limbus for 360°. Total superficial keratectomy is performed that extends over the limbus to remove all corneal epithelium and damaged anterior stroma, together with any abnormal conjunctiva that surrounds the corneal limbus.

The depth of the keratectomy depends upon how deep the abnormal corneal tissue is and how much visual improvement may be expected without a subsequent penetrating keratoplasty. For example, if the scar tissue is very deep and extensive, the primary goal of conjunctival transplantation may be to restore the ocular surface and the superficial keratectomy may be shallow. If the scar tissue can be completely removed by superficial keratectomy, however, then the superficial keratectomy should be deep enough to remove all this tissue.

Obtain healthy conjunctiva from the opposite eye. Tent up the conjunctiva with smooth forceps and remove the tissue with scissors. Pieces may be 3 mm in diameter. Close the excision sites with nonabsorbable sutures.

Place grafts around the periphery of keratectomized cornea, leaving visual axis bare. Take care that the shiny epithelial side is up. Suture grafts to the limbus with 10-0 sutures. Pass 10-0 nylon suture through apices of conjunctival graft to hold the grafts against the corneal stromal surface. This suture does not pass into the cornea at all. Place a soft contact lens over the cornea. Antibiotics and a cycloplegic are used postoperatively.

Visual outcome is in the 20/80 to 20/200 range, and the cosmetic result is good. With a contact lens, visual acuity may improve to 20/40. In addition, the patient is able to function without the need for frequent follow-up, frequent medication, etc.

Complications include perforation of the cornea at the time of keratectomy, and possible infection. If perforation occurs, glue may be used at the time of surgery. However, avoiding this complication with careful attention to detail of stromal depth and with mapping of thickness prior to surgery is the best course of action.

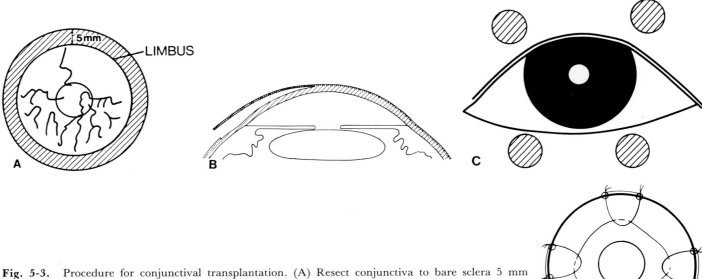

**Fig. 5-3.** Procedure for conjunctival transplantation. (A) Resect conjunctiva to bare sclera 5 mm outside the limbus. (B) Superficial keratectomy to remove epithelial layer and abnormal scar and neovascularization. (C) Grafts are taken from opposite eye. (D) Placement of conjunctival grafts. Sutures anchor grafts at the limbus and another suture holds the grafts in apposition but does not enter the corneal stroma. (Reproduced with permission from Thoft, RA: Conjunctival transplantation. Arch Ophthalmol 95:1425, 1977.)

Conjunctival flap is usually reserved for eyes in which the prognosis for vision is poor.[19] Placing a flap makes it difficult to observe the healing process, but it brings in an immediate source of vessels and fibroblasts. This leads to rapid corneal healing and ocular comfort. It is particularly useful in treating nonhealing, infected corneal ulcers with corneal thinning. Because the optical and cosmetic results of a flap are poor, consideration should be given to other forms of therapy prior to the use of a flap.

Conditions in which a flap is particularly useful include herpetic stromal melting, neuroparalytic keratitis, keratitis sicca that has failed all other forms of therapy, peripheral corneal ulcerations, and unresponsive bacterial or fungal ulcers when all else fails.[19] In all these conditions, conjunctival flaps may be useful for the control of pain, infection, and stromal ulceration. Although the visual and cosmetic results of a flap are poor, the arrest of progressive corneal melting with impending perforation occurs rapidly. Later, the conjunctival flap may be removed, and consideration may be given to corneal transplantation to restore vision.

The following technique for a Gundersen conjunctival flap is illustrated in Figure 5-4.[19] Local anesthesia with lid and retrobulbar injections is performed. All of the corneal epithelium and necrotic tissue of the perforated area should be removed to assure flap adherence and prevent future retraction of the conjunctival flap.

Undermine and mobilize a large area of conjunctiva. Since the flap is easier to create from the superior bulbar area, the eye may be rotated downward by a traction suture in the cornea below the 12 o'clock position.

A 360° conjunctival peritomy is cut as close to the limbus as possible with undermining of the inferior conjunctiva for a few millimeters. The conjunctival flap is meticulously

dissected over the entire superior aspect of the globe. A subconjunctival injection may elevate the conjunctiva from the globe and make dissection easier. All underlying tissue is separated so that the flap is thin.

Once the flap is thinned and stretched over the entire cornea without excess tension, a relaxing incision is made in the superior fornix. Great care should be taken not to perforate the area of the conjunctiva that will cover the cornea. Any inadvertent "button-holes" of the flap are repaired at once. These open sites may serve as areas for flap retraction and exposure of the underlying cornea.

The flap is smoothed down over the cornea and closed over its entire open edge with interrupted 10-0 nylon sutures. The horizontal intact bridges are maintained so as to provide flap nutrition via its vascular supply. The superior conjunctiva is left bare since the epithelium will rapidly cover this bare surface. If an attempt is made to close this defect, ptosis may result.

Antibiotic and cycloplegic drops are applied and the sutures removed in 1–2 weeks. Topical therapy for the underlying corneal disease may be stopped because the flap is impermeable to medication. Gradual whitening or thinning of the flap occurs over the next month and the flap often becomes translucent enough to actually allow rough anterior segment inspection at a later time.

There are few complications associated with conjunctival flaps. Ptosis may occur and may result from too vigorous dissection high in the fornix. Usually the benefits of conjunctival flap outweigh the side effect of ptosis. Conjunctival cyst may result, and occasionally it may require excision or unroofing. It results from infolding of the conjunctival edges or from remnants of corneal epithelium that proliferate on the back side of the conjunctival flap. Rarely, corneal perfo-

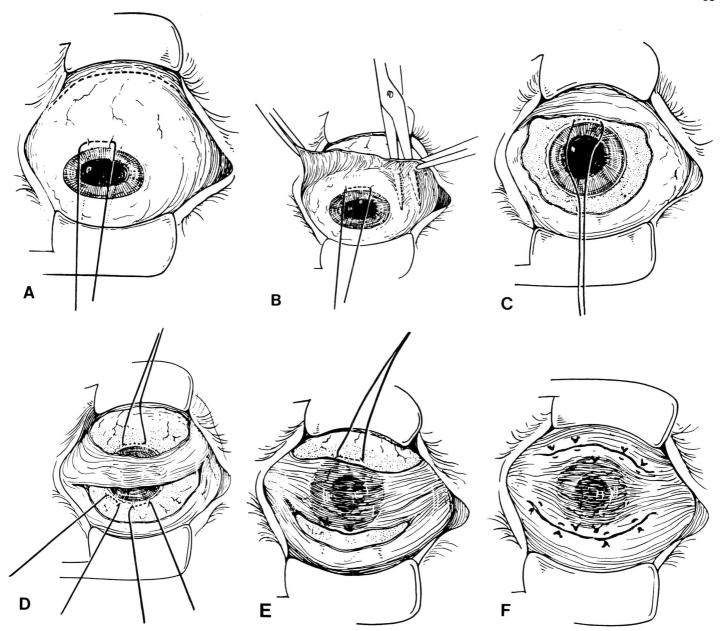

**Fig. 5-4.** Gundersen conjunctival flap. (A) Expose superior conjunctiva by a traction suture placed through the upper limbus. (B) Incise conjunctiva. (C) Complete peritomy. (D)(E) Spread flap over cornea and suture in place. (F) Final result. (Reproduced with permission from Gundersen, T: Conjunctival flaps in the treatment of corneal disease with reference to a new technique of application. Arch Ophthalmol 60:880, 1958.)

ration may occur under a conjunctival flap. This may be very difficult to assess, and the best method is to grossly assess the intraocular pressure.

Correction of lid malposition is important when this is contributing to the underlying corneal problem.[10,11] Entropion or ectropion surgery may be the factor that allows a corneal epithelial defect to heal under certain circumstances. The lids are crucial for the proper distribution of tears over the corneal epithelium. If there is exposure or inadequate spreading of tears over the cornea by the lids, a chronic corneal epithelial defect may result.

Other lid problems that may require surgical correction include trichiasis and distichiasis, the abnormal positioning of lashes that may rub on the corneal surface and cause a nonhealing corneal epithelial defect. Cryotherapy may be effective if abnormal lashes are extensive, and epilation may be adequate if there are few abnormal lashes.

Microdiathermy has been recently advocated as a therapy for chronic corneal epithelial defects.[47] It presumably acts by causing damage to the basement membrane/stroma leading to new connective tissue secretion by the epithelium and stromal fibroblasts. This new tissue then may serve as a suitable substrate to which the epithelium can adhere. Multiple puncture wounds to Bowman's layer has also been advocated for the treatment of recurrent erosion.[26] The mechanism of action may be similar.

The creation of scar tissue to allow epithelial adhesion may be useful, but these treatments are controversial and require careful scrutiny before widespread usage.

## REFERENCES

1. Baumgartner SD, Binder PS: Refractive keratoplasty: Histopathology of clinical specimens. Ophthalmology 92:1606–1615, 1985

2. Berman MB: Collagenase and corneal ulceration, in Woolley DE, Evanson JM (eds): Collagenase in Normal and Pathological Connective Tissues. New York, Wiley, 1980, pp 141–174

3. Burns RP: Meesman's corneal dystrophy. Trans Am Ophthalmol Soc 66:530–635, 1968

4. Cavanagh HD: Herpetic ocular disease: Therapy of persistent epithelial defects. Int Ophthalmol Clin 15:67–88, 1975

5. Cavanagh HD, Colley A, Pihlaja DJ: Persistent corneal epithelial defects. Int Ophthalmol Clin 19:197–206, 1979

6. Cogan DG, Donaldson DD, Kuwabara T, et al.: Microcystic dystrophy of the corneal epithelium. Trans Am Ophthalmol Soc 62:213–225, 1964

7. Daniele S, Frati L, Fiore C, et al.: The effect of the epidermal growth factor (EGF) on the corneal epithelium in humans. Graefes Arch Ophthalmol 210:159–165, 1979

8. Deg JK, Zavala EY, Binder PS: Delayed corneal wound healing following radial keratotomy. Ophthalmology 92:734–740, 1985

9. Dohlman CH, Boruchoff SA, Mobilia EF: Complications in use of soft contact lenses in corneal disease. Arch Ophthalmol 90:367–371, 1973

10. Dryden RM, Doxanas MT: Eyelid malpositions, part I: Lid retraction, facial nerve paralysis, trichiasis, in McCord CD (ed): Oculoplastic Surgery. New York, Raven Press, 1981, pp 97–120

11. Dryden RM, Doxanas MT: Eyelid malpositions, part II: Ectropion and entropion, in McCord CD (ed): Oculoplastic Surgery. New York, Raven Press, 1981, pp 121–149

12. Fogle JA, Kenyon KR, Stark WJ: Damage to epithelial basement membrane by thermokeratoplasty. Am J Ophthalmol 83:392–401, 1977

13. Fogle JA, Kenyon KR, Stark WJ, et al.: Defective epithelial adhesion in anterior corneal dystrophies. Am J Ophthalmol 79:925–940, 1975

14. Foidart JM, Bere EW, Yaar M, et al.: Distribution and immunoelectron microscopic localization of laminin, a noncollagenous basement membrane glycoprotein. Lab Invest 42:336–342, 1980

15. Foulks GN, Thoft RA, Perry HD, et al.: Factors related to corneal epithelial complications after closed vitrectomy in diabetics. Arch Ophthalmol 97:1076–1078, 1979

16. Fujikawa LS, Foster CS, Harrist TJ, et al.: Fibronectin in healing rabbit corneal wounds. Lab Invest 45:120–129, 1981

17. Fujikawa LS, Foster CS, Gipson IK, et al.: Basement membrane components in healing rabbit corneal epithelial wounds: Immunofluorescent and ultrastructural studies. J Cell Biol 98:128–138, 1984

18. Grayson M, Wilbrandt H: Dystrophy of the anterior limiting membrane of the cornea (Reis-Bücklers type). Am J Ophthalmol 61:345–349, 1966

19. Gundersen T: Conjunctival flaps in the treatment of corneal disease with reference to a new technique of application. Arch Ophthalmol 60:880–887, 1958

20. Holly FJ, Lemp MA: Tear physiology and dry eyes. Surv Ophthalmol 22:69–87, 1977

21. Karr DJ, Grutzmacher RD, Reeh MJ: Radial keratotomy complicated by sterile keratitis and corneal perforation. Ophthalmology 92:1244–1248, 1985

22. Kenyon KR: Recurrent corneal erosion: Pathogenesis and therapy. Int Ophthalmol Clin 19:169–195, 1979

23. Kenyon KR: Morphology and pathologic responses of the cornea to disease, in Smolin G, Thoft RA (eds): The Cornea: Scientific Foundations and Clinical Practice. Boston, Little, Brown, 1983, pp 43–75

24. Khodadoust AA, Silverstein AM, Kenyon KR, et al.: Adhesion of regenerating corneal epithelium. Am J Ophthalmol 65:339–348, 1968

25. Laterra J, Silbert JE, Culp LA: Cell surface heparan sulfate mediates some adhesive responses to glycosaminoglycan-binding matrices, including fibronectin. J Cell Biol 96:112–123, 1983

26. McLean EN, MacRae SM, Rich LF: Recurrent erosion: Treatment by anterior stromal puncture. Ophthalmology 93:784–787, 1986

27. Mobilia E, Dohlman CH, Holly F: A comparison of various soft contact lenses for therapeutic purposes. Contact Intraocul Lens Med J 3:9–15, 1977

28. Mutasim DF, Takahashi Y, Labib RS, et al.: A pool of bullous pemphigoid antigen(s) is intracellular and associated with the basal cell cytoskeleton-hemidesmosome complex. J Invest Dermatol 84:47–53, 1985

29. Nishida T, Nakagawa S., Awata T, et al.: Fibronectin eyedrops for traumatic recurrent corneal erosion. Lancett ii:521–522, 1983

30. Nishida T, Tanaka H, Nakagawa S, et al.: Fibronectin synthesis by the rabbit cornea: Effects of mouse epidermal growth factor and cyclic AMP analogs. Jpn J Ophthalmol 28:196–202, 1984

31. Nishida T, Nakagawa S, Manage R: Clinical evaluation of fibronectin eyedrops on epithelial disorders after herpetic keratitis. Ophthalmology 92:213–222, 1985

32. O'Connor GR: Calcific band keratopathy. Trans Am Ophthalmol Soc 70:58–81, 1972

33. Pfister RR, Murphy GE: Corneal ulceration and perforation associated with Sjogren's syndrome. Arch Ophthalmol 98:89–94, 1980

34. Rice N, Ashton N, Jay B, et al.: Reis-Bücklers' dystrophy: A clinico pathological study. Br J Ophthalmol 52:577–603, 1968

35. Savage CR, Cohen S: Proliferation of corneal epithelium induced by epidermal growth factor. Exp Eye Res 15:361–366, 1973

36. Stanley JA: Strong alkali burns of the eye. N Engl J Med 273:1265–1266, 1965

37. Stanley JR, Woodley DT, Katz SI, et al.: Structure and function of basement membrane. J Invest Dermatol 79:69s–72s, 1982

38. Stark WJ, Bruner WE, Maumenee AE: Surgery of the cornea, in Rice TA, Michels RG, Stark WJ (eds): Ophthalmic Surgery. St. Louis, C.V. Mosby, 1984, pp 115–137

39. Suda T, Nishida T, Ohashi Y, et al.: Fibronectin appears at the site of corneal stromal wounds in rabbits. Curr Eye Res 1:553–556, 1981/1982

40. Thiel HJ, Behnke H: Eine bisher unbekannte subepitheliale hereditare hornhautdystrophie. Klin Monatsbl Augenheilkd 150:862–874, 1967

41. Thoft RA: Conjunctival transplantation. Arch Ophthalmol 95:1425–1427, 1977

42. Thoft RA: Conjunctival transplantation as an alternative to keratoplasty. Ophthalmology 86:1084–1091, 1979

43. Thoft RA: Indications for conjunctival transplantation. Ophthalmology 89:335–339, 1982

44. Tseng SCG, Maumenee AE, Stark WJ, et al.: Topical retinoid treatment for various dry-eye disorders. Ophthalmology 92:717–727, 1985

45. Vannas A, Hogan MJ, Wood I: Salzmann's nodular degeneration of the cornea. Am J Ophthalmol 79:211–219, 1975

46. Weise RA, Mannis MJ, Vastine DW, et al.: Conjunctival transplantation: Autologous and homologous grafts. Arch Ophthalmol 103:1736–1740, 1985

47. Wood TO, McLaughlin BJ, Boykins LG: Electron microscopy of corneal surface microdiathermy. Curr Eye Res 4:885–895, 1985

48. Yaoita H, Foidart JM, Katz SI: Localization of the collagenous component in skin basement membrane. J Invest Dermatol 70:191–193, 1978

# 6

# Corneal Edema

## Richard L. Abbott    Walter E. Beebe

Corneal edema remains a significant problem in ophthalmology. Although infrequent in occurrence, it is nevertheless encountered by general ophthalmologists as well as subspecialists. It is a source of visual morbidity and ocular discomfort to the patient and often occurs bilaterally. Fortunately, great progress has been made in recent years in both the medical and surgical management of the disease. This chapter first reviews the pathophysiology of corneal edema and discusses some of the more common etiologies. This knowledge is then utilized to better understand the various medical and surgical approaches to the problem. In addition, modern advances in penetrating keratoplasty are considered.

## PATHOPHYSIOLOGY OF CORNEAL EDEMA

### Regulation of Corneal Hydration

Maintenance of a clear cornea necessitates a constant regulation of stromal and epithelial hydration. This regulation of corneal water content is dependent upon many factors, including stromal swelling pressure, the endothelial active transport system, epithelial and endothelial barrier functions, intraocular pressure, and evaporation. Each affects corneal hydration by working to either increase or decrease the total water content. The final equilibrium that is reached determines whether the cornea remains thin and transparent or becomes edematous (Fig. 6-1).

### Stromal Swelling Pressure

The normal corneal stroma possesses a relatively high water content of approximately 78 percent. This is by and large the result of the water-binding capacities of the proteoglycans, keratin sulfate and chondroitin sulfate, which occupy the stromal space between the collagen fibers.[23] Although they make up only a small percentage of the total stromal weight, these glycosaminoglycans are responsible for

the tendency of the stroma to swell in the absence of the endothelium and epithelium. This is known as the stromal swelling pressure and may be measured experimentally.[8,15] The imbibition pressure (IP) of the stroma is defined as the difference between the intraocular pressure (IOP) and the swelling pressure (SP) of the stroma (IP = IOP − SP). Under normal conditions the imbibition pressure value is between 30–40 mm Hg.

### Epithelial and Endothelial Barrier Function

The epithelium and endothelium in the healthy state function as semipermeable membranes and act as a barrier to discourage the influx of water into the stroma. This barrier action is more a function of the high degree of resistance of these layers to the diffusion of electrolytes than to a resistance to water flow across the barrier. Permeation of small ions through the endothelium is 800 times less than through the stroma and 1700 times less than diffusion in aqueous solution. Additionally, the epithelium is 100 times less permeable than the endothelium.[22] Thus, these two layers function to successfully maintain normal corneal hydration. In disease states that alter the normal hexagonal endothelial mosaic and its junctions, however, or in conditions that disrupt the epithelial surface, the effectiveness of these two layers is diminished.

### Endothelial Pump

The barrier function of the limiting layers of the cornea is unable by itself to counteract the swelling pressure of the stroma. In order to have effective deturgescence of the stroma, an active transport mechanism that constantly removes water from the stroma is felt to be operative. Classical experiments involving temperature reversal and the use of metabolic inhibitors support this theory. The pump is believed to exist primarily in the endothelium and to involve a Na-K ATPase dependent bicarbonate pump.[16]

SURGICAL INTERVENTION IN CORNEAL AND EXTERNAL DISEASES
ISBN 0-8089-1850-8

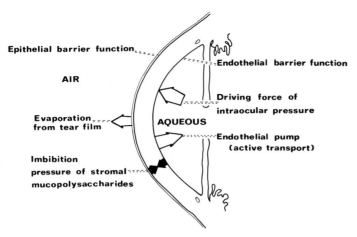

**Fig. 6-1.** Diagrammatic representation of the dynamics of corneal hydration.

## Intraocular Pressure

In the normal state intraocular pressure has been shown to have very little effect on stromal thickness or epithelial edema. In fact this is true for intraocular pressures ranging from essentially zero to 40 mm Hg.[31] In cases where the intraocular pressure exceeds the imbibition pressure of the stroma, however, epithelial edema occurs. This may result when either the intraocular pressure is high, as in acute glaucoma, or when the intraocular pressure is normal and the imbibition pressure is altered, such as in endothelial dysfunction.

## Evaporation

Evaporation of the aqueous component of the precorneal tear film occurs between each blink of the eyelids. This results in a hypertonic state of the tear film, which acts to draw water out of the cornea. This fluid loss is minimal, is probably readily replaced by aqueous, and is of little clinical significance.

## Summary

Many factors are responsible for the maintenance of a clear cornea. Stromal swelling pressure and the intraocular pressure tend to increase stromal hydration while the barrier function of the endothelium and epithelium, the endothelial pump, and evaporation all work to maintain corneal deturgescence. The equilibrium of these factors in each individual will determine the ultimate state of hydration of the cornea.

## SEQUELA OF CORNEAL EDEMA

Corneal edema may lead to corneal morbidity, often bilaterally, and can occur in eyes with previously good visual acuity. The adverse effects usually include chronic inflammation and severe intermittent ocular pain caused by the chronic epithelial breakdown. In addition, epithelial edema causes a compromised surface that is prone to ocular infections.

Most distressing to the patient is the detrimental effect on visual acuity. Swelling of the epithelium creates an irregular surface that results optically in an irregular astigmatism. In addition, it is known from optical theory that the refractive elements of the cornea must be less than one half of the wavelength of light (approximately 2000A) to preserve transparency. The corneal collagen fibers normally satisfy this criterion. In the presence of stromal edema, however, the separation becomes too great and transparency is impaired.[12]

## PROCESSES LEADING TO CORNEAL EDEMA

Corneal edema may result from a variety of pathologic conditions that adversely affect one of the regulatory mechanisms of corneal hydration that have been previously discussed. Although diverse in etiology, the pathophysiology usually involves either primary or secondary endothelial cell dysfunction, causing deficient pump and barrier functions. In addition, problems relating to increased intraocular pres-

**Table 6-1**
Common Causes of Corneal Edema

I. *Endothelial cell decompensation*
Dystrophies/degenerations
    Fuchs' endothelial dystrophy
    Congenital hereditary endothelial dystrophy (CHED)
    Posterior polymorphous dystrophy (rarely)
    Iridocorneal endothelial syndrome
        Chandler's syndrome
        Essential iris atrophy
        Iris–nevus (Cogan-Reese) syndrome
Trauma
    Penetrating and nonpenetrating injuries
    Retained anterior chamber foreign bodies
Cataract surgery
    Aphakic and pseudophakic bullous keratopathy
    Vitreous touch syndrome
    Stripped Descemet's membrane
    Preexisting endothelial disease
Inflammatory
    Graft rejection
    Herpes simplex keratitis and keratouveitis
    Acute iridocyclitis
Rupture of Descemet's membrane
    Birth trauma (forceps delivery)
    Congenital glaucoma
    Hydrops (keratoconus)
Graft failure
II. *Increased intraocular pressure*
    Acute glaucoma
    Chronic glaucoma—mild or moderate pressure elevation
    in the presence of compromised endothelium

sure that overwhelms the capacity of the pump can also cause corneal edema. Often the edema may be a result of a combination of both factors. Some of the more important entities causing corneal edema are listed in Table 6-1.

## MEDICAL TREATMENT

The medical treatment of corneal edema has several goals: to maximize the functioning state of the endothelial cells (thereby minimizing the degree of stromal edema), to reduce epithelial edema, and to provide the greatest degree of patient comfort possible. Although not successful in abolishing the underlying disease, these measures often temporize the condition and allow the avoidance or postponement of complex surgical procedures.

## Suppression of Inflammation

The presence of inflammation in the cornea or anterior chamber may compromise the endothelial cell function enough to be a contributing factor to corneal edema. Inflammation may adversely affect the metabolism of the endothelial pump as well as cause compromise of the barrier function.

Corticosteroid administration in animal models of intraocular inflammation has been efficacious in preventing the loss of endothelial pump sites as well as in preventing an increase in endothelial permeability (barrier function).[20,21] Consideration of a trial of topical corticosteroids should therefore be given in instances of corneal edema accompanied by significant intraocular inflammation. Many conditions such as homograft rejection, acute and chronic iridocyclitis, and Herpes simplex keratitis and keratouveitis may respond favorably.

## Reduction of Intraocular Pressure

Elevated intraocular pressure is a force that drives aqueous fluid through the endothelium and into the anterior corneal structures. Hence, any maneuver that lowers the intraocular pressure may lessen the degree of clinical edema that is present. Although it has been shown that pressure elevation of up to 40 mm Hg has little effect on corneal hydration in the normal eye,[31] pathologic states render the cornea acutely sensitive to even minimal pressure elevations or sometimes even borderline normal pressures. This is most evident in states of compromised endothelium (i.e., Fuchs' dystrophy, aphakic and pseudophakic bullous keratopathy, Chandler's syndrome, and borderline grafts) and in cases of markedly elevated intraocular pressure (acute glaucoma). Experienced clinicians have all observed instances of prolonged corneal deturgescence and patient comfort by simply lowering the intraocular pressure from 20 to 15 mm Hg in these individuals. In other diseases such as Chandler's syndrome, in which both glaucoma and pathologic endothelium exist, medical and/or surgical glaucoma treatment may be necessary to avoid the need for corneal transplantation.

## Hyperosmotic Agents

It is well known that clinical corneal edema is somewhat reduced during the waking hours by changes in tear film tonicity that occurs from evaporation while the eyelids are open. Similarly, agents that render the precorneal tear film hypertonic will extract fluid from the epithelium and lessen the amount of epithelial edema that is present. Hot, dry air such as that from an electric hair dryer held at arm's length may be very successful in the treatment of early epithelial edema. Patients must be cautioned on its use, however, as serious ocular surface effects may occur if misused. Although a variety of topical hypertonic agents, such as glycerine, Karo syrup, EKG gel (10% NaCl), etc., have been used, the mainstay of modern therapy remains 5% NaCl.[5,19] Traditionally, this is administered as a drop 4 times daily and as an ointment at bedtime. Many individuals will have edema that is worse in the morning. These patients may profit from frequent instillation of the medication for the first several hours of the day and then as needed as the day progresses. Many patients will maintain functional vision on hyperosmotic agents for prolonged periods of time.

It must be realized that hypertonic agents are only successful in reducing epithelial edema and will have very little effect on stromal edema. This is because the volume of fluid present in the edematous stroma is many times larger than the tear film volume. The small amount of stromal fluid that is extracted by these agents is readily replaced by aqueous that enters through the abnormal endothelium.

## Bandage Contact Lens

When ocular discomfort can no longer be controlled with the above means, consideration may be given to fitting the patient with a bandage hydrophilic contact lens.[11] First introduced to ophthalmologists in the late 1960s, many lenses are now available in a variety of thicknesses, base curves, diameters, and water contents. Table 6-2 lists these various parameters for currently available therapeutic contact lenses. It is a rare patient who cannot be successfully fit with one of the modern-day bandage contact lenses.

The use of bandage contact lenses in bullous keratopathy is limited primarily to the palliation of the associated ocular discomfort prior to keratoplasty or when good vision in the fellow eye allows postponement of surgery to a later date. Although therapeutic contact lenses provide a regular surface and may lessen some of the irregular astigmatism that is present, they rarely improve vision significantly because they may cause mild worsening of the stromal edema. However, when properly fit, most patients will experience greatly improved ocular comfort.

In general the choice of a particular bandage contact lens is not of great importance in bullous disease. Attention should instead be paid to achieving the best possible fit. Although controversial, many physicians use a topical antibiotic concomitantly, such as tobramycin drops twice daily, due to the vulnerability to infection of the diseased epithelium. The benefits of this prophylaxis, however, remain

**Table 6-2**
Characteristics of PLANO Therapeutic Contact Lenses*

| Lens | Manufacturer | Water Content (%) | Polymer | Base Curve (mm) | Diameter (mm) | Center Thickness (mm) |
|---|---|---|---|---|---|---|
| *High Water Content* | | | | | | |
| Permalens T-lens | CooperVision | 71 | Poly (HEMA†/vinyl pyrrolidone) | 9.0 | 15.0 | 0.24 |
| Permalens XL | CooperVision | 71 | Poly (HEMA/vinyl pyrrolidone) | 8.3 | 14.5 | 0.23‡ |
| Sauflon PW | Vision Tech | 79 | Poly (methyl methacrylate/vinyl pyrrolidone) | 8.1, 8.4, 8.7 | 14.4 | 0.16 |
| Softcon EW | Ciba Vision Care Framingham | 55 | Poly (HEMA/vinyl pyrrolidone) | 8.1, 8.4, 8.7 8.7 | 14.0 14.5 | 0.12 |
| *Intermediate* | | | | | | |
| Plano-T | Bausch & Lomb | 38.6 | HEMA | N/A | 14.5 | 0.15 |
| *Thin Lenses* | | | | | | |
| U | Bausch & Lomb | 38.6 | HEMA | N/A | 12.5 | 0.07 |
| U3 | Bausch & Lomb | 38.6 | HEMA | N/A | 13.5 | 0.07 |
| 04 | Bausch & Lomb | 38.6 | HEMA | N/A | 14.5 | 0.06 |
| B4 | Bausch & Lomb | 38.6 | HEMA | N/A | 14.5 | 0.12 |
| CSI-T | Sola-Syntex | 38.5 | Poly (glyceryl methacrylate/methyl methacrylate) | 8.0, 8.3, 8.6, 8.9, 8.6, 8.9, 9.35 | 13.8 14.8 | .035 |
| Soft-site | Soft-site | 45 | Poly (HEMA/vinyl thyrodidone) | 8.6 9.5, 9.8 | 13.5 15.5 | 0.07–0.10 |

* Table compiled May, 1986.
† HEMA = hydroxyethyl methacrylate.
‡ Center thickness is for a −3.00 power lens.

unproven. Complications with these continuous-wear lenses are infrequent with proper fitting and adequate follow-up examinations. Such complications may occur, however, and include corneal infections, sterile infiltrates, lens deposits, lens loss, and stromal vascularization.[7]

## SURGICAL TREATMENT

### Penetrating Keratoplasty

Corneal edema usually develops as a result of either primary or secondary endothelial cell dysfunction and is one of the leading indications for penetrating keratoplasty.[1,2] The most common conditions encountered within this group are aphakic and pseudophakic corneal edema and phakic Fuchs' dystrophy. The surgical approach to each of these clinical conditions is discussed in the following sections.

#### Preoperative Evaluation

Prior to performing penetrating keratoplasty on a patient with corneal edema careful preoperative planning and attention must be given to several potential problems. In aphakic and pseudophakic eyes the following potential problems are of particular importance:

1. The presence of irregular thinning or thickening and neovascularization of the host cornea.

2. The presence of loose vitreous in the anterior chamber.
3. The presence of anterior and/or posterior synechia.
4. The status of the pupil and the size and location of the peripheral iridectomy.
5. The presence and/or status of the intraocular lens implant.
6. The increased incidence of elevated intraocular pressure.
7. The increased incidence of cystoid macular edema.
8. The status of the opposite eye (phakic, aphakic, or pseudophakic).

The surgical technique of aphakic and pseudophakic keratoplasty may vary depending on these findings. It is the obligation of the corneal surgeon to recognize these potential problems preoperatively so that the surgical approach can be appropriately tailored for best results. In addition, thorough familiarization with anterior vitrectomy techniques and instrumentation should be accomplished prior to performing this type of surgery.

#### Technique in Aphakic Corneal Edema

Surgery may be done under general endotracheal anesthesia or with retrobulbar and seventh nerve regional anesthesia combined with intravenous analgesic and hypnotic medication administered by a stand-by anesthesiologist. If general anesthesia is employed, a nonpolarizing muscle relaxant (i.e., pancuronium) may be used to prevent any

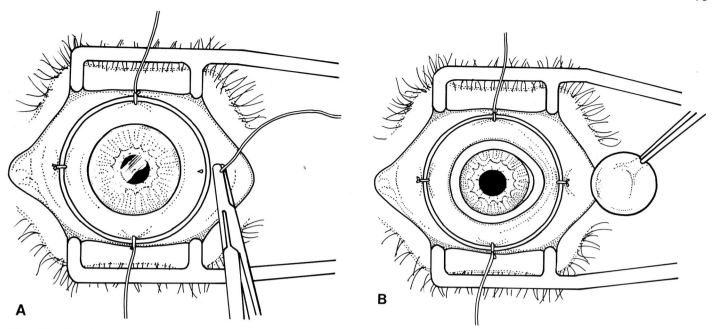

**Fig. 6-2.(A)** Suturing of the scleral support ring prior to corneal trephination. (B) Inadvertent, unequal placement of the scleral ring fixation sutures resulting in distortion of the graft bed when the recipient cornea is removed.

"bucking" or possible movement of the patient during surgery. Prior to draping, attention should be given to the positioning of the patient on the operating table. Tilting the table in a slight reverse Trendelenberg position and avoiding significant hyperextension of the neck helps to decrease positive vitreous pressure in the aphakic eye. Turning the patient's head slightly to the side opposite the eye to be operated on increases exposure and helps decrease any interference from the patient's nose during surgery. In some cases, intravenous 20% mannitol (1.5–2.0 gm/kg) may be started 45 minutes prior to surgery to soften the eye and minimize vitreous bulging once the cornea has been trephined. The operating microscope with coaxial illumination and foot controls for focus, zoom, and x-y translation is then positioned over the patient and adjusted for height and surgical field. A microsurgical vitrectomy instrument is prepared for possible use during surgery. After a routine sterile washing and draping of the patient are performed, the operation is ready to commence.

A wire or solid blade lid speculum is inserted between the lids and carefully checked to insure that there is no pressure on the globe. Either a single- or double-Flieringa ring may be fixed to the globe using sutures of 6-0 Mersilene (Ethicon, Inc., Somerville, NJ) on a spatula-type needle to avoid inadvertent scleral perforation (Fig. 6-2A). The 12 and 6 o'clock sutures are left long for stabilization of the globe by the assistant during the trephination. Extreme care must be taken in the placement of the scleral support ring because unequal placement of the fixation sutures can cause irregularity in the graft recipient bed and marked graft astigmatism (Fig. 6-2B). Because of this problem, many corneal surgeons have discontinued using the Flieringa ring and simply place a bridle suture beneath the superior and inferior

rectus muscles using 5-0 silk suture. These two sutures provide a means for stabilization of the globe during trephination (Fig. 6-3). If proper care is taken in the preoperative positioning of the patient, softening of the globe, and placement of the lid speculum, there seems to be less need for the scleral support ring.

At this time the eye is carefully inspected through the operating microscope. Attention is specifically directed to the status of the cornea and presence of neovascularization or anterior synechiae. The anterior chamber and iris are examined to confirm preoperative findings of vitreous involvement, secondary membranes, posterior synechiae, and the status of the pupil. Using a hand-held trephine of suitable diameter (either disposable or re-useable) a mark is made on the surface of the cornea that will serve as a guide to help choose the appropriate graft size. This mark is best seen if

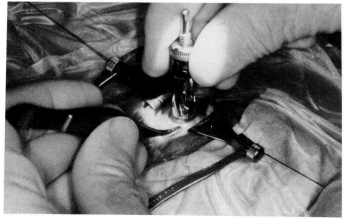

**Fig. 6-3.** Sutures placed beneath the superior and inferior rectus muscles providing a means for stabilization of the globe during trephination.

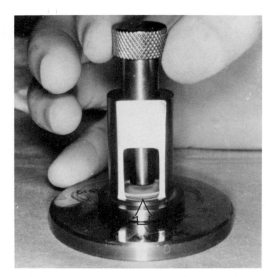

**Fig. 6-4.** Donor corneal tissue (arrow) is centered on the teflon block beneath the punch trephine.

the cornea is blotted dry. If the epithelium is edematous and loose, it may be removed with a cellulose sponge at this time. The graft tissue should be large enough to replace a significant portion of the edematous cornea, but not so large that peripheral anterior synechiae and secondary glaucoma become an increased postoperative risk. In addition, attention must be paid to other important findings (position of the pupil, presence of peripheral iridectomy, location of deep corneal neovascularization) in determining the final size and position of the new corneal graft. Almost all trephine incisions in aphakic cases have been 7.5–8.5 mm in diameter.

At this point attention is directed away from the recipient eye to a separate table where the donor cornea is prepared. A corneal protector is placed over the patient's eye and the microscope light turned off. The donor cornea with a 2 mm scleral rim is transferred from a small vial containing tissue culture #199-dextran (McCarey-Kaufman) medium with gentamicin and placed on a dry teflon cutting block with the epithelial surface facing down. Extreme care is taken to minimize trauma to the endothelial cells.

The donor cornea is carefully centered on the teflon block beneath the punch trephine to avoid cutting an oval button or creating a shelved edge (Fig. 6-4). A disposable trephine blade is used, usually 0.2–0.5 mm larger than the recipient graft bed. A slightly larger donor button is punched to avoid the disparity that is created by trephining the recipient from the epithelial surface and donor from the endothelial surface with the same size blade.[4,18] Firm, steady pressure is applied to the punch trephine to allow it to pass through the donor tissue into the teflon block (Fig. 6-5). When the trephine has passed through the donor corneal tissue and engages the cutting block, there is a sudden change in resistance and a distinct "crunching" sound is heard. If a clean through-and-through cut has been made, the donor button should remain on the teflon block when the punch trephine is removed (Fig. 6-6). A drop of BSS or TC-199 is carefully placed on the endothelial surface to prevent drying. The donor button is then put into a moist

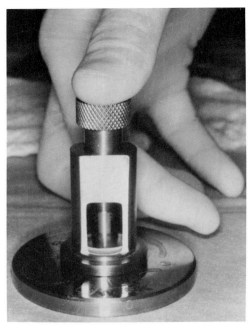

**Fig. 6-5.** Downward pressure is applied to the punch trephine, allowing it to pass through the donor tissue.

chamber for temporary storage by covering the teflon block with a moistened medicine glass or transferring the donor tissue into a moistened petri dish. The tissue is then brought back to the recipient·table for later use.

Attention is now directed back to the patient where the corneal protector is removed, the eye and the recipient cornea are once again carefully inspected, and the epithelium is lightly marked with the trephine. If a guarded trephine is used, it should be set for cutting 80 percent depth. The assistant holds the superior and inferior rectus sutures and the surgeon grasps the horizontal limbal tissue at 9 or 3 o'clock with 0.12 or 0.3 tooth forceps to stabilize and prevent rotary motion of the globe (Fig. 6-3). The trephine blade is then set within the previous mark on the cornea surface. After ensuring that there is not any undue pressure on the

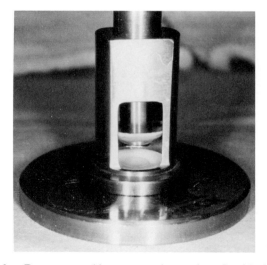

**Fig. 6-6.** Donor corneal button remains on the teflon block as the punch trephine is elevated.

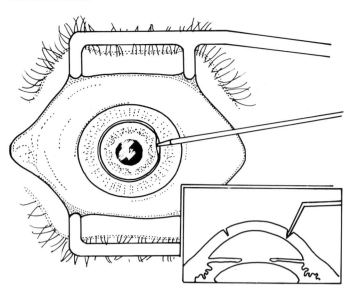

**Fig. 6-7.** After the corneal trephination has been completed, the depth of the incision is checked with the microcyclodialysis spatula.

globe and the trephine is perpendicular to the corneal surface, the cutting of the corneal tissue is carefully begun. The surgeon gently rotates the trephine in a circular motion attempting to apply equal pressure on all edges of the cutting surface so that uniform depth is obtained. Care should be taken to avoid uncontrolled entry into the anterior chamber at this time.

The trephine is removed and the depth of the incision is checked with the microcyclodialysis spatula (Fig. 6-7). In vascularized corneas, partial-thickness trephination allows bleeding and rapid spasm of the superficial and midstromal blood vessels, avoiding hemorrhage into the anterior chamber. If the incision depth is found to be unequal, the trephine may be placed within the previous cut by "skating" the trephine on the corneal surface and feeling the blade enter into the deeper portions of the incision. Extreme care must be taken to avoid creating a "double cut" in the corneal tissue. This step can be repeated as often as necessary until a deep cut is obtained in all areas. Beveling of the incision

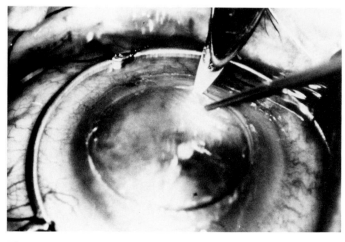

**Fig. 6-8.** Anterior chamber is entered through the trephine incision close to the point of fixation.

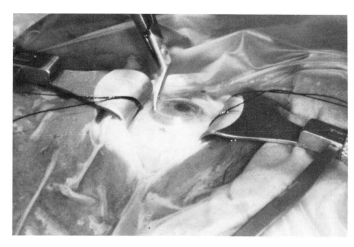

**Fig. 6-9.** Curved corneal scissors are kept perpendicular to the plain of the iris in removal of the recipient cornea.

through the stroma should be avoided to allow precise fitting of the donor button within the recipient bed.

The anterior chamber is slowly entered with a disposable miniblade, a razor blade fragment, or a diamond knife within the incision close to the point of fixation (Fig. 6-8). Approximately a 3–4 mm incision is made to allow easy entrance of the angulated curved microcorneal scissors. The blades of the scissors are kept perpendicular to the plane of the iris, leaving a narrow rim of endothelium and Descemet's membrane on the posterior margin of the recipient bed (Fig. 6-9). As the cutting of the cornea is completed, attention should be directed to its endothelial surface where vitreous attachments or iris adhesions may have to be cut prior to removal of the corneal tissue. In addition, any adventitious tissue should be removed from the wound with the Vannas scissors (Fig. 6-10).

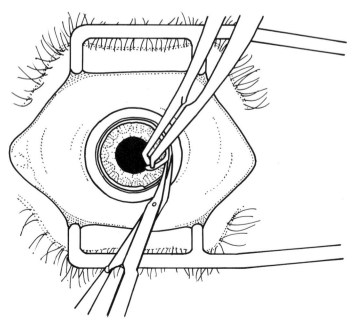

**Fig. 6-10.** A narrow rim of Descemet's membrane is trimmed from the wound with the Vannas scissors.

Once the recipient cornea has been removed from the eye, several different approaches may be taken depending on the preoperative and intraoperative findings. These may be divided into four separate groups and are discussed separately:

1. Aphakia with hyaloid face intact,
2. Aphakia with loose vitreous in the anterior chamber,
3. Pseudophakia with hyaloid face intact, and
4. Pseudophakia with loose vitreous in the anterior chamber.

## Aphakia with Hyaloid Face Intact

If the hyaloid face is intact and away from the cornea, the pupil may be constricted with acetylcholine to help maintain this state. The decision regarding whether to insert an intraocular lens into this eye is based on the following considerations.

1. Whether the other eye is phakic or has an intraocular lens.
2. Whether the other eye is aphakic and a contact lens is successfully worn.
3. The physical needs and activities of the patient.
4. Whether there is an inability to wear a contact lens.
5. The overall health of the involved eye for tolerating a secondary implant.
6. The relative risk of insertion and possible vitreous involvement.

If an intraocular lens is to be inserted into the eye, a small amount of viscoelastic material is first placed over the pupil and on the surface of the iris to help act as a "cushion" for the underlying vitreous. Using a flexible-loop anterior chamber-style lens with 3-point fixation, the insertion can be performed through a 7.5 mm or larger recipient bed opening without difficulty. Once the lens is in appropriate position, additional viscoelastic material as well as balanced salt solution are used to fill the remainder of the anterior chamber. The donor button is then transferred to the recipient bed and sutured in place (see below).

## Aphakia with Loose Vitreous in the Anterior Chamber

During preoperative evaluation of the patient, attempts should be made to determine the presence of loose vitreous in the anterior chamber. If vitreous is present or highly suspected, plans should be made prior to surgery to prepare and have ready a guillotine-type vitreous cutting and aspirating instrument. The mechanical vitreous cutting instrument in these cases reduces vitreous traction and iris inflammation associated with the technique of removal by cellulose sponge absorption.[3] Some surgeons have also advocated the evacuation of fluid vitreous through the pars plana prior to entry into the anterior chamber.[10]

If formed vitreous is encountered in the anterior chamber at the time of removal of the corneal button, care must be

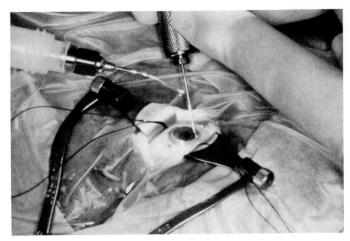

**Fig. 6-11.** "Open-sky" vitrectomy is performed through the pupil and peripheral iridectomy with a mechanical vitreous cutting instrument.

taken to cut any adhesions from the posterior surface of the cornea. Once the cornea has been removed, an "open-sky" vitrectomy is performed with the mechanical vitreous instrument held within the center of the pupil or in the peripheral iridectomy using low suction (4–6 mm Hg) and a rapid cutting rate (300–400 cuts/minute) (Fig. 6-11). Balanced salt solution may be gently dripped into the anterior chamber as needed during vitrectomy. The vitrectomy is considered adequate when the iris has dropped posteriorly well back from the recipient bed and there is no formed vitreous left in the anterior chamber. This can be checked with a cellulose sponge, carefully touching the surface of the iris.

Attempts should be made to free the pupil from vitreous adhesions and secondary membranes as well as removing any strands of vitreous to the peripheral cornea. After this has been completed, the anterior chamber is filled with balanced salt solution prior to placement of the donor tissue within the recipient bed. If indicated, consideration for a secondary lens implant may be given prior to placement of the donor graft tissue (see list in previous section).

A vitrectomy should not be performed if the vitreous face is unbroken and does not protrude anteriorly because there is an increased risk of cystoid macular edema and retinal detachment following this procedure.[17]

## Pseudophakia with Hyaloid Face Intact

The presence of an intraocular lens in a patient with corneal edema requires careful clinical examination and planning prior to surgery. Several important factors must be considered in performing surgery on these patients. If the hyaloid is unbroken or the posterior capsule is intact, the style of the implant and its affect on the eye primarily determine the surgical approach. Indications for removing the intraocular lens at the time of keratoplasty are as follow:

1. Patient history of pain, and signs of recurrent hyphema, uncontrolled glaucoma, or persistent uveitis

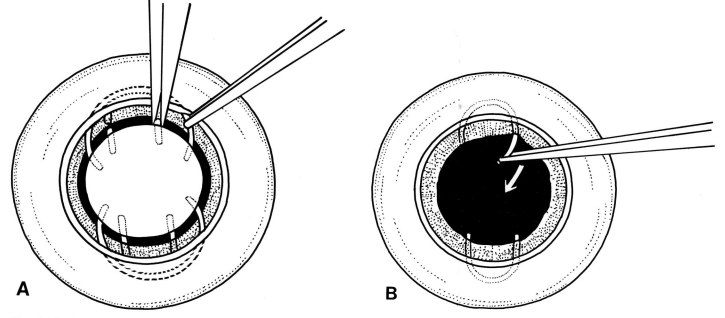

**Fig. 6-12.(A)** Supporting haptic loops are amputated from the lens optic. (Redrawn with permission from Leibowitz HM: Corneal Disorders—Clinical Diagnosis and Management. Philadelphia, W.B. Saunders Co., 1984.) (B) Following removal of the optic portion of the IOL, the haptic loops are rotated free from the dense fibrous tissue in the angle or ciliary sulcus. (Redrawn with permission from Leibowitz HM: Corneal Disorders—Clinical Diagnosis and Management. Philadelphia, W.B. Saunders Co., 1984.)

2. Endothelial touch
3. Dislocated loops and unstable lens
4. Metal haptic materials
5. Presence of chronic cystoid macular edema
6. Iris sphincter erosion

If the pseudophakos must be removed, plans for an anterior vitrectomy must be made even if the hyaloid face previously had been undisturbed. Depending on the lens style and length of time that it has been in place, frequently there are strong adhesions to the angle, iris, vitreous, capsular bag, or ciliary sulcus. Removal of these lenses can be extremely difficult and traumatic to the eye and requires familiarity with the many styles of lenses that have been available for insertion over the years.[27] Various forms of iris clips and loops must be opened or cut prior to lysis of iris and vitreous adhesions that surround the implant. The use of blunt and sharp dissection in the removal of these lenses is required and care must be taken to preserve as much iris tissue as possible. In some cases, supporting haptics must be cut from the optic and then carefully rotated free from dense fibrous tissue in the angle or ciliary sulcus (Figs. 6-12A and B).

After removal of the implant, the anterior vitrectomy is performed in a similar fashion as described in the previous section. Consideration for implantation of a different style pseudophakos (usually a flexible-loop anterior chamber lens with 3-point fixation) can be given if this is indicated (Table 3-2).

If the pseudophakos can be retained, the operation in some regards may actually be less complicated than the usual aphakic keratoplasty. The miotic pupil and intraocular lens help provide a barrier to the prolapse of vitreous through the pupil when the posterior capsule is not intact. The more recent use of posterior chamber lenses has decreased the incidence of uveitis, secondary glaucoma, and corneal-related problems, and frequently allows the implant to remain in place at the time of keratoplasty.[30] Considerations for leaving the intraocular lens in place include evaluating whether:

1. The lens is in a satisfactory position and appears stable,
2. The eye is quiet,
3. There is no low-grade inflammation, and
4. The pupil is mobile.

## Pseudophakia with Loose Vitreous in Anterior Chamber

In patients with pseudophakic corneal edema and loose vitreous involving the anterior segment, the course of action is mainly determined by the type of implant present. In most cases, plans should be made for removal of the pseudophakos combined with a partial anterior vitrectomy at the time of keratoplasty. The style of the implant and its position in the eye will help determine the surgical approach.

In general, iris plane lenses should be removed, however, anterior chamber lenses that appear stable can frequently be left in place, performing the vitrectomy beneath the lens (Fig. 6-13). Similar problems are encountered in removal of these lenses as discussed in the previous section; however, vitreous involvement may be more extensive and

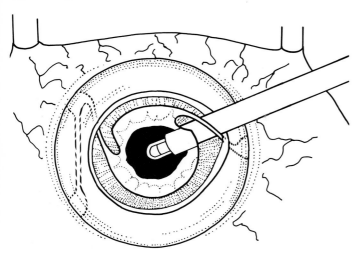

**Fig. 6-13.** Partial anterior vitrectomy is performed beneath a well positioned anterior chamber lens implant.

may require a partial vitrectomy prior to lens removal. Placement of a different style lens implant in these eyes should only be considered in patients who absolutely cannot tolerate a contact lens or aphakic spectacles.

## Technique in Phakic Corneal Edema

In patients undergoing penetrating keratoplasty for phakic corneal edema, careful attention must be directed to the lens. During the preoperative examination the lens is closely examined, if possible, to determine its status. If it is

felt that the lens is clear and should not be removed, pilocarpine 1% drops are instilled about 30 minutes prior to surgery to constrict the pupil. If the lens is cataractous and necessitates removal, however, the pupil is widely dilated prior to surgery. In cases in which the status of the lens is not known because of diffuse corneal edema, the pupil is only partially dilated with 2.5% phenylephrine and intraoperative evaluation is performed after removal of the recipient cornea. Unfortunately, assessment of lens transparency through the operating microscope is difficult to carry out. It is probably most helpful to use only the coaxial illumination light of the microscope in a darkened room to examine the lens against the red fundus reflection. If the lens must be removed, mydriatics may be supplemented by instillation of nonpreserved epinephrine to the iris surface.

The cataract extraction can be performed with either an intracapsular or extracapsular technique through a 7.5-mm graft incision without difficulty. Using the intracapsular technique, the cryoprobe is applied to the anterior lens surface and lens delivery is performed using a gentle upward and rocking motion. In some cases, alpha-chymotrypsin may be used to facilitate lens removal. A peripheral iridectomy should be done to prevent pupillary block.

Placement of a flexible-loop anterior chamber lens may be performed through the trephine opening. Instillation of acetylcholine to constrict the pupil and the use of a viscoelastic substance in the anterior chamber help protect the intact vitreous face during lens insertion. While supporting the lens by the superior haptic with a fine, smooth forcep, it is guided through the trephine opening placing the inferior haptic into the inferior angle. The optic is gently stabilized and maintained in position with the smooth-angled forceps while the superior haptic is grasped at its end and maneuvered in a downward, central direction through the trephine opening into the superior angle (Fig. 6-14A). The use of additional

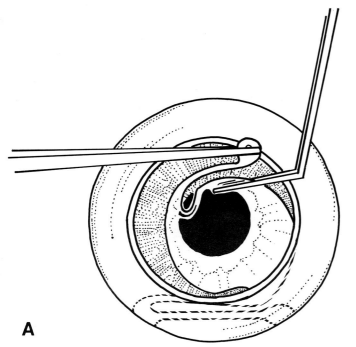

A

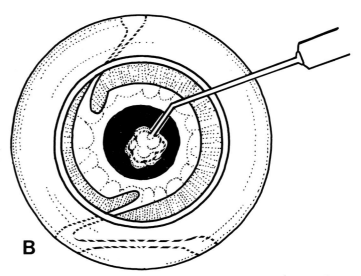

B

**Fig. 6-14.** (A) Insertion of a flexible loop anterior chamber lens implant through the trephine opening. (Redrawn with permission from Leibowitz HM: Corneal Disorders—Clinical Diagnosis and Management. Philadelphia, W.B. Saunders Co., 1984.) (B) Sodium hyaluronate is placed over the anterior surface of the intraocular lens as added protection for the endothelium during suturing of the graft. (Redrawn with permission from Leibowitz HM: Corneal Disorders—Clinical Diagnosis and Management. Philadelphia, W.B. Saunders Co., 1984.)

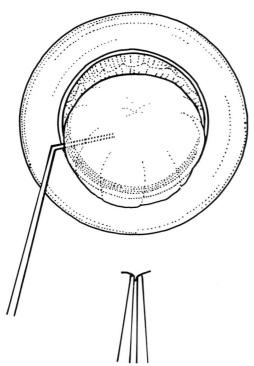

**Fig. 6-15.** Nucleus of the lens is prolapsed from the globe by applying gradual downward pressure over the insertion of the superior rectus muscle. The nucleus is guided out of the eye with a microcyclodialysis spatula.

sodium hyaluronate over the anterior surface of the lens is helpful to prevent contact with the endothelium during suturing of the graft (Fig. 6-14B).

Planned extracapsular cataract extraction is likewise performed with an open sky technique through the corneal trephine opening. Following the anterior capsulotomy with a bent, sharp, disposable needle or other instrument, the nucleus is gently loosened and dislodged into the anterior chamber by any of a variety of techniques. One approach is to apply gradual pressure with a fine-tooth forcep directed downward toward the middle of the eye over the insertion of the superior rectus muscle. As the nucleus moves anteriorly, it is manipulated out of the eye with either a lens loop or a microcyclodialysis spatula (Fig. 6-15).

Another method that works well is to use a cryoprobe to gently deliver the nucleus through the corneal opening. The remaining cortex is aspirated using either a mechanical or manual irrigating aspiration handpiece or a manual double-bore needle. Because this is performed in an open sky fashion, a relatively high flow of balanced salt solution is required to allow adequate suction to develop and maintain a deep anterior chamber. Peripheral cortical material is engaged in the aspiration port behind the iris and stripped centrally away from the capsule. Once all of the cortex has been removed, the posterior capsule is gently polished with a fine diamond dusted irrigation cannula.

If desired, insertion of a posterior chamber lens implant is now performed over the intact posterior capsule. This is accomplished by grasping the superior edge of the lens optic with smooth-angled forceps and guiding the inferior loop into the inferior capsular bag or ciliary sulcus (Fig. 6-16A). Spreading the capsular bag leaflets with a viscoelastic sub-

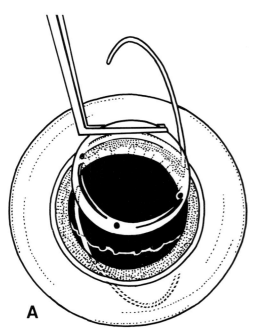

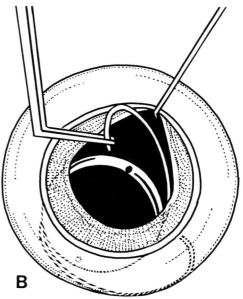

**A**                    **B**

**Fig. 6-16.** (A) Insertion of a posterior chamber lens implant into the inferior capsular bag of ciliary sulcus. (Redrawn with permission from Leibowitz HM: Corneal Disorders—Clinical Diagnosis and Management. Philadelphia, W.B. Saunders Co., 1984.) (B) Placement of the superior haptic loop with the help of a small iris hook. (Redrawn with permission from Leibowitz HM: Corneal Disorders—Clinical Diagnosis and Management. Philadelphia, W.B. Saunders Co., 1984.)

stance prior to insertion of the lens is often helpful in visualizing the capsular bag. The superior loop is grasped at its tip, bent centrally toward the optic and inserted behind the iris. If the pupil is not widely dilated, a small iris hook may be used to retract the pupillary margin to facilitate placement of the superior loop (Fig. 6-16B). The implant is carefully rotated to center the optic and avoid inadvertent tucking of the iris. Once the implant is in satisfactory position, acetylcholine is dripped on the iris to constrict the pupil and viscoelastic substance is placed on the surface of the lens for added protection of the donor endothelium during suturing of the graft.

### Suturing of The Donor Button

The donor graft, which has been temporarily stored in a moist chamber on the mayo stand, is now transferred by the surgeon to the recipient bed. This is accomplished either by grasping the anterior edge of the button with a fine 0.12-mm forceps or by using a corneal spatula to invert the graft onto the recipient bed. Depending on the condition of the anterior chamber, either a large air bubble, BSS, or a visoelastic substance will be present beneath the graft. If a pseudophakos is present, it is imperative that the endothelium does not come in contact with it during the suturing of the graft.

Wound closure is accomplished with 10-0 monofilament nylon suture approximately 23–27 microns in diameter. A spatula-shaped, side-cutting needle with a radius of curvature of 160°–175° facilitates small deep suture bites that easily penetrate corneal tissue. The suturing technique attempts to evenly secure the donor button to the recipient corneal bed and may be accomplished in several ways: multiple interrupted sutures, a single running suture, a combination of interrupted and running sutures or a double-running suture. Care must be taken in the placement of the first corneal suture at 12 o'clock because the graft is freely mobile and can easily be displaced causing possible damage to the endothelium. It is recommended, therefore, that this first suture be placed primarily to anchor the graft in position and can easily be removed and replaced later with a deeper suture if necessary. All sutures should be placed at least

three-quarters depth within donor and host tissue without taking too long a bite.

The most important suture to be placed by the surgeon is the second cardinal suture at 6 o'clock. It is this suture that most affects the final position of the donor graft within the recipient bed and careful attention should be paid to the alignment of this suture. It is recommended that the surgeon leave the needle in place after it has been passed through both the donor and host tissue to check the graft edges at 3 and 9 o'clock for override or gaping of the wound (Fig. 6-17A). If this is detected, then the needle can easily be backed out of the wound and repositioned, thus correcting the possible wound disparity (Fig. 6-17B). The 3 and 9 o'clock sutures are then placed equidistant between the 12 and 6 o'clock sutures. The graft surface is dried to better observe the diamond crease that forms between the four cardinal sutures. If the sutures have been placed equidistant from each other, each side of the diamond will be equal and additional sutures may now be placed. Cardinal sutures may have to be repositioned, however, if the sides of the "diamond" are not aligned, causing malposition of the donor graft (Fig. 6-18).

Once satisfactory placement of the initial four cardinal sutures has been completed the anterior chamber should be redeepened with either BSS or viscoelastic material using a 2-cc syringe attached to a 30-gauge angulated cannula. Closure of the wound is now completed with one of the above-mentioned suturing techniques.

On completion of suturing, the anterior chamber is carefully examined to make sure that there are no synechiae present, that the pseudophakos (if present) is in good position, and that large amounts of air or viscoelastic substance have been removed. The integrity of the wound is checked by applying gentle pressure with a dry cellulose sponge between each suture on the host cornea. If any fluid escapes, a suture is either added or replaced to achieve satisfactory wound closure. The eye is left normotensive at the completion of the case. The bridle sutures are removed and the subconjunctival injections of antibiotic (tobramycin, 20 mg and cefazolin, 100 mg) are give inferiorly.

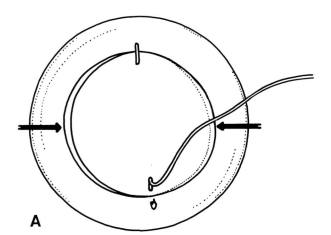
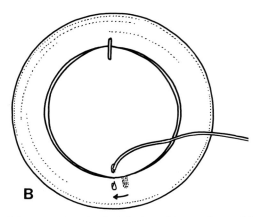

**Fig. 6-17.** (A) Initial placement of the 6 o'clock cardinal suture. Note gaping of the wound at the 9 o'clock position and override at the 3 o'clock position (arrows). (B) Repositioning of the 6 o'clock cardinal suture allowing better wound apposition of the corneal graft.

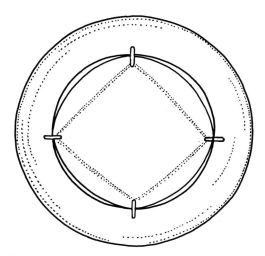

**Fig. 6-18.** Following placement of the four cardinal sutures, the diamond crease on the corneal surface is observed to be unequal, representing malposition of the donor graft.

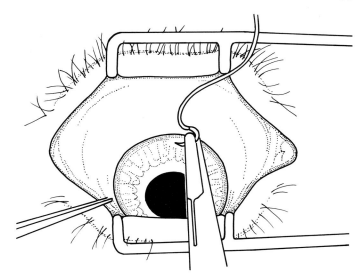

**Fig. 6-19.** Placement of superior traction suture at the corneal limbus.

Subconjunctival injection of a corticosteroid is given when there has been a vitrectomy or significant manipulation of the iris at the time of surgery. If interrupted sutures have been used, a bandage therapeutic soft contact lens may be placed over the cornea to help promote epithelialization of the graft and provide additional patient comfort.[28] Several drops of a combined antibiotic–corticosteroid medication are given, the lids are closed and a monocular bandage applied.

## Conjunctival Flap Graft

Due to the modern advances in microsurgical technique, the current success rate with penetrating keratoplasty, and the wide availability of therapeutic contact lenses, the frequency of other surgical procedures in the treatment of bullous keratopathy has declined. Nevertheless, there will continue to be individuals with good vision in their fellow eye and poor visual potential in the involved eye who are excellent candidates for surgical procedures to eliminate their ocular discomfort.

One such procedure is the use of a conjunctival flap graft. Although conjunctival techniques were described by Scholer in 1877,[26] modern techniques revolve around the classical description of Gundersen[13,14] with later modifications by numerous authors.[24,29] The technique is not difficult to learn but is tedious and requires meticulous attention to detail. It is aided greatly by the help of an able assistant. The success of the procedure depends on the observation of several fundamental principles, including (1) complete removal of the corneal epithelium and debridement of any necrosis that is present, (2) creation of a mobile, thin, conjunctival flap that is devoid of Tenon's capsule and any conjunctival adhesions, (3) absence of any conjunctival buttonholes that may lead to flap retraction, (4) and the absence of any traction of the flap at its margins.

General anesthesia may be employed but local anesthesia with retrobulbar and lid block for adequate akinesia is usually sufficient. The procedure is begun by placing a trac-

tion suture of 5-0 nylon on a spatula needle through the cornea limbus at the 12 o'clock position (Fig. 6-19). This is used for subsequent positioning of the eye as necessary. A small needle, usually 27- or 30-gauge, is then used to inject 1% lidocaine with epinephrine (1:100,000) into the subconjunctival space at the lateral and medial margin of the desired flap (Fig. 6-20). The entry site of the needle should be away from the proposed flap to avoid having a needle hole that may enlarge into an actual buttonhole.

The injection will balloon the conjunctiva superiorly and provide a natural separation from underlying Tenon's fascia and facilitate subsequent flap dissection. The conjunctiva between the upper limbus and upper fornix is now inspected and a slightly curved horizontal incision made with blunt Wescott scissors. The incision usually starts 15–18 mm above the superior limbus and extends for a horizontal distance of approximately 30 mm (Fig. 6-21). This extra tissue (the vertical cornea usually measures only 11–12 mm) allows

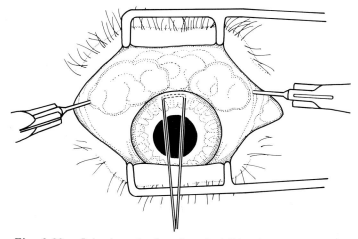

**Fig. 6-20.** Injection of subconjunctival lidocaine with epinephrine. Note entry of needle is well away from the eventual flap site.

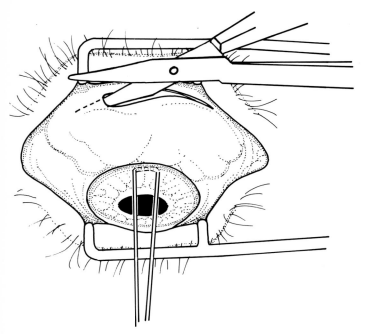

**Fig. 6-21.** Flap preparation is initiated with a curvilinear incision through the superior conjunctiva.

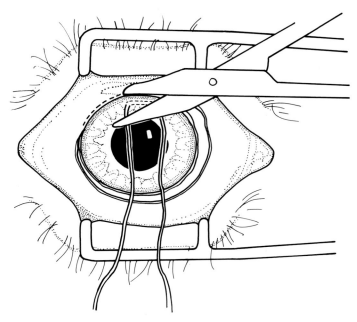

**Fig. 6-23.** A 360° limbal perimetry is performed.

for some later contraction of the flap. Care must be taken not to include Tenon's fascia with this initial incision because this may interfere with the definition of the dissection plane. Using blunt Wescott scissors and a delicate, nontoothed forcep the flap dissection is now carried inferiorly until the superior limbus is reached (Fig. 6-22). It is important that this dissection of conjunctiva from the underlying Tenon's fascia be carefully performed under direct visualization to prevent any inadvertent conjunctival perforation. It is a useful exercise to visualize the scissor tips prior to making each

cut to insure that no conjunctival tissue is included. Once the limbus is reached, a 360° peritomy is performed (Fig. 6-23). At this point additional undermining of the flap is accomplished to relieve all tension and traction and to allow the conjunctival bridge flap to cover the entire cornea and rest without traction. This is very important because any tension may cause future flap retraction. The flap preparation is now complete and attention is turned to preparing the corneal surface.

Gundersen advocated 1/3–1/2 thickness lamellar keratectomy for this purpose,[14] whereas Sugar[29] and others later utilized a more superficial keratectomy involving Bowman's

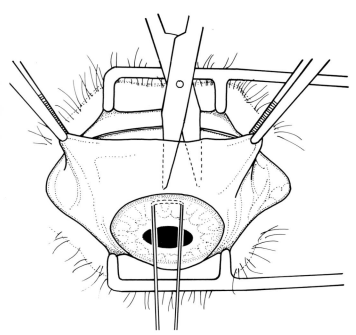

**Fig. 6-22.** Flap dissection is continued by separating conjunctiva from Tenon's fascia until superior limbus is reached.

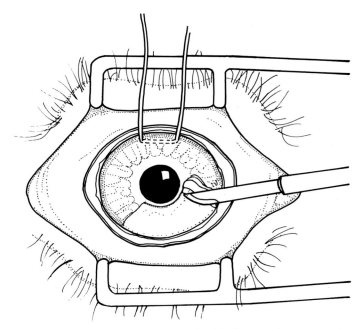

**Fig. 6-24.** Gentle debridement of epithelium and any necrotic tissue with #64 Beaver® blade.

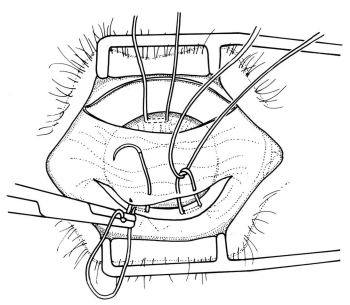

**Fig. 6-25.** Lower edge of bridge flap is secured to episclera with two interrupted mattress sutures.

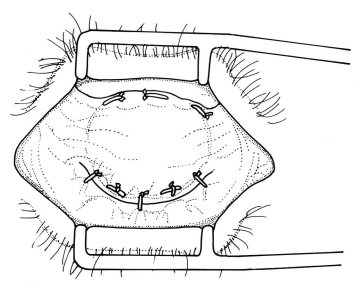

**Fig. 6-27.** Appearance of completed conjunctival flap graft.

layer and superficial stroma for this purpose. Most ophthalmologists have found that removal of the epithelium along with any necrotic stroma that may be present is adequate. As the epithelium in bullous disease is quite loosely adherent, this is easily accomplished with the use of a #64 Beaver® blade and gentle scraping (Fig. 6-24).

The flap is then positioned over the prepared cornea and sewn into place. This may be accomplished by any number of ways. We prefer to begin by placing two double-armed mattress sutures of 6-0 vicryl in the episclera at the 5 and 7 o'clock positions 2 mm from the limbus. Both ends are brought through the conjunctival edge of the lower border of the flap and secured to the episclera (Fig. 6-25). The original

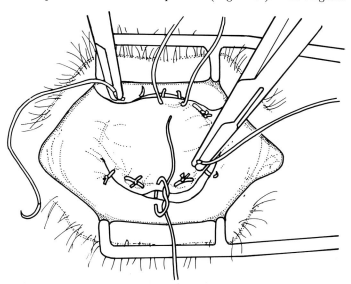

**Fig. 6-26.** Lower edge of bridge flap and inferior conjunctiva are approximated with interrupted sutures as needed. Superior conjunctiva is secured to episclera with three interrupted mattress sutures.

conjunctiva of the lower limbus is then approximated to the lower border of the bridge flap and closed with several interrupted sutures (Fig. 6-26). usually one or two sutures on either side of the mattress sutures suffices. The upper border of the bridge flap is then secured to the superior episclera with similar double-armed mattress sutures at the 11 and 1 o'clock positions and the corneal traction suture is remove (Fig. 6-27). The procedure is now complete and the eye is dressed with an antibiotic–steroid ointment and mild pressure dressing.

The postoperative course is usually uneventful. The residual inflammation subsides in several weeks and the flap continually thins over several months (Fig. 6-28; see color insert following page 139). The patient characteristically experiences marked improvement from the preoperative pain and photophobia. The amount of vision that returns can be surprising and depends largely on the obtained thinness of the flap and the preoperative status of the cornea and retina. The complications are relatively few:

1. Hemorrhage underneath flap
2. Retraction of flap
3. Enlargement of flap
4. Epithelial inclusion cysts
5. Postoperative ptosis
6. Infection (rare)

By far the most deleterious to the function of the conjunctival flap are undetected buttonholes that enlarge and cause retraction of the flap. If detected intraoperatively an attempt to close them with interrupted 10-0 nylon suture may be made. Although not considered a true complication, a graft that has failed is virtually impossible to revise because the additional conjunctiva necessary is not readily available.

In summary, conjunctival flaps offer a reasonable alternative to penetrating keratoplasty in a patient for whom the alleviation of pain is the prime objective. In addition, a conjunctival graft does not preclude additional corneal surgery in the future. The graft can be taken down and a penetrating keratoplasty performed at a later date if visual improvement becomes necessary.

## Salleras Procedure

The Salleras procedure (cautery of Bowman's layer) remains a very useful procedure as an alternative to penetrating keratoplasty in selected individuals. These are usually patients with painful bullous keratopathy in whom other visual disorders such as optic nerve or retinal disease preclude a sight-restoring keratoplasty. Vision is usually good in the fellow eye and a bandage contact lens is either poorly tolerated or inappropriate due to poor hygiene or inadequate follow-up potential. In addition, many individuals may find this procedure more cosmetically acceptable than conjunctival flap grafting.

First described by Salleras in Argentina,[25] this technique was introduced in the United States by DeVoe in 1966.[6] It may be performed with topical anesthesia although we have found retrobulbar anesthesia to be far more satisfactory to both the patient and the surgeon. The loosely adherent epithelium is first removed from the cornea with a #64 Beaver® blade. The cauterization is then carried out with a standard Bovie electrosurgical unit in the diathermy mode. A blunt-tip diathermy probe is used to deliver the cautery by continuously depressing the control foot pedal and gently touching the probe tip to Bowman's layer. The power is set initially on zero and gradually increased. The desired endpoint is reached when application of the diathermy probe causes small stellate contractions ("splintering") in Bowman's layer as well as the formation of a thin coagulum (Fig. 6-29). After the proper power setting is ascertained it usually remains constant for the remainder of the procedure.

Small burns are now placed in a circular fashion starting first in the corneal periphery and working centrally until the entire corneal surface is covered (Fig. 6-30). Usually 400–500 applications are required. If only segmental edema is present, then burns are delivered to the affected area only. Because significant corneal contraction may occur and cause elevation of the intraocular pressure, it is necessary at the end of the procedure to perform tonometry. If the pressure is elevated an anterior chamber paracentesis is performed and a short course of oral acetazolamide is initiated.

An appropriate bandage contact lens is placed on the cornea intraoperatively to aid epithelialization (see Table 3-2). Additionally, a topical steroid-antibiotic drop is prescribed. Postoperatively a thin eschar initially forms but then disappears in several days. Complete epithelialization usually is accomplished within 2–3 weeks and is greatly aided by the presence of the therapeutic contact lens. Multiple small subepithelial opacities are evident for several months and correspond to the sites of diathermy delivery (Fig. 6-31). They gradually diminish in density.

Histologic studies[9] reveal that subepithelial connective tissue forms between the epithelium and Bowman's layer. In areas where interruption of Bowman's layer has occurred stromal connective tissue fills the gap and becomes continu-

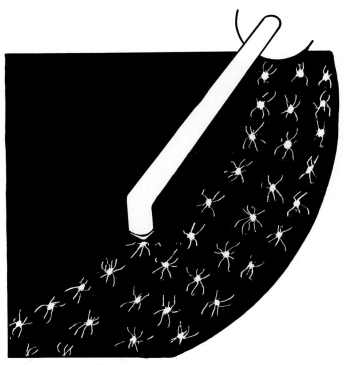

**Fig. 6-29.** A properly applied diathermy burn results in the formation of a thin coagulum and "splintering" of Bowman's layer.

ous with the anterior subepithelial connective tissue. Clinically, it is felt that this superficial scarring provides a very effective connective tissue barrier to the flow of fluid through the cornea and therein lies the success of this procedure in the treatment of bullous keratopathy.

Complications are rare but include perforation, desmetocoele formation, elevation of intraocular pressure, and failure of epithelialization.

Success is the general rule, and symptomatic improvement may be expected in over 90 percent of individuals.[9] If

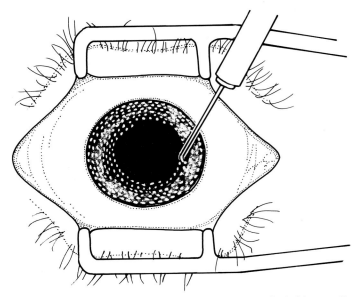

**Fig. 6-30.** Small burns are applied in a systematic fashion until the entire corneal surface has been treated.

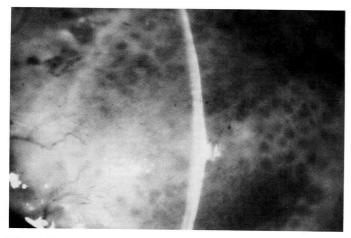

**Fig. 6-31.** Appearance of a cornea 2 months after a Salleras procedure. Subepithelial opacities are still evident but will continue to fade with time.

not successful with the initial treatment, the applications may be repeated. If treatment is initially successful but relapse occurs, additional treatment may be performed at a later date with renewed success. We have seen patients retreated up to five times over the course of several years with satisfactory results on each occasion. Glaucomatous eyes have a slightly poorer response than normotensive eyes due to persistent stromal edema as a result of the chronic elevation of intraocular pressure.

## ACKNOWLEDGMENTS

Portions of this chapter are reproduced with permission from Abbott, RL: Techniques of Aphakic and Pseudophakic Keratoplasty, in Brightbill, F. (ed): Corneal Surgery: Theory, Technique and Tissue. St. Louis, C.V. Mosby Co., 1986.

## REFERENCES

1. Arentsen JJ, Morgan B, Green WR: Changing indications for keratoplasty. Am J Ophthalmol 81:313–318, 1976
2. Bernth-Petersen P: A change in indications for cataract surgery? A 10 year comparative epidemiologic study. Acta Ophthalmol 59:206–210, 1981
3. Boruchoff SA: Therapeutic keratoplasty, in Smolin G, Thoft RA (eds): The Cornea. Boston, Little Brown, 1983, pp 437–453
4. Casey TA, Mayer DJ: Corneal Grafting-Principles and Practice. Philadelphia, Saunders, 1984, p 131
5. Cogan DG, Kinsey VE: The cornea vs. physiologic aspects. Arch Ophthalmol 28:661–669, 1942
6. DeVoe AG: Electrocautery of bowman's membrane. Trans Am Ophthalmol Soc 64:109–122, 1966
7. Dohlman CH, Boruchoff SA, Mobilia EF: Complications in the use of soft contact lenses in corneal disease. Arch Ophthalmol 90:367–371, 1973
8. Dohlman CH, Hedbys BO, Mishima S: The swelling pressure of the corneal stroma. Invest Ophthalmol 1:158–162, 1962
9. Farris RL, Iwamoto T, DeVoe AG: Cautery of Bowman's membrane. Am J Ophthalmol 77:548–554, 1974
10. Fine, M: Keratoplasty in aphakia, in King JH Jr, McTigue JW (eds): The Cornea World Congress. Washington, Butterworths, pp 538–552, 1965
11. Gassett AR, Kaufman HE: Bandage lens in the treatment of bullous keratoplasty. Am J Ophthalmol 69:252–259, 1970
12. Goldman JN, Benedek GB: The relationship between morphology and transparency in the non-swelling corneal stroma of the shark. Invest Ophthalmol 6:574, 1967
13. Gundersen T: Conjunctival flaps in the treatment of corneal disease with reference to a new technique of application. Arch Ophthalmol 60:880–888, 1958
14. Gundersen T: Surgical treatment of bullous keratoplasty. Arch Ophthalmol 64:260–267, 1960
15. Hedbys BO, Dohlman CH: A new method for the determination of the swelling pressure of the corneal stroma in vitro. Exp Eye Res 2:122–129, 1963
16. Hodson S, Miller F: The bicarbonate ion pump in the endothelium which regulates the hydration of rabbit cornea. J Physiol 163:563–577, 1976
17. Kramer SG: Cystoid macular edema after aphakic penetrating keratoplasty. Ophthalmol 88:782–787, 1981
18. Kramer SG: Keratoplasty techniques. Trans Pac Coast Otoophthalmol Soc Annu Meet 64:39–43, 1983
19. Luxenberg MN, Green K: Reduction of corneal edema with topical hyperosmotic agents. Am J Ophthalmol 71:847–853, 1971
20. MacDonald JM, Edelhauser HF: The corneal endothelial barrier—The effect of anti-inflammatory agents during intraocular inflammation. Invest Ophthalmol Vis Sci (ARVO Abstr, Suppl) 26(3):320, 1985
21. MacDonald JM, Geroski DH, Edelhauser HF: Pump site density of the corneal endothelium during intraocular inflammation. Invest Ophthalmol Vis Sci (ARVO Abstr, Suppl) 27(3):174, 1986
22. Mishima S: Corneal thickness. Surv Ophthalmol 13:57–96, 1968
23. Mishima S, Hedbys BO: Physiology of the cornea. Int Ophthalmol Clin 8:527–560, 1968
24. Paton D, Milauskas AT: Indications, surgical technique, and results of thin conjunctival flaps on the cornea. Int Ophthalmol Clin 10:329–345, 1970
25. Salleras A: Bullous keratoplasty, in King JH, Jr, McTigue JW (eds): The Cornea World Congress. Washington, Buttersworths, pp 292–299, 1965
26. Scholer KW: Jahresberichte über die wirksamkait der augenklinik, in den jahren 1874–80. Berlin: H. Peters, 1875–1881.
27. Stamper RL, Sugar A: The intraocular lens. Am Acad Ophthalmol, San Francisco, 1982
28. Stark, WJ, Terry AC, Worthen D, et al.: Update of intraocular lenses implanted in the United States. Am J Ophthalmol 98:238–239, 1984
29. Sugar HS: The use of Gundersen flaps in the treatment of bullous keratoplasty. Am J Ophthalmol 57:977–983, 1964
30. Taylor DM, Atlas BF, Romanchuk KG, et al.: Pseudophakic bullous keratoplasty. Ophthalmology 90:19–24, 1983
31. Ytteborg J, Dohlman CH: Corneal edema and intraocular pressure, II clinical results. Arch Ophthalmol 74:477–484, 1965

## 7

# Noninfected Corneal Perforations

## Sid Mandelbaum        Ira J. Udell

Options in the management of corneal perforations have substantially increased in the past 20 years with the introduction of tissue adhesive, improvements in soft contact lenses, and refinements in surgical instrumentation, sutures, and techniques. These are welcome additions, but they have complicated the therapeutic decision-making process by introducing new variables. The primary purpose of this chapter and the next is to discuss the modalities available for treating corneal perforations in detail, with specific attention to the reasoning involved in choosing the optimum approach for a particular clinical setting.

Determination of the etiology of the corneal perforation is important in the management of this problem. There are multiple factors that may result in corneal stromal melting; differences in etiology may dictate differences in therapy. If the predisposing condition is not addressed, the process may recur despite an initially effective treatment for the perforation. Corneal ulcerations can broadly be divided into those that result from infectious agents (bacteria, fungi, viruses, or parasites) and those that are not infected.

The most common causes of corneal ulcerations and perforations are microbial agents. All corneal ulcers should be suspected of being infected and should be cultured; most should also be treated initially with topical antibiotics pending culture results. Infection cannot be ruled out by clinical signs alone. The cornea may be infected despite the absence of biomicroscopically visible stromal infiltrate. The infecting agent may be so indolent that an inflammatory response is not elicited, or the eye may be too immunocompromised to mount visible inflammation. Special considerations involved in the treatment of perforations associated with infectious agents will be discussed in Chapter 8.

Classic teaching suggests that peripheral ulcers occur in relation to conjunctival and systemic diseases, whereas central corneal ulceration is more typically a result of exogenous microbial infection.[74] While this generalization is often true, any classification based solely on location is somewhat artificial and is subject to many exceptions. Keratitis due to *Neisseriae gonorrhea,* for example, has a predeliction for the corneal periphery where it may rapidly progress to perforation. It should be emphasized that whether the ulceration occurs centrally, midperipherally, or peripherally, it is imperative to rule out a microbial etiology with appropriately performed cultures.

The more common nonmicrobial causes of corneal melting are listed in Table 7-1. Determination of the etiology of noninfected corneal ulceration requires a combination of careful ocular examination, systemic history, general physical examination, and directed laboratory studies, keeping in mind the specific diseases in Table 7-1. Although evaluation by an internist may be helpful, the ophthalmologist should communicate to the internist those diseases that are of particular concern. While in some cases an underlying systemic disease is already recognized (frequently the case with rheumatoid arthritis), corneal melting may occasionally be the presenting sign of a systemic disorder. It is particularly important to identify a condition such as Wegener's granulomatosis for example, which is fatal if untreated but in which remission rates of as high as 90 percent can be obtained with systemic immunosuppressive agents.[25] Systemic evaluation is also essential before making the diagnosis of Mooren's ulcer, which, by definition, should be made only when extensive and repeated testing for underlying systemic disorders is negative.

## OBJECTIVES OF THERAPY

The primary objective in managing a patient with a corneal perforation is to re-establish the structural integrity of the globe as rapidly as possible. This minimizes intraocular inflammation and the risks of intraocular infection and epithelial downgrowth. Restoration of normal intraocular fluid dynamics by sealing the leak will limit the development of peripheral anterior synechiae and lens opacification, and resolve choroidal effusions resulting from hypotony. The ultimate purpose, of course, is to restore useful vision. This may require a staged approach, however, with initial therapy

SURGICAL INTERVENTION IN CORNEAL AND EXTERNAL DISEASES
ISBN 0-8089-1850-8

**Table 7-1**
Etiologies of Non-infectious Corneal Melts

| | |
|---|---|
| Postinfectious | Bacterial[42] |
| | Fungal[42] |
| | Herpes simplex[19] or zoster[56] |
| Immunologic | Hypersensitivity (eg staph)[74] |
| | Collagen vascular diseases |
| |    rheumatoid arthritis[22,26] |
| |      Wegener's granulomatosis[15] |
| |      periarteritis nodosa[17] |
| |      others (less commonly) |
| | Sjogren's syndrome[48,63] |
| | Pemphigoid[55] |
| | Stevens-Johnson syndrome[20] |
| | Mooren's ulceration[11] |
| | Vernal conjunctivitis ("shield ulcer")[41] |
| | Graft-versus-host disease[32] |
| Exposure | VII nerve paralysis, lid abnormalities[34] |
| | Nocturnal lagophthalmos[43] |
| | Exophthalmos (eg dysthyroid opthalmopathy)[31] |
| Neurotropic | V nerve lesions[28,52] |
| | Post herpes zoster[80] |
| | Familial dysautonomia (Riley Day)[51] |
| Traumatic | Chemical injuries[62,73] |
| | Thermal burns[73] |
| Dermatologic | Rosacea[13] |
| | Atopic dermatitis[67] |
| Miscellaneous | Post cataract extraction[1,18,33] |
| | Vitamin A deficiency[64] |
| | Post irradiation[54] |
| | Topical anesthetic abuse[24] |

**Table 7-2**
Treatment of Corneal Perforations

Medical
  Patching
  Therapeutic soft contact lens
  Tissue adhesive
Surgical
  Suture closure
  Lamellar graft
  Penetrating keratoplasty
  Conjunctival flap

to be familiar with all of the techniques described below since several different modalities may be required in the course of treatment.

## MEDICAL TREATMENT OF CORNEAL PERFORATIONS

### Patching

The application of a semi-pressure patch may allow a pinpoint perforation to seal. Adding a topical cycloplegic may be helpful by moving the lens–iris diaphragm posteriorly, thus deepening the chamber. The beneficial effect of patching may be in maintaining the upper lid in a position to bridge the defect, thereby encouraging the deposition of fibrin and/or the sliding of adjacent epithelium to cover the site of the leak. No matter how carefully the patch is applied, however, it also puts some pressure on the globe, which may partially counteract its benefit. While it is in position, topical medications cannot be applied. Another fundamental problem with patching is the inability to determine its effectiveness for the initial 24 hours or so that the patch should be left in place. We recommend this approach primarily for dealing with very small leaks that may occur in the immediate postoperative period after anterior segment surgery. In this situation, if patching has not been effective after 24 hours, the operative wound should be secured with additional sutures. When there is a significant loss of tissue, patching is usually ineffective and delays institution of more definitive therapy.

### Therapeutic Soft Contact Lens

When a therapeutic soft lens is applied over a small corneal perforation, the lens is utilized as a mechanical splint and scaffold. The lens may act to trap fibrin and epithelial debris in the perforation site, thus plugging it. The epithelium adjacent to the perforation is protected from the action of the lids with each blink, thus encouraging epithelial sliding. On occasion, corneal epithelium has been observed to bridge a stromal defect by initially adhering to the posterior surface of a bandage soft lens before eventually adhering to the corneal surface.[50] The lens probably causes slight swelling of the cornea adjacent to the perforation that may also help in decreasing aqueous leakage.

directed towards preservation of the eye and secondary visual rehabilitative procedures reserved until the eye is quiet.

Unfortunately, the tendency to focus on the corneal perforation itself may overshadow the critical role of adjunctive therapy in the overall management. The rational use of specific antimicrobials to control the infecting organisms, of cycloplegics to decrease the relative pupillary block often present, and the cautious use of anti-inflammatory agents are important to the outcome even though they are not the modalities that will seal the leak. Many cases of corneal perforations share the common feature of poor ocular surfacing. Use of lubricants, a therapeutic soft lens, punctal occlusion, or partial tarsorrhaphy are frequently necessary to maintain an intact epithelium and prevent re-ulceration and re-perforation. Measures for promoting and maintaining the epithelial surface are discussed in detail in Chapter 5.

Medical and surgical approaches to perforations are listed in Table 7-2. The major determinants of the therapeutic modality selected are the underlying cause of the perforation, its size and location, the status of the adjacent cornea, whether the anterior chamber is partially formed or flat, other ocular abnormalities, and the general medical condition and prognosis of the patient. It is prudent for the ophthalmologist managing a patient with a corneal perforation

The fit is important if a soft lens is to achieve these goals when used to treat a perforation. The lens should be relatively large and fit snugly, with minimal movement. Both the base curve and diameter can be adjusted to achieve this fit. Available lens center thicknesses vary by a factor of 10 from 0.035mm (CSI Therapeutic) to 0.30mm (Softcon). Sometimes, too thin a lens may not provide the desired stabilizing effect. It is useful to have lenses of different parameters available, so that an optimum fit can be achieved for a particular eye. FDA approved therapeutic soft lenses include low water content lenses (38 percent: Bausch and Lomb, CSI), medium water content (55 percent: Softcon, Softsite, and Hydrocurve) and high water content (71 percent: Permalens and 79 percent: Sauflon).

All patients fit with a therapeutic lens should be examined several hours and approximately 24 hours after the lens is applied because of the possibility of significant lens tightening during this period. We supply a protective shield to be worn at night, to keep the patient from inadvertently rubbing the eye overnight or upon awakening. If the lens does come out overnight, the patient may be able to find it in the shield in the morning. Lubricating drops are helpful particularly upon awakening, and are mandatory if the eye is dry. If frequent lubrication is required, nonpreserved tears such as unit dose Refresh® (Allergan) may help avoid potential preservative-induced epithelial toxicity. Bacterial keratitis is of particular concern with a therapeutic soft lens,[10] because the corneal surface requiring such a lens is compromised. It is not known whether prophylactic topical antibiotics reduce the incidence of microbial keratitis in this setting. We tend to empirically prescribe a bactericidal topical antibiotic 2–4 times a day after we apply a therapeutic lens for a corneal perforation, but there are no firm data that support this approach. We prefer to avoid neomycin-containing preparations both because of the epithelial toxicity and the relatively high incidence of allergic reactions associated with this antibiotic.

A soft lens should be utilized as the sole treatment only for very small perforations with healthy adjacent tissue, or in small, virtually self-sealed corneal lacerations whose edges are already well apposed and aligned.[49] If the perforation has not completely sealed within 24 or at most 48 hours, additional therapy is indicated. Because of the availability of tissue adhesives, we very rarely treat perforations with a therapeutic soft lens alone. If the perforation is an appropriate size for treatment with a soft lens, then the application of adhesive prior to placing the lens provides much greater certainty that the perforation will be immediately sealed.

## Tissue Adhesives

Tissue adhesives represent a major advance in the treatment of corneal perforations. The first human patients with perforations treated with tissue adhesives were reported by Webster and coworkers in 1968.[77] Since then, numerous reports have verified the therapeutic efficacy and safety of tissue adhesives when used for this purpose.[7,27,37–40,53,65,76,78] Adhesives allow convenient, immediate closure of a perfora-

tion, generally without the necessity of surgical intervention. The cornea will frequently heal while the glue is in position—in many cases, when the glue spontaneously comes off or is removed weeks to months after application, the perforation remains sealed.

In order to achieve good results with tissue glue, appropriate case selection and attention to the details of application are critical. Indiscriminate use or sloppy application of the adhesive may result not only in failure of closure of the perforation, but also possible additional complications. The perforations for which glue is most effective are small (less than 1.5 mm or at most 2 mm in diameter at the level of Descemet's) with fairly solid surrounding tissue. If the tissue peripheral to the perforation to which the adhesive is applied is soft and necrotic, the glue is not likely to remain in position for very long even if the actual perforation is small. This is frequently a problem in severe microbial keratitis where a perforation develops within a large necrotic ulcer. If the eye is aphakic and vitreous presents through the perforation, glue is relatively contraindicated. Even if the glue would adhere, there is the risk of causing traction on the vitreous and therefore on the retina. Surgical repair of the cornea incorporating an anterior vitrectomy is usually recommended in this situation.

A flat chamber complicates, but does not contraindicate use of tissue adhesive. Considerable care must be taken with its application, however, because the glue can adhere to intraocular structures directly under the perforation. We are aware of cases of adhesive applied to central perforations where the glue adhered to the anterior lens capsule or to an intraocular lens. Lens extractions (or IOL removal) were ultimately required in these situations. Iris directly under a perforation poses less of an anatomic problem; it is preferable not to apply the glue directly to the iris, however. If the perforation is otherwise suitable for adhesive, the anterior chamber can be slightly formed in the area of the perforation with a small air bubble or with sodium hyaluronate.[37,39,53] If even a small separation can be achieved between critical intraocular structures and the perforation, adhesive can be safely applied. With a soft eye and a flat chamber (especially if the eye is phakic) it is dangerous to attempt a limbal stab incision. The air or sodium hyaluronate should be placed into the anterior chamber via the perforation site using a blunt-tipped, small gauge cannula on a syringe. The cannula should be carefully held at the level of the perforation with the opening directed towards the AC, rather than attempting to insert the cannula into the eye. The purpose is to locally create a small separation. No attempt should be made to completely form the anterior chamber in this way. We prefer to try an air bubble first; if not effective, a small amount of sodium hyaluronate can be instilled. Excess hyaluronate should be wiped away from the perforation site with sterile surgical spears before applying the adhesive.

### Techniques of Application

There are numerous techniques that have been utilized for application of tissue glue to the cornea. Our experience has been using Histoacryl Blue (B. Braun Melsungen AG,

Melsungen, Germany). We will present three different application techniques with which we have personally had success, and will discuss the situations in which we prefer each method. Certain aspects and considerations are independent of the technique utilized. As thin a layer of glue as possible should be applied. The most common mistake we have seen in use of this modality is the application of too much glue. The less glue applied, the less elevated above the adjacent cornea it will be when polymerized. A flat application of glue is less disturbing to tear flow and to the lids, thus better resisting dislodgment. All necrotic tissue and debris should be carefully removed prior to glue placement to facilitate its adherence. If the glue is applied over epithelium, it will usually separate within several days as the underlying epithelium continues to replicate. A platinum spatula or a blade may be used to gently debride the epithelium for 1–2 mm adjacent to the perforation site—this can be done at the time corneal cultures are being taken. Alternatively, the epithelium adjacent to the perforation can be softened and loosened using a cut surgical spear soaked in cocaine. A dry spear can then be used to push the epithelium peripherally. The edge of the epithelium can be lifted with a jeweler's forceps and trimmed with a fine scissors to several millimeters peripheral to the ulcer bed.

The glue is polymerized by free anions, which are present in tissue fluids including aqueous humor.[76] The area to which the glue is being applied should thus be carefully dried with surgical spears prior to its application. The glue does not adhere to conjunctiva long-term, because the presence of surface conjunctival epithelium and the mobility of the conjunctiva both tend to dislodge it. For these reasons, if the perforation is just within the limbus, the glue should be placed in such a manner to allow as little of it as possible onto the conjunctiva. Occasionally, a local peritomy and conjunctival recession may be necessary to allow optimum glue adherence if the perforation is very close to the limbus.

If there is any question as to the adequacy of the adhesive closure after glue is applied, Seidel's test can be performed by "painting" the cornea just adjacent to the adhesive with a slightly moistened fluorescein strip. If a leak is present, the glue should be removed and carefully reapplied so that the seal is watertight. To prevent constant irritation to the upper palpebral conjunctiva by the polymerized glue, and to minimize the tendency to dislodgment of the glue by upper lid blinking, we always apply a therapeutic soft lens as soon as the glue has polymerized. The lens should completely cover the glue; if the application has been successful in achieving a very thin film of adhesive, a very thin lens can be used. Thicker applications of glue can sometimes be salvaged with a thicker, steeper lens that will better protect the glue from movement of the upper lid than a thinner lens.

*Drip technique of adhesive application.* If the long nose of the plastic container in which the glue is supplied is cut off at the level indicated in Figure 7-1, the taper of the remaining portion will seat well in the hub of a standard needle. A 27 or 30 gauge needle can be used to dispense a very small drop of glue directly from the container. The drop from a 30 gauge needle is smaller, but the diameter of the needle is so small

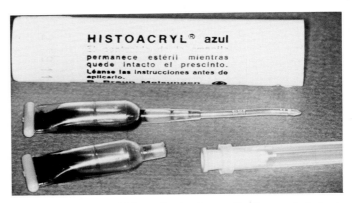

**Fig. 7-1.** Histoacryl Blue adhesive is supplied in a sealed plastic tube. If the tube is cut as shown, the taper of the remaining portion fits well into the hub of a 27 gauge needle. This provides a convenient way of dispensing appropriately small drops of the liquid.

that the glue may polymerize in its shaft before it can be dispensed. If a 27 gauge needle is used, only part of a drop need be applied. The glue can be stored refrigerated with the capped needle left on the plastic vial, and is useful as long as it remains liquid. When the glue is next used, the needle on the vial should be replaced.

Dripping a very small amount of glue directly into the perforation is most effective in slow-leaking, localized, crater-like perforations with nearly full thickness adjacent corneal walls (as in Fig. 7-2). Such perforations are not infrequently seen in patients with rheumatoid arthritis. A single drop of glue may be dripped into this type of perforation directly from the glue container using a 27 or 30 gauge needle. If the drop of glue is small, it will be nearly flush with the surrounding corneal surface once it polymerizes. This is easiest to accomplish with the patient supine, and the head and eye positioned in such a way that gravity keeps the glue at the perforation site rather than allowing it to drip away. An assistant or a lid speculum is used to maintain the lids open. The base of the perforation is dried with a surgical spear held in one hand just prior to dripping the single drop of glue into the site with the other hand. Polymerization will occur in seconds, during which time the eye should remain open and immobile. A soft contact lens is then applied. This

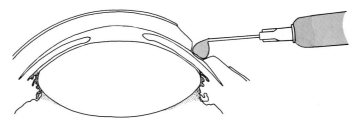

**Fig. 7-2.** Drip technique of adhesive application. A small drop of cyanoacrylate adhesive is being dripped directly into a slowly-leaking perforation with full thickness walls. When the glue polymerizes, it should be almost flush with the anterior surface of the cornea. The epithelium was removed from the edges of the perforation prior to applying the glue.

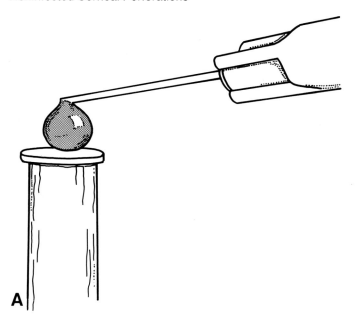

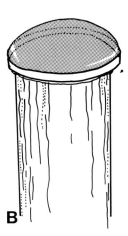

**Fig. 7-3.** (A) A 3 mm plastic disc maintained on the end of a wooden applicator stick by a small amount of ointment. A single drop of adhesive is being dispensed onto the surface of the disc using a 27 or 30 gauge needle attached to the glue container. (B) Glue on the plastic disc ready for application to the eye. Prior to polymerization, the glue will not adhere to the plastic disc.

technique is easy and rapid, but useful only if the leak is slow and the perforation crater-like.

*Disc technique of adhesive application.* With a brisk aqueous leak, glue dripped into the perforation will stream out of the perforation site along with the aqueous, polymerizing along the way. This usually results in an unacceptably elevated, irregular, mound of glue. To avoid this, a small air bubble can be injected locally into the anterior chamber, which may internally seal the leak sufficiently to allow adhesive application. Alternatively, the disc technique originally described by Refojo can be used.[65] The disc technique is also useful if a large area of cornea adjacent to the perforation is thin. Use of the disc will flatten the adhesive applied, resulting in a thinner layer of glue than if it were dripped into the perforation site. A circular disc is cut from the plastic backing removed from an eye drape. Since it is difficult to uniformly cut small discs by hand, we prefer to punch out 3 and 4 mm diameter discs in advance using trephines; in our experience, these are the optimum size. We place several of these discs on a colored background for better visualization, gas sterilize them, and keep them available in the clinic in individual packages.

A tiny amount of any ophthalmic ointment is placed on the end of a wooden applicator stick. A small forceps is used to transfer a disc to the ointment. The ointment will hold the disc to the applicator while it is being manipulated but will allow it to separate from the applicator when pressed into position. A tiny drop of the adhesive delivered through a 27 or 30 gauge needle is placed on the plastic disc (Fig. 7-3). Prior to polymerization, the glue will not adhere to the plastic disc.

At the slit lamp, with the patient upright and the lids separated, the perforation site is dried and the disc and glue

are precisely pressed into position over the perforation (Fig. 7-4). Usually, the disc will adhere to the glue as it polymerizes; it will separate easily from the applicator because of the ointment. The contact lens usually rides smoothly over these discs (Fig. 7-5). An advantage of round discs prepared with a trephine is that there are no sharp edges to catch the lens and elevate the glue as there might be if the discs were fashioned with scissors. This technique can also be utilized with the patient supine under an operating microscope.

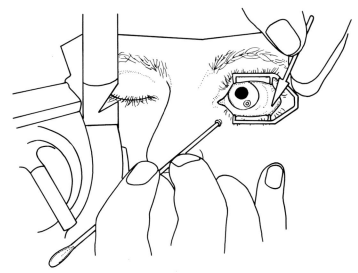

**Fig. 7-4.** Disc technique of adhesive application. The patient's lids are maintained open by a wire speculum and the slit-lamp is used for visualization. The perforation has just been dried with a surgical spear. The applicator stick with the plastic disc and glue on its end is about to be pressed directly onto the perforation.

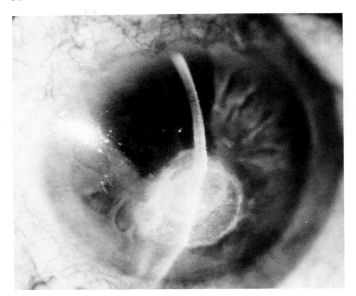

Fig. 7-5. Slit-lamp photograph taken about 24 hours after application of adhesive to a corneal perforation using the disc technique. Although the 3 mm plastic disc is still present on the surface of the glue, the slit beam shows the minimal elevation of the glue and disc above the corneal surface. A therapeutic soft lens is in position, fitting well over the adhesive and disc. The anterior chamber has reformed.

*Microapplicator technique of adhesive application.* A microapplicator (B. Braun Melsungen, available though Trihawk International, Montreal Canada, Fig. 7-6) is partially filled with adhesive. With the patient at the slit lamp, a circular motion of the microapplicator is used to apply a thin layer of glue just peripheral to the perforation (Fig. 7-7A). After allowing about a minute for polymerization, the central ulcer bed is again dried with a surgical spear. A light streaking motion with the microapplicator is then used to superficially bridge the perforation site from the previously glued peripheral area (Fig. 7-7B). Sometimes a thin strand of adhesive polymerizes as the applicator is withdrawn; this may be trimmed with a fine scissors. The adhesive is dispensed from the microapplicator by capillary action. The applicator must therefore be moved fairly quickly to prevent too much glue from being discharged. If the glue in the applicator tip polymerizes prematurely, the tip can be cut about 1 mm back, thus re-establishing adhesive flow. Practice with the microapplicator to learn the optimum rate of motion for dispensing a fine layer of adhesive is essential. Once mastered, this technique can be utilized to deal with most of the perforations to which glue is applicable.

Once glue has been successfully applied, we usually leave it in position until it spontaneously comes off, generally weeks to several months after application. The granular character and blue color of the polymerized adhesive prevents clear visualization through it, making slit-lamp determination of the thickness of underlying cornea difficult. As the cornea heals, the glue will begin to lift slightly around the edges. The bed may become vascularized. We do not recommend mechanically removing the adhesive unless the oph-

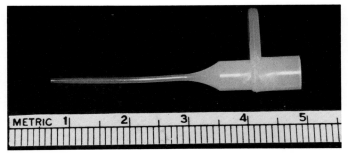

Fig. 7-6. Microapplicator, which may be partially filled with cyanoacrylate adhesive. The glue is dispensed by capillary action; occluding the wider end of the microapplicator with a fingertip will decrease the flow of adhesive at the tip.

thalmologist is reasonably certain that the underlying perforation has sealed.

The mechanism of action of tissue adhesive is uncertain. Certainly, one component of its effect is the ability to seal the leak and provide structural support to the area of melted cornea. The beneficial effect of adhesive in this situation probably extends beyond this, however. Experimental evidence indicates that ulcerating corneas to which glue has been applied are nearly devoid of acute inflammatory cells, compared to the intense intrastromal inflammation present in ulcerating corneas that have not been glued.[45] Fogle and coworkers have postulated that the adhesive provides a barrier to the influx of neutrophils, which probably exacerbate stromal ulceration.[27] The migration of early regenerating epithelium that may release chemotactic factors or stimulate inflammatory cells is also inhibited by the adhesive.[27]

### Complications of Adhesive Use

The tissue adhesives principally used in ophthalmology are the higher alkyl cyanoacrylate derivatives. These derivatives appear to degrade more slowly than the lower order derivatives (e.g. methyl cyanoacrylate) and appear to be better tolerated by living tissue.[66] Reports of the ocular toxicity of these adhesives have varied depending on the system in which they were studied, the amount used, the manner and location of application, and the endpoint of the response.[66] When tissue adhesives are used clinically in the manner we have described, toxic reactions to the glue itself are very uncommon. It is important to differentiate true toxic reactions from complications related to the application technique, and from complications related to the underlying disease process.

Most complications we have recognized are due to the basic condition that necessitated the gluing. Persistent stromal melting may occur despite the glue, especially in diseases characterized by aggressive and widespread rather than localized ulceration. In some cases, the eye may remain formed without progressive corneal melting, but the stroma may not heal despite the glue, and the perforation may still be present once the glue is removed months later. We have encountered this situation in melts of multiple etiologies including neurotrophic keratitis, herpetic keratitis, Stevens-Johnson syndrome, alkali burns, cicatricial pemphigoid, and

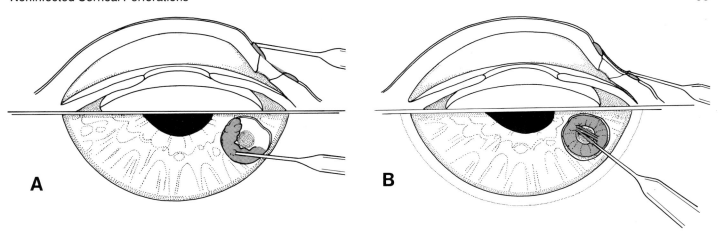

**Fig. 7-7.** Microapplicator technique of adhesive application. (A) A circular motion of the microapplicator is used to apply a thin layer of adhesive around the perforation after the epithelium, if present, has been removed. The glue is allowed to polymerize. (B) After the perforation site is again dried with a surgical spear, a back-and-forth streaking motion with the microapplicator applies glue to bridge the perforation and seal it.

melting associated with atopic keratoconjunctivitis. This represents a lack of effectiveness of the glue in a particular clinical setting, and should not be considered a complication of its use. In general, the vascularization that may be elicited by the adhesive is a welcome response, since this often accompanies healing of the underlying defect. Once the perforation is sealed and the glue is no longer present the vessels may diminish in caliber. Vascularization may complicate penetrating keratoplasty, if subsequently required, by increasing the risk of homograft rejection.

Corneal infiltrates, usually due to secondary infection, may occur adjacent to the adhesive despite the use of prophylactic topical antibiotics. Weiss and associates reported that 7 of the 80 eyes they treated with adhesive developed corneal infiltrates; 5 of these 7 were culture positive for bacteria.[78] We have not noted as high an incidence of this complication but have seen it on several occasions. It is unlikely that the glue is the source of the infection. In vitro, the cyanoacrylates have been shown to be mildly bacteriostatic for Gram-positive organisms for a short time after polymerization.[23] In all cases, the microbial keratitis appeared many weeks after the application of the glue rather than immediately, as would be expected if the glue were the source of the infecting organisms. The disease processes resulting in corneal melting locally immunocompromise the cornea making it more susceptible to bacterial superinfection. The presence of the therapeutic soft lens placed over the adhesive also may predispose to bacterial keratitis.[10]

Rapid progression of a cataract has occasionally been noted after closure of a perforation with adhesive.[35] Since the flat anterior chamber and intraocular inflammation present before the glue is applied predispose to cataract formation, the lens swelling and opacification in these cases may be multifactorial. The rarity of this occurrence, however, makes it unlikely that cataract formation is a direct result of adhesive properly applied to the cornea.

On occasion, intraocular pressure may markedly rise after the perforation is sealed with adhesive. Several mechanisms may be responsible for this phenomenon. The trabecular meshwork of some eyes seems to require several days after the perforation is sealed to regain its normal level of function. In other cases, large choroidal effusions that developed when the eye was open may push the ciliary body and lens forward resulting in relative ciliary and/or pupillary block. Pupillary block may also be increased if the lens swells because of aggravation of a preexisting cataract.

Tissue adhesive has been discussed in great detail because we believe it has a critically important role in the management of corneal perforations. Unfortunately, despite having been used in ophthalmology for this purpose for nearly 2 decades, cyanoacrylate is considered an investigational device by the Food and Drug Administration. As such, an Investigational Device Exemption (IDE) is legally required for its use. Medical grade cyanoacrylate adhesive is therefore not available in this country, although it is available outside the United States, including Canada. At the present time devices do not fall under the Orphan Products Act, and hence manufacturers do not enjoy the same incentives offered to orphan drugs under this act. The Food and Drug Administration is actively working with the American Academy of Ophthalmology and the Health Industry Manufacturer's Association to alter the current situation by attempting to obtain sponsorship, to have the necessary studies done, and thus to put the cyanoacrylates in a position for obtaining FDA approval for use in corneal perforations.

While tissue adhesive has been a major addition to the armementarium for dealing with corneal perforations, there are situations where it is not likely to be, or has not been, effective. Large perforations (greater than 2 mm in diameter), particularly if complicated by vitreous prolapse, or perforations that have not healed despite well-applied glue generally require surgical intervention.

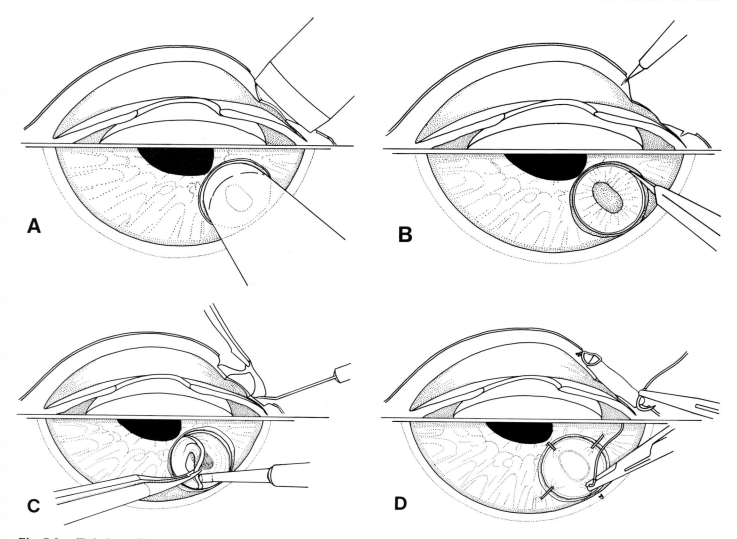

**Fig. 7-8.** Technique of lamellar patch graft. (A) A trephine which surrounds the perforation is used to lightly mark the corneal surface. (B) A sharp blade is used to cut the cornea along the circular mark for its entire circumference. (C) The circumscribed cornea is lamellarly dissected and removed. (D) The donor button is secured in position. A total of eight sutures will be used in this case; sutures near the visual axis are intentionally shorter. The donor button is slightly thicker than the host defect, as the overhydrated donor tissue will thin.

## SURGICAL TREATMENT OF CORNEAL PERFORATIONS

### Suture Closure

Closing a perforation with sutures is very rarely useful in cases of corneal ulceration. The combination of tissue loss, irregular edges, and soft corneal stroma due to aqueous imbibition make good approximation of the edges difficult. Even if a watertight closure can be achieved initially, sutures placed under considerable tension may cheesewire through the cornea resulting in recurrence of the leak. Large reactive sutures such as silk may be less prone to cut through adjacent stroma, but tend to aggravate the situation by increasing corneal stromal inflammation and ultimately ulceration. If the patient is being brought to the operating theater, a more definitive procedure should be planned. We can only recom-

mend suture closure for immediate postoperative cases that are leaking, where better edge apposition will provide a watertight seal, but where there is no tissue deficit.

### Lamellar Patch Graft

A lamellar patch graft is particularly useful in peripheral perforations. The ulceration is usually narrowest at Descemet's membrane and wider anteriorly. It is difficult and not necessary to shape the donor plug to precisely fit the perforation; the critical aspect is that the donor corneal patch fit well into the anterior portion of the perforation. A partial thickness corneal patch generally is better for this purpose than a full thickness one. A bed must be fashioned into which the donor tissue is sewn so that the anterior surfaces of the donor and adjacent host cornea will be of approximately equal heights once the cornea heals. The easiest approach is to first mark the surface of the cornea with a circular trephine that surrounds the corneal perforation (Fig. 7-8A). The

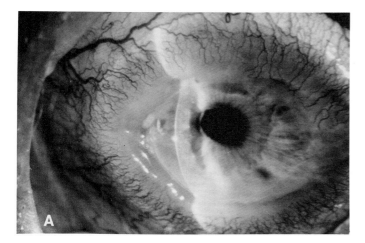

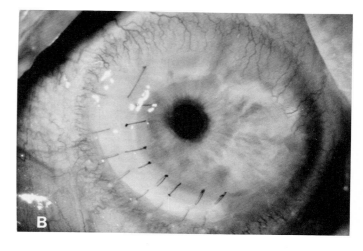

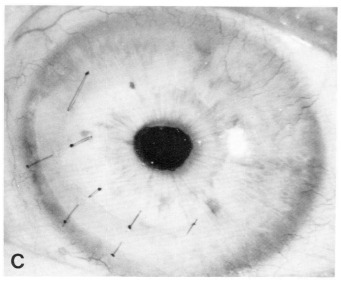

**Fig. 7-9.** (A) An approximately 3 mm wide midperipheral corneal melt extending from 5:30 to 10:00 o'clock in the left eye of a 76-year-old female with severe rheumatoid arthritis. The considerable loss of tissue and a perforation within the melted zone have combined to cause extensive collapse of the cornea. (B) Three days after surgical repair with a crescentic lamellar patch graft. The anterior chamber is well formed. (C) Two months postoperatively. Approximately one-half of the sutures initially placed have been removed. Visual acuity is 20/40 with aphakic correction. The patient was found to have high levels of circulating immune complexes. She was placed on prednisone and methotrexate for control of her systemic disease, and to prevent further corneal ulceration.

diameter of the trephine should be larger than the perforation and extend to an area where the stroma is not necrotic and is at least half normal thickness. Only nondisposable trephines are available between 1 and 5 mm diameters in 1 mm increments. Sharper disposable trephine blades are manufactured in diameters greater than 6 mm. In perforations requiring these larger grafts, however, it is likely that penetrating rather than lamellar keratoplasty would be performed since the visual axis would be involved. Usually the eye is too soft to allow enough pressure to be placed on the trephine to cut the stroma—it is, however, very useful to make a circular mark in the epithelium. The sharpest available blade is then used to carefully cut the cornea along the entire circumference of the mark to at least half stromal thickness, providing a substantial peripheral ledge into which the donor can be sewn (Fig. 7-8B). A diamond blade is excellent for cutting the cornea of a soft eye; certainly a sharp razor blade can also be used. Once the tissue along the circular mark has been circumscribed, it is lamellarly dissected and removed from the bed (Fig. 7-8C). A slightly larger diameter circular donor button is then prepared, and secured in position with 6–12 interrupted 10/0 nylon sutures, depending on the size of the button (Fig. 7-8-D). The donor lamellar button may be slightly thicker than the defect in the

host as the donor tissue is usually overhydrated and can be expected to thin.

For dissecting a lamellar patch, it is easiest to work from the anterior surface of the donor material; a whole globe is therefore optimum. If a whole globe is not available, the patch graft must be punched from the endothelial side of the donor tissue. It is important to allow for the fact that tissue prepared in this fashion is slightly smaller than if cut from the anterior cornea. Posterior layers of stroma may be dissected from the donor cornea until it is of appropriate thickness. It is helpful to have an assistant stabilize the tissue when this is performed.

The donor and host grafts are easiest to prepare, match, and secure in a watertight fashion if they are both circular. If the corneal melt and perforation are peripheral to the visual axis but are of a shape that cannot be repaired with a circular graft, a lamellar patch is still the preferred approach. It is helpful to delineate as much of the donor with circular trephines as possible, completing the remainder freehand and rounding the edges to avoid sharp points of tissue. An example is shown in Figure 7-9A: an arcuate midperipheral corneal melt extending from 5:30 to 10:00 o'clock and approximately 3 mm in maximal width developed in a patient with long-standing rheumatoid arthritis. In the operating room,

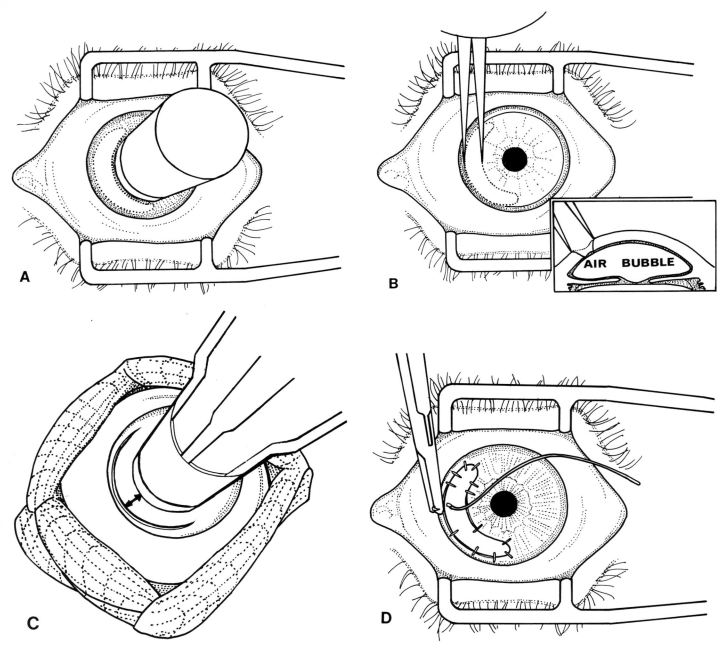

**Fig. 7-10.** Technique of crescentic lamellar patch graft. (A) After an air bubble is injected into the anterior chamber to expand the central cornea to approximately its normal curvature, the two trephines that most closely match the inner and outer curvatures of the melt are selected. (B) The width of the melt is measured in several locations with calipers. (C) The previously selected trephines are used to make partial-thickness arcuate cuts into a donor globe. The distance between these cuts is 0.5 mm greater than the width of the melt. A blade is used to complete excision of the tissue. (D) The patch graft removed from the donor cornea is sutured into the host. The edges are shaped to match the melted cornea.

an air bubble was placed in the anterior chamber to dome the cornea to approximately normal curvature. Trephines were selected whose curvatures matched the inner and outer margins of the arcuate melt (Fig. 7-10A). The width of the melt was measured in several locations with calipers (Fig. 7-10B). The trephines previously selected were then used to trephine partial thickness into the cornea of a whole globe so the donor tissue was approximately 0.5 mm wider than the width of the melt in the patient (Fig. 7-10C). A razor blade

was used to dissect along the trephine marks, removing donor tissue of approximately the same thickness as the host defect. The patch graft was then sutured in position (Fig. 7-10D), rounding the ends to match the defect in the host. The outcome in this patient is shown in Figures 7-9B and 7-9C.

Lamellar patch grafts have a larger area of contact with the host cornea than do penetrating grafts. The donor tissue extends beyond the edge of the perforation and overlies a deep lip of host cornea, making it easier to achieve a water-

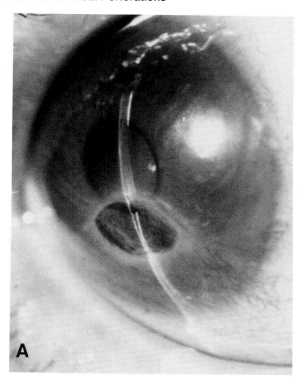

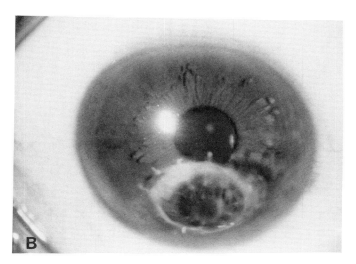

**Fig. 7-11.** (A) Inferior corneal melt and perforation in the right eye of a 36-year-old female with a history of recurrent episodes of right ocular irritation, and topical steroid use for many years. The anterior chamber is flat. At surgery, the cornea peripheral to the melt was too thin and soft to allow for the dissection necessary for a lamellar patch graft. A 4 mm full-thickness eccentric keratoplasty was performed. (B) Same eye, 5 months after surgical repair. With a $-2.25 +2.00 \times 150°$, visual acuity is 20/20−. Since the graft is peripheral to the visual axis, good visual acuity should be maintained even if it opacifies.

tight closure than with a full thickness graft. Another advantage of lamellar grafts is that the quality of the donor tissue is not critical. The status of the donor endothelium makes no difference since little if any of it is transplanted. Once the graft heals, the host endothelium will dehydrate the donor stroma even if it was very edematous at the time of surgery. A rehydrated glycerine-preserved cornea can be used. Even fresh or glycerine-preserved sclera can be used as a lamellar patch if corneal tissue cannot be obtained.

Lamellar grafts heal more rapidly than do full thickness grafts because there is a larger area of contact between donor and host corneal stroma. Sutures can be removed when they loosen, when the area vascularizes, or when a visible cicatrix forms at the donor/host junction. Depending on the situation, a localized conjunctival flap can be placed over a peripheral patch graft at the time of surgery to prevent further ulceration.

## Penetrating Keratoplasty

### Peripheral

Despite the advantages of a lamellar patch graft, it may be necessary to perform a full thickness graft even for a peripheral perforation if the perforation is surrounded by a zone of corneal thinning, softening, or necrosis of such size that it precludes preparing a bed into which to sew a lamellar

patch. Such perforations can be handled with an eccentric full-thickness keratoplasty. If a 3 or 4 mm donor button is of sufficient size to replace the perforated and surrounding thin cornea, and if it can be placed in such a way as to be outside the visual axis, then this approach is generally preferable to a large central keratoplasty (Fig. 7-11). The smaller donor tissue will heal more quickly. The quality of the endothelium is not critical, since the host usually has sufficient endothelial reserve to repopulate such a small donor graft. Most importantly, since the graft remains outside the visual axis, vision will be preserved even if it is immunologically rejected. A disadvantage of peripheral grafts is that they may cause moderate, occasionally irregular astigmatism, although most patients in whom we have performed these grafts have had refractive errors correctable by spectacle lenses.

In performing a peripheral full thickness keratoplasty it is again easiest to match a circular donor graft to a circular host bed if the shape of the perforation will allow. Because the eye is soft, the trephine is useful only for marking the epithelium. Sodium hyaluronate instilled into the anterior chamber through the perforation is helpful in providing a firmer cornea to cut against, and in separating the cornea from the iris. The sharpest available blade is used to dissect through the corneal stroma along the circular trephine mark and to enter the anterior chamber. Short radius keratoplasty scissors (because of the sharp curvature of the small graft) are used to excise the button. Care must be taken not to snag the

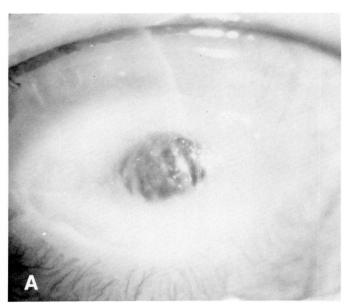

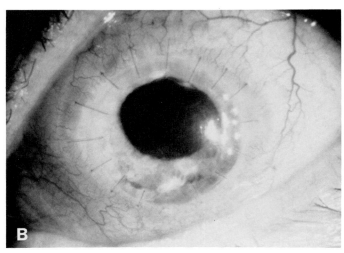

**Fig. 7-12.** (A) Central corneal perforation within a zone of corneal stromal opacification and thinning in the aphakic left eye of an 81-year-old female with a history of prior ophthalmic herpes zoster and recent topical steroid use. Vitreous is present at the perforation site. The fellow eye was blind. (B) Same eye 3 weeks after slightly eccentric penetrating keratoplasty (8.5 mm donor, 8.0 mm host bed) and anterior vitrectomy. There was no growth from cultures of the excised cornea.

iris when the scissors are introduced and manipulated. Six to 12 interrupted 10/0 nylon sutures are used to secure the donor button in position.

### Central

A central therapeutic keratoplasty is indicated in large central or paracentral perforations, or in cases of diffuse stromal melting where enough relatively normal peripheral corneal tissue remains to which the graft can be anchored (Fig. 7-12). If a paracentral or central perforation has been glued for several months and no healing has occurred, keratoplasty would be the reasonable next step. It is also worth considering in central perforations where the chamber has not reformed despite proper application of adhesive, as the only hope for reforming the chamber angle.

We utilize general anesthesia when performing therapeutic penetrating grafts. The orbital vascular dilatation usually present in these cases makes it difficult to achieve good anesthesia using a retrobulbar block because of rapid diffusion of anesthetic from the area. It also increases the risk of hemorrhage if a retrobulbar injection is attempted. Since a perforated eye would likely be substantially damaged should a retrobulbar hemorrhage occur, we believe general anesthesia is safer. If the patient's cardiac status will permit, we intravenously infuse 1–2 Gm/kg of a 20 percent mannitol solution over 30 minutes just before surgery in order to dehydrate the vitreous and minimize bulging of the intraocular contents that so frequently occurs in these eyes.

*Techniques of trephination.* Even though tissue glue may not be a viable alternative for the long-term management of the perforation, it can sometimes be helpful in temporarily closing the perforation in the operating room. This may allow sufficient formation of the anterior chamber to make trephination of the globe easier. Again, the minimum

amount of glue should be used, keeping it localized to the perforation site so that it will not interfere with the trephine blade. The same cautions regarding intraocular structures and vitreous as previously noted apply. We generally do not use a Flieringa ring in these cases because of the difficulty in suturing a ring to a soft eye and the conjunctival and episcleral bleeding which occurs. If the perforation has been intraoperatively closed with adhesive and intraocular pressure has increased to a normal range, a Flieringa ring can be used if the surgeon prefers.

In our hands, the optimum trephine for central therapeutic keratoplasty is the Hessburg-Barron vacuum trephine (Jedmed, St. Louis, MO. Fig. 7-13). This disposable trephine has a peripheral suction ring connected to a syringe by plastic tubing. An inner circular blade, which is turned by the finger wheel, cuts the cornea. Initially, the cutting blade is aligned so that it is even with the inner portion of the suction ring, using the operating microscope for visualization. The cutting blade must then be backed up 3–5 quarter turns of the finger wheel so the blade does not contact the corneal surface while the trephine is being applied. For the trephine to adhere well, loose epithelium must be removed from the cornea in the area where the suction ring attaches; wetting the peripheral cornea also facilitates adherence. Since the suction ring of the trephine limits visualization peripherally, the trephine must be carefully centered by sighting through its central opening. The assistant fully depresses the plunger of the syringe. The surgeon places the trephine on the cornea, evenly pressing it in position sufficiently to slightly indent the anterior cornea. The assistant then releases the syringe plunger—the spring action of the plunger generates suction that secures the trephine to the cornea. The surgeon should verify that the trephine is attached to the cornea by gently wiggling it.

The trephine can then be used to slightly elevate the

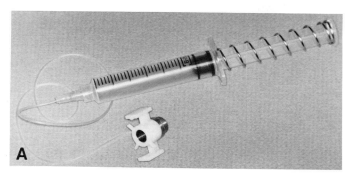
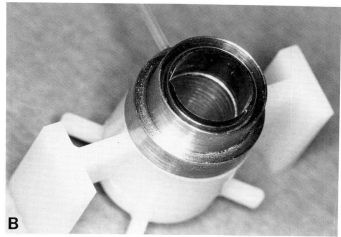

**Fig. 7-13.** Hessburg-Barron vacuum trephine. (A) Syringe with spring-loaded plunger (used to generate suction) is connected to outer ring of the trephine via plastic tubing. The two plastic posts are used to hold the trephine. The four spoke finger wheel turns the inner cutting blade. (B) Higher magnification view of underside of the trephine. The trephine attaches to the cornea by suction delivered between the outer and middle metal rings. The inner circular cutting blade has been extended beyond the suction rings.

cornea, separating it from critical intraocular structures. Trephination is performed by rotating the plastic finger wheel, which advances the trephine blade approximately 0.06–0.07 mm for each quarter turn. The blade is of band steel formed into a circle, which can be machined much thinner and therefore sharper than the circular blades of standard disposable trephines. Entering the anterior chamber (AC) with the Hessburg trephine is not safe or necessary because the chamber is usually flat and one cannot rely on the usual gush of aqueous to signal AC penetration. The blade is so sharp that it can be inadvertently advanced through the iris and the anterior lens capsule. For this reason, we recommend deep, but not full thickness trephination. Initially the blade is advanced the same number of quarter turns it was previously retracted, thus bringing it flush with the corneal surface. Continuing to rotate the finger wheel in a clockwise direction past this point advances the cutting blade into the cornea. If the trephination is being performed in a zone of normal corneal thickness, 6 or 7 quarter turns beyond the zero point will provide a sufficiently deep cut. If the midperipheral cornea is thinner than normal, the blade should not be advanced as much. Prior to removing the trephine from the cornea, suction should be released by completely depressing the plunger of the syringe.

If the trephine is attached close to the limbus, a portion of the suction ring may be occluded by conjunctiva. This keeps the trephine from being flush with the corneal surface in this region, resulting in a locally shallower cut. It may also result in loss of suction while trephination is being performed. To avoid these difficulties, a localized conjunctival peritomy may be necessary if the trephine must be placed eccentrically and near the limbus.

Suction trephines are currently available in 6.5–9.0 mm diameters in 0.5 mm diameter increments. If a larger keratoplasty is required to encompass the corneal pathology, or if a suction trephine is not available, a standard circular trephine is used. Disposable circular trephine blades are available

from several manufacturers in 0.25 mm size increments up to 9.5 mm diameter; 10.0 and 11.0 mm diameter disposable blades are also available from Edward Weck & Co. (Research Triangle Park, NC). For larger grafts, nondisposable trephines must be used. On an open eye, a standard trephine blade is useful primarily for marking the epithelium. Unless the perforation can be closed intraoperatively with tissue adhesive, the pressure required to actually cut the stroma with the trephine is more than is safe to exert on an open eye. After the ocular surface is marked with the trephine, a diamond blade or the sharpest available razor blade is used to slowly cut through the cornea in a location where the iris can be well visualized. When the anterior chamber is entered, we inject sodium hyaluronate into the anterior chamber directing it under the cornea marked with the trephine. This separates the iris from the cornea to allow safer insertion of the corneal scissors. Additional hyaluronate is injected as the cutting proceeds to new areas, progressively separating iris from cornea. Care must be taken to make certain the anterior chamber is actually entered each time, so that injection of the hyaluronate or insertion of the scissors does not detach Descemet's membrane.

*Operative technique—additional considerations.* Once the cornea to be excised has been entirely circumscribed with a scissor cut, it should be gently and slowly elevated. There are frequently adhesions between the cornea and iris, especially adjacent to the perforation site. These should be gently teased apart with a cyclodialysis spatula, or carefully cut. Any adherent vitreous should be cut with scissors as the cornea is removed. We routinely bisect the excised cornea, sending one half for pathologic examination and placing the other half directly on an agar plate for culture. There is frequently a dense fibrin membrane on the surface of the iris and lens. Once an edge is located, this membrane can usually be peeled off the surface of the iris. Even if such a membrane is not present, the iris surface should be carefully inspected because Descemet's membrane may iatrogenically detach when the corneal button is removed. Posterior synechiae are broken with the cyclodialysis spatula. Several radial sphincterotomies may be required if the pupil is very small. These sphincterotomies should not be made too large since the tension of a central iris ring may help in keeping the peripheral iris from adhering to the peripheral cornea, thus limiting development of peripheral anterior synechiae (PAS). In an inflamed eye, the tendency to synechiae formation is such that it is wise to fashion several iridectomies or iridotomies if the patient is phakic. If the bleeding from the iris that results from these maneuvers does not spontaneously stop, bleeding sites can be lightly coagulated with a wet-field cautery.

If the patient is phakic and the lens is not densely cataractous, we prefer not to remove it even though this may make the anterior chamber slightly more difficult to form. We do not recommend lens removal solely to control a bulging lens–iris diaphragm in this clinical setting. Usually, a bulging posterior capsule (which is prone to rupture) results. The protruding lens–iris complex will tend to return to its normal position once the donor cornea is secured. If the cataract is dense or mature, then it is reasonable to remove it at the time of the keratoplasty, preferably extracapsularly.

If the patient is already aphakic and the vitreous face is broken, an open-sky vitrectomy with an automated cutter is indicated. Extreme care is necessary in performing the vitrectomy because the choroidal effusions frequently present in a soft eye with a corneal perforation bring the peripheral retina towards the center of the virtreous cavity (Fig. 7-14). If the excised corneal button is eccentric, the vitreous cutter should be inserted towards the center of the globe rather than the center of the corneal opening to keep the cutter as far from the vitreous base as possible. Vitreous must also be meticulously removed from the surface of the iris to prevent subsequent formation of peripheral anterior synechiae.

We oversize the donor buttons for large therapeutic grafts by at least 0.5 mm. For grafts 10.0 mm or larger, it is necessary to oversize by a full millimeter since trephines in 0.5 mm increments are not available. A larger graft allows for better formation of the anterior chamber angle. Since the host button is often excised following only a mark on the corneal surface, the cut may be irregular; the additional tissue of a larger donor facilitates donor-host apposition. The full-thickness donor button is punched from the endothelial side using a circular disposable or nondisposable trephine, depending on the size required.

Prior to suturing the donor button in place, we have found it worthwhile to carefully separate the peripheral iris from the peripheral cornea for 360° using either dry surgical spears or a cyclodialysis spatula. There is sometimes an inflammatory membrane joining the peripheral iris and cornea that can be transected or removed with the spatula. A small amount of sodium hyaluronate can then be injected into the angle recess; this will keep the iris and cornea apart at least initially. These maneuvers are probably helpful in limiting synechiae formation. Care must be used in separating the peripheral iris from the cornea because if bleeding is

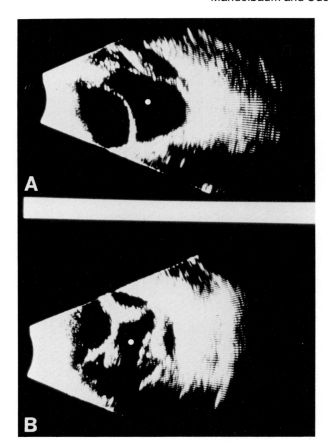

**Fig. 7-14.** Two B scan ultrasounds of the eye shown in Figure 7-12. Large choroidal effusions are present. The vitreous cavity is identified by a white dot. Lower photograph represents an ultrasonic frontal section through the globe near the ora serrata. This view shows the large choroidal effusions about as they would appear when looking into the eye at surgery. Ultrasonography on an open eye should be performed only by an ophthalmologist or experienced ultrasonographer through closed lids to avoid placing any pressure on the globe.

induced, it will increase the likelihood of PAS formation. A small amount of hyaluronate should also be placed on the anterior surface of the lens or implant if one is present, to protect the central donor corneal endothelium when the button is placed in position.

We prefer the use of interrupted nylon sutures to secure the donor button. Multiple interrupted sutures provide better apposition in areas where the donor and host opening are not perfectly matched. There are usually differential rates of healing and vascularization; interrupted sutures allow individual removal of those sutures that vascularize or loosen early. If the donor tissue is being secured into cornea, 10/0 nylon sutures are best. When the opening is so large or eccentric that the button is being secured directly to sclera, we have found 9/0 sutures preferable, although the needle is not as sharp as that on the 10/0 suture. If the location of the perforation is such that the sutures securing the donor graft will need to be placed into sclera, a conjunctival peritomy should be fashioned prior to removing the host cornea. Approximating the donor and host tissues often requires that the initial four sutures be pulled very tightly; this is particularly true if there is considerable bulging of the iris and lens through the host opening. As the graft is secured in place, the lens-iris diaphragm is forced posteriorly. At least 16 interrupted sutures are required. For grafts larger than about 8.5 mm, we generally use 24 rather than 16 sutures, because of the greater circumference of the button.

In cases where a graft is performed for a perforation, it is helpful to place a paracentesis tract in clear paralimbal cornea. The tract allows access to the anterior chamber without manipulating the graft-host junction. It is a particularly useful site through which to form the anterior chamber, to lyse synechiae, and to manipulate the peripheral iris once the donor button has been secured in position. If there is a localized area where the peripheral iris and cornea are not in contact, the tract may be placed there. If the eye is very soft and the anterior chamber is flat, particularly in a phakic patient, it is safer not to create a peripheral tract unless one is required for a specific purpose. If it does become necessary, the peripheral keratotomy is best performed after the graft has been partially secured and the chamber partially formed.

### Choroidal Effusions

Choroidal effusions are frequently present in eyes which have been hypotonous as a result of a corneal perforation. Usually, these effusions are serous and will resolve rapidly once the perforation is sealed and normal intraocular fluid dynamics are restored. It is not necessary to drain small serous choroidal effusions. Performing a sclerotomy and attempting to drain a soft and inflamed eye may result in conversion of a serous effusion to a more dangerous hemorrhagic effusion. Rarely, the effusions are so large as to be "kissing" (Fig. 7-15). In such cases, drainage of the choroidal effusions is necessary to separate the retina and avoid development of interretinal adhesions. If choroidal effusions

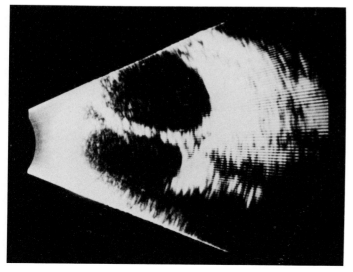

**Fig. 7-15.** B scan ultrasound showing "kissing" choroidals in an eye with a corneal perforation. The vitreous cavity is essentially obliterated by the huge choroidal effusions.

of the size seen in Figure 7-15 are not drained intraoperatively, it will be extremely difficult if not impossible to adequately reform the anterior chamber once the graft is sewn in position. In the rare cases where drainage of choroidals is necessary, we fashion a circumferential sclerotomy approximately 4 mm posterior to the limbus, scratching carefully through the sclera with a 64 Beaver blade or equivalent until the choroid is reached. The edges of the sclera are manually separated to obtain good drainage from the choroid. Sclerotomies may be required in several locations to obtain adequate drainage. When planning the surgical approach, it is helpful to be aware of the extent and location of choroidal effusions to determine whether and where a sclerotomy should be performed. Preoperative ultrasound examination gently performed through closed lids can provide this information.

### Postoperative Care

Careful attention must be paid to intraocular pressure in the immediate postoperative period. The pressure may be very low due to large choroidal effusions and aqueous hyposecretion. On the other hand, closure of the leak sometimes results in marked elevation of pressure. In some eyes it seems as if the lack of aqueous flow through the trabecular meshwork during the time the perforation site is open results in decreased function of the meshwork for several days after the perforation is closed. We have seen pressures as high as 70 mm in the early postoperative period with angles that are gonioscopically open. If the pressure can be controlled for several days, the situation will often equilibrate, presumably due to a return of normal meshwork function or normal levels of aqueous secretion. We generally monitor intraocular pressure in these eyes at least twice daily for several days after closure of the perforation. Tactile tensions may be inaccurate, and useful mires often cannot be obtained with the Goldmann applanator; optimally, a pneumatonometer or similar device should be available for measuring intraocular pressure.

In addition to careful monitoring and maintenance of intraocular pressure within a normal range, the substantial intraocular inflammation usually present postoperatively must be controlled. A major risk of this inflammatory response is the development of extensive PAS. Often the anterior chamber is virtually filled with fibrin after a therapeutic graft. Frequent topical corticosteroids are usually administered, as often as hourly depending on the extent of inflammation and the clinical setting. Occasionally, the inflammatory response is so exuberant that a short course of systemic steroids may be warranted.

A critical aspect of postoperative care is maintenance of an intact epithelial surface to avoid repeat ulceration. Optimum lid position is crucial to maintaining the ocular surface. Ectropion, entropion, and lagophthalmos should be corrected at the time of the keratoplasty. Punctal occlusion, lateral tarsorrhaphy, or a partial conjunctival flap may be necessary in cases where the eye is too dry to be lubricated by drops and ointments alone. A therapeutic contact lens may be considered as a short term approach to aid in resurfacing

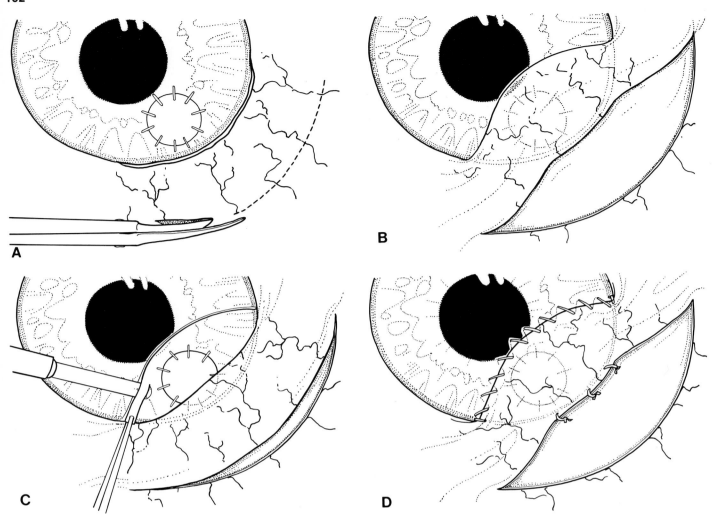

**Fig. 7-16.**   Technique for fashioning a peripheral conjunctival flap. (A) A limbal peritomy is performed in the appropriate quadrant. An arcuate relaxing incision is made parallel to the limbus. (B) The bridge of conjunctiva is dissected from Tenon's and moved into the desired position to verify that there is no tension on it. (C) A shallow ledge of cornea is removed at the central-most extent of the intended position of the flap. (D) After all corneal epithelium has been removed in this quadrant, the central edge of the conjunctival flap is joined to the shelf of cornea with a running monofilament suture. The other side of the flap is secured just beyond the limbus with several absorbable sutures.

the cornea, but should not be relied upon as a permanent solution. Depending on the configuration of the cornea postoperatively, a contact lens may be difficult to fit.

## Conjunctival Flap

A conjunctival flap by itself is no longer considered satisfactory treatment for a corneal perforation. The flap may not reform the anterior chamber; persistence of a flat chamber will result in permanent PAS and intractable glaucoma. A large conjunctival bleb may develop if the flap does not adhere to the edges of the perforation site. If the ulceration is caused by bacteria or fungi, the microbial agent may not be eliminated by the flap, and appropriate antibiotic therapy is hampered by its presence. A conjunctival flap will ultimately thin, but initially it precludes examination of anterior segment structures.

Although we are opposed to use of a conjunctival flap for primary treatment of a corneal perforation, it may be extremely helpful when used in combination with other modalities. We frequently place partial conjunctival flaps over peripheral lamellar or full thickness grafts to prevent re-ulceration, especially in patients with severe dry eyes or exposure. Occasionally, despite all attempts at maintaining the epithelial surface, a therapeutic graft itself is subject to progressive melting. In these cases, a total conjunctival flap may stabilize the situation.

To fashion a peripheral conjunctival flap, the conjunctiva in the quadrant where the flap is to be placed is dissected from Tenon's extending from the limbus peripherally. Once sufficient conjunctiva has been mobilized, an arcuate relaxing incision parallel to the limbus is made (Fig. 7-16A), which allows a bridge of conjunctiva to be pulled onto the cornea without tension (Fig. 7-16B). A shallow ledge of 5–10 percent corneal thickness is dissected in the cornea central to where the corneal patch graft has previously been secured (Fig. 7-16C). All residual corneal epithelium is removed from the donor and host cornea in this quadrant either mechanically or by using a surgical spear moistened with cocaine or absolute alcohol. The central edge of the flap is joined to the shelf created in the cornea with a running monofilament suture, and the peripheral edge is tacked to the episclera just beyond the limbus with several absorbable sutures (Fig. 7-16D). Joining the edge of conjunctiva to a corneal shelf maintains the conjunctiva flush with the adjacent cornea, minimizing disruption of the tear flow and trauma to the edge of the flap by the lids. The running suture can be removed in 7–14 days. Should a total flap be required, it may be fashioned as described initially by Gundersen (see Chapter 6).[36,60]

## PREVENTION OF CORNEAL PERFORATION

While we have directed our attention in this chapter to the treatment of an existing corneal perforation, it is obviously preferable to stop corneal ulceration before a perforation develops. When faced with a melting cornea, all efforts should be aimed at halting progression of the process and preventing development of a perforation.

### Pathogenesis and General Therapy

The following factors have been implicated in the pathogenesis of corneal ulceration:

1. Persistent epithelial defect[70]
2. Products of bacterial and fungal organisms[42]
3. Collagenase[5]
4. Plasminogen activator-plasmin system[6]
5. Polymorphonuclear leukocyte-derived lytic enzymes[16,68]
6. Scorbutic anterior segment of alkali burned eyes[62]
7. Neurotrophic corneas lack of "trophic" substances[28,52]
8. Immune mechanisms[12,57]
9. Ischemia[2]

Regardless of the specific cause, common to all ulceration is a persistent epithelial defect.[70] It is unclear why only some eyes with longstanding epithelial defects develop progressive stromal loss.

The pathophysiology of corneal melting is incompletely understood. Berman's studies suggest a complex interaction between cellular and humoral factors.[6] Tissue collagenase, which cleaves stromal collagen fibrils, is thought to be derived from damaged epithelium, stromal fibroblasts, and stromal keratocytes (latent collagenase).[5] Brown has demonstrated that the conjunctiva adjacent to Mooren's ulcer also exhibits collagenolytic activity.[8] The injured cornea releases plasminogen activator, which may promote chemotaxis of polymorphonuclear leukocytes.[6] In turn, the polyps may release the many lytic enzymes (including collagenase, elas-

Table 7-3
General Measures for Treating Noninfectious Corneal Ulceration*

Promote Epithelialization
    Lubrication (drops, ointments)
    Punctal occlusion (temporary, permanent)
    Correct abnormal lid position, trichiasis
    Decrease exposure (patching, tarsorrhaphy)
    Therapeutic soft contact lens
    Topical retinoic acid
    Fibronectin
    Conjunctival transplantation
    Keratoepithelioplasty
Prevent Progressive Stromal Ulceration
    Oral tetracycline
    Acetylcysteine
    Medroxyprogesterone
    Topical and systemic steroids
    Ascorbate, citrate
    Tissue adhesive
    Conjunctival resection
    Lamellar patch graft
    Conjunctival flap (partial or total)
    Systemic immunosuppressive agents

*See text for comments, references.

tase, and cathepsin) contained in their lysosomes, further aggravating stromal destruction.[44] Kenyon and coworkers have emphasized the significant role of these host-derived acute inflammatory cells in actively melting corneas.[16,45,46]

Therapy of corneal ulceration should be directed towards the maintenance or restoration of the epithelial surface and limitation of stromal ulceration. To effectively accomplish this, it is vital to determine the cause of corneal ulceration so that specific therapy can be directed towards reversing the primary disease process. The multiple precipitating causes of stromal ulceration are listed in Table 7-1. In addition to therapy specifically directed to the underlying disease, however, general measures to promote epithelialization and prevent stromal ulceration are appropriate. These are listed in Table 7-3 and briefly discussed below.

The condition of the lids, conjunctiva, and preocular tear film is often overlooked. Subtle lagophthalmos, intermittent entropion, and misdirected lashes are frequent causes of epithelial defects. The benefits of topically applied lubricants and punctal occlusion should not be underestimated in patients with keratoconjunctivitis sicca. Palpebral conjunctival damage and keratinization, which may occur as a result of ocular pemphigoid or drug toxicity, may cause a chronic epithelial defect. Lubricant ointments or application of a therapeutic contact lens may allow healing of the corneal epithelium in this situation by keeping the offending conjunctiva away from the cornea. Topical retinoic acid shows promise both for healing chronic corneal epithelial defects and reversing squamous metaplastic changes of the conjunctiva, which may have contributed to their development.[75] Autologous fibronectin has been reported to be a useful adjunct in the therapy of trophic corneal ulcers.[59] A multicenter collaborative trial has been organized to study its role in refractory corneal epithelial defects. If an epithelial defect does not heal with medical therapy, Thoft has described two surgical procedures that may be useful: conjunctival transplantation[69,71] and keratoepithelioplasty.[72]

A variety of pharmacologic agents have been suggested for stopping progressive stromal ulceration; unfortunately, few have actually been shown to be effective. Although topical corticosteroids are helpful in suppressing the acute inflammatory response, their continued use may potentiate ulceration by impeding normal corneal repair.[44] Whether they also enhance the effect of collagenase has been debated.[14,44] Medroxyprogesterone has been suggested to reduce inflammation without suppressing wound repair;[58] this hypothesis has yet to be proven in human studies. Acetylcysteine (Mucomyst) has been recommended for topical use on the theory that it would inhibit proteolytic enzymes[4]; unfortunately, most who have used this agent do not feel that it is effective in this setting.[21,63] Oral tetracycline has been clinically effective in inhibiting corneal melting associated with rosacea keratitis. Recently, its use has been advocated in other causes of corneal melting on the theory that it inhibits collagenase activity;[61] again this has not been proven. Subconjunctivally administered heparin has been suggested as a means of limiting stromal ulceration, but its use has generally been abandoned. Ascorbate and citrate have decreased stromal ulceration in the chemically injured animal cornea but have not yet been proven effective in man.[62]

The application of tissue adhesive to an ulcerating but nonperforated cornea does, in many cases, appear effective in stabilizing the melt before a frank perforation develops.[27] When used in this fashion, the adhesive appears to promote corneal healing, presumably by the same mechanisms as when applied to a perforation. Care must be used if the adhesive is applied to a large descemetocele—an irregular protrusion of glue may act as a lever, tearing Descemet's membrane and resulting in a leak. Finally, certain surgical procedures described above (such as a localized conjunctival flap[60] or a lamellar patch graft) may be considered if glue has not been effective for a progressively ulcerating but not yet perforated cornea. Conjunctival resection is another surgical approach that is applicable in specific corneal melts as described below.

## Conjunctival Resection

Resection of paralimbal conjunctiva adjacent to a region of peripheral corneal melting may reverse the process in certain marginal melting syndromes. This approach has been advocated principally for Mooren's ulcer[3,9,11,47] and for rheumatoid arthritis.[22,26] It appears to be more effective for the less aggressive variety of Mooren's ulcer where only one eye at a time is involved, as opposed to the usually more aggressive bilateral simultaneous form of the condition.[11] It is postulated that removal of adjacent conjunctiva eliminates the humoral, enzymatic, and cellular factors that mediate the corneal melting.[8,9] Under local anesthesia, a strip of conjunctiva 3–4 mm wide beginning at the limbus adjacent to the

melt is resected. Our experience with this technique has confirmed its beneficial effect in these milder cases of Mooren's ulceration. Prior to proceeding with conjunctival resection, topical corticosteroids should be tried, as they may occasionally control the corneal melting of Mooren's ulcer.

The improvement resulting from conjunctival resection may be temporary, with recurrence of the melting in the same or a different location weeks to months later. Conjunctival resection can be repeated, again usually with a beneficial effect. Some authors have advocated combining cryotherapy to the ulcerating cornea with conjunctival resection[3]; it is uncertain whether the results of this combined approach are any better than conjunctival resection alone. If neither topical steroids, conjunctival resection, nor a combination of the two resolves the melting in a severe progressive bilateral Mooren's ulceration, we would recommend systemic immunosuppressive therapy as advocated by Foster.[29]

Conjunctival resection has also been found effective by several authors in cases of peripheral corneal melts associated with rheumatoid arthritis.[22,26,79] We feel that conjunctival resection is a logical approach for peripheral corneal melting when the adjacent conjunctiva is inflamed. Rheumatoid corneal melts may, however, occur in white, relatively quiet eyes in a paracentral location. Although our experience with conjunctival resection in rheumatoid arthritis is limited, we suspect that it is less likely to be effective in this group of patients than in eyes where the conjunctiva is clinically inflamed. In the clinical setting of a quiet eye with rheumatoid ulceration, we recommend increased lubrication, a trial of a therapeutic soft lens, and application of tissue adhesive if the melting is progressive and threatening perforation. Topical steroids may potentiate corneal melting in this particular situation[48] and should thus generally be avoided. A trial of systemic corticosteroids or an increase in dosage if the patient is already maintained on systemic steroids may be beneficial. Progressive peripheral noninfectious corneal melting associated with collagen vascular disorders that is not responding to these measures should be considered for systemic immunosuppressive therapy.[29,30] We have seen remarkable arresting of the melting process when these agents have been employed. Foster has stressed the association between peripheral ulcerative keratitis and systemic vasculitis (which may be unrecognized); in this clinical setting immunosuppressive therapy appears to have beneficial systemic as well as ocular effects.[30] Immunosuppressive agents are potentially lethal, and should thus be administered only by physicians familiar with their use and side effects. Local measures (e.g. soft contact lens, tissue adhesive, conjunctival resection) may still be required to limit progressive stromal ulceration during the lag period between initiation of systemic immunosuppressives and clinical evidence of a positive response to their administration.

## REFERENCES

1. Arentsen JJ, Christiansen JM, Maumenee AE: Marginal ulceration after intracapsular cataract extraction. Am J Ophthalmol 81:194–197, 1976

2. Aronson SB, Elliot JH, Moore TE Jr, et al: Pathogenetic approach to therapy of peripheral corneal inflammatory disease. Am J Ophthalmol 70:65–90, 1970

3. Aviel E: Combined cryoapplications and peritomy in Mooren's ulcer. Br J Ophthalmol 56:48–51, 1972

4. Berman MB: Collagenase inhibitors: rationale for their use in treating corneal ulceration. Int Ophthalmol Clin 15(4):49–66, 1975

5. Berman M: Regulation of collagenase; therapeutic considerations. Trans Ophthalmol Soc UK 98:397–405, 1978

6. Berman M, Leary R, Gage J: Evidence for a role of the plasminogen activator-plasmin system in corneal ulceration. Invest Ophthalmol Vis Sci 19:1204–1221, 1980

7. Boruchoff SA, Refojo MF, Slansky H, et al: Clinical applications of adhesives in corneal surgery. Ophthalmology 73:499–504, 1969

8. Brown SI: Mooren's ulcer; histopathology and proteolytic enzymes of adjacent cornea. Brit J Ophthalmol 59:670–674, 1975

9. Brown SI: Mooren's ulcer; treatment by conjunctival excision. Br J Ophthalmol 59:675–682, 1975

10. Brown SI, Bloomfield S, Pearce DB, et al: Infections with the therapeutic soft lens. Arch Ophthalmol 91:275–277, 1974

11. Brown SI, Mondino BJ: Therapy of Mooren's ulcer. Am J Ophthalmol 98:1–6, 1984

12. Brown SI, Mondino BJ, Rabin BS: Autoimmune phenomenon in Mooren's ulcer. Am J Ophthalmol 82:835–840, 1976

13. Brown SI, Shahinian L Jr: Diagnosis and treatment of ocular rosacea. Ophthalmology 85:779–786, 1978

14. Brown SI, Weller CA: The pathogenesis and treatment of collagenase-induced diseases of the cornea. Ophthalmology 74:375–382, 1970

15. Bullen CL, Liesgang TJ, McDonald TJ, et al: Ocular complications of Wegener's granulomatosis. Ophthalmology 90:279–290, 1983

16. Burnett JM, Smith LE, Prause JU, et al: Acute inflammatory cells and collagenase in tears of human melting corneas. Invest Ophthalmol Vis Sci 20 (Suppl):173, 1981

17. Cogan DG: Corneoscleral lesions in periarteritis nodosa and Wegener's granulomatosis. Trans Am Ophthalmol Soc 53:321–342, 1955

18. Cohen KL: Sterile corneal perforation after cataract surgery in Sjogren's syndrome. Br J Ophthalmol 66:179–182, 1982

19. Coster DJ: Herpetic keratitis and corneal destruction. Trans Ophthal Soc UK 98:372–376, 1978

20. Dohlman CH, Doughman DJ: The Stevens-Johnson syndrome, in Symposium on the Cornea; Transactions of the New Orleans Academy of Ophthalmology. St. Louis, CV Mosby, 1972, pp 236–252

21. Easty DL, Madden P, Jayson MIV, et al: Systemic immunosuppression in marginal keratolysis. Trans Ophthal Soc UK 98:410–417, 1978

22. Eiferman RA, Carothers DJ, Yankeelov JA: Peripheral rheumatoid ulceration and evidence for conjunctival collagenase production. Am J Ophthalmol 87:703–709, 1979

23. Eiferman RA, Snyder JW: Antibacterial effect of cyanoacrylate glue. Arch Ophthalmol 101:958–960, 1983

24. Epstein DL, Paton D: Keratitis from misuse of corneal anesthetics. N Engl J Med 279:396–399, 1968

25. Fauci AS, Wolff SM: Wegener's granulomatosis; studies in 18 patients and a review of the literature. Medicine 52:535–561, 1973

26. Feder RS, Krachmer JH: Conjunctival resection for the treatment of the rheumatoid corneal ulceration. Ophthalmology 91:111–115, 1984

27. Fogle JA, Kenyon KR, Foster CS: Tissue adhesive arrests stromal melting in the human cornea. Am J Ophthalmol 89:795–802, 1980

28. Foster CS: Ocular surface manifestations of neurological and systemic disease. Int Ophthalmol Clin 19(2):207–242, 1974

29. Foster CS: Immunosuppressive therapy for external ocular inflammatory disease. Ophthalmology 87:140–150, 1980

30. Foster CS, Forstot SL, Wilson LA: Mortality rate in rheumatoid arthritis patients developing necrotizing scleritis or peripheral ulcerative keratitis. Ophthalmology 91:1253–1263, 1984

31. Foster CS, Yee M: Corneoscleral manifestations of Graves' disease, the acquired connective tissue disorders, and systemic vasculitis. Int Opthalmol Clin 23(1):131–157, 1983

32. Franklin RM, Kenyon KR, Tutschuka PJ, et al: Ocular manifestations of graft-versus-host disease. Ophthalmology 90:4–13, 1983

33. Gelender H: Descemetocele after intraocular lens implantation. Arch Ophthalmol 100:72–76, 1982

34. Grayson M: Diseases of the Cornea (ed 2). St. Louis, CV Mosby, 1983, p 530

35. Gudas PP Jr, Altman B, Nicholson DH, et al: Corneal perforations in Sjogren's syndrome. Arch Ophthalmol 90:470–472, 1973

36. Gundersen T: Conjunctival flaps in the treatment of corneal disease with reference to a new technique of application. Arch Ophthalmol 60:880–888, 1958

37. Hirst LW, DeJuan E Jr: Sodium hyaluronate and tissue adhesive in treating corneal perforations. Ophthalmology 89:1250–1253, 1982

38. Hirst LW, Smiddy WE, Stark WJ: Corneal perforations; changing methods of treatment, 1960–1980. Ophthalmology 89:630–635, 1982

39. Hirst LW, Stark WJ, Jensen AD: Tissue adhesives: new perspectives in corneal perforation. Ophthalmic Surg 10:58–64, 1979

40. Hyndiuk RA, Hull DS, Kinyoun JL: Free tissue patch and cyanoacrylate in corneal perforations. Ophthalmic Surg 5:50–55, 1974

41. Jones BR: Vernal keratitis. Trans Opthal Soc UK 81:215–228, 1961

42. Jones DB: Pathogenesis of bacterial and fungal keratitis. Trans Ophthal Soc UK 98:367–371, 1978

43. Katz J, Kaufman HE: Corneal exposure during sleep (nocturnal lagophthalmos). Arch Ophthalmol 95:449–453, 1977

44. Kenyon KR: Decision-making in the therapy of external eye disease; noninfected corneal ulcers. Ophthalmology 89:44–51, 1982

45. Kenyon KR, Berman MB, Hanninen L: Tissue adhesive prevents ulceration and inhibits inflammation in the thermal-burned rabbit cornea. Invest Ophthalmol Vis Sci 18 (Suppl):196, 1979

46. Kenyon KR, Berman M, Rose J, et al: Prevention of stromal ulceration in the alkali burned rabbit cornea by glued-on contact lens. Evidence for the role of polymorphonuclear leukocytes in collagen degradation. Invest Ophthalmol Vis Sci 18:570–587, 1979

47. Kogbe OI, Abiose A: Mooren's ulcer: treatment by limbal conjunctivectomy. J Ocul Ther Surg 4:74–79, 1985

48. Krachmer JH, Laibson PR: Corneal thinning and perforation in Sjogren's syndrome. Am J Ophthalmol 78:917–920, 1974

49. Leibowitz HM: Hydrophilic contact lenses in corneal disease IV. Penetrating corneal wounds. Arch Ophthalmol 88:602–606, 1972

50. Leibowitz HM, Rosenthal P: Hydrophilic contact lenses in corneal disease I. Superficial, sterile, indolent ulcers. Arch Ophthalmol 85:163–166, 1971

51. Leibman SD: Riley-Day syndrome. Arch Ophthalmol 58:188–192, 1957

52. Mackie IA: Role of corneal nerves in destructive disease of the cornea. Trans Ophthal Soc UK 98:343–347, 1978

53. Maguen E, Nesburn A, Macy JI: Combined use of sodium hyaluronate and tissue adhesive in penetrating keratoplasty of corneal perforation. Ophthalmic Surg 15:55–57, 1984

54. McFaul PA, Bedford MA: Ocular complications after therapeutic irradiation. Br J Ophthalmol 54:237–247, 1970

55. Mondino BJ, Brown SI: Ocular cicatricial pemphigoid. Ophthalmology 88:95–100, 1981

56. Mondino BJ, Brown SI, Mondzelewski JP: Peripheral corneal ulcers with herpes zoster ophthalmicus. Am J Ophthalmol 86:611–614, 1978

57. Mondino BJ, Brown SI, Rabin BS: Autoimmune phenomenon of the external eye. Ophthalmology 85:801–817, 1978

58. Newsome DA, Gross J: Prevention by medroxyprogesterone of perforation in the alkali-burned rabbit cornea: inhibition of collagenolytic activity. Invest Ophthalmol Vis Sci 16:21–31, 1977

59. Nishida T, Ohashi Y, Awata T, et al: Fibronectin; a new therapy for corneal trophic ulcer. Arch Ophthalmol 101:1046–1048, 1983

60. Paton D, Milauskis AT: Indications, surgical technique, and results of thin conjunctival flaps on the cornea. Int Ophthalmol Clin 10:329–345, 1970

61. Perry HD, Kenyon KR, Lamberts DW, et al: Systemic tetracycline in the treatment of persistent epithelial defects. Ophthalmology 92 (Suppl):77, 1985

62. Pfister RR: Chemical corneal burns. Int Ophthalmol Clin 24(2):157–?, 1984

63. Pfister RR, Murphy GE: Corneal ulceration and perforation associated with Sjogren's syndrome. Arch Ophthalmol 98:89–94, 1980

64. Pirie A: Effect of vitamin A deficiency on the cornea. Trans Ophthal Soc UK 98:357–360, 1978

65. Refojo MF, Dohlman CH, Ahmad B, et al: Evaluation of adhesives for corneal surgery. Arch Ophthalmol 80:645–656, 1968

66. Refojo MF, Dohlman CH, Koliopoulos J: Adhesives in ophthalmology: a review. Surv Ophthalmol 15:217–236, 1971

67. Rich LF, Hamifin JM: Ocular complications of atopic dermatitis and other eczemas. Int Ophthalmol Clin 25(1):61–76, 1985

68. Snip RC, Kenyon KR: Acute inflammatory cells in melting human corneas. Invest Ophthalmol Vis Sci 17(Suppl):252, 1978

69. Thoft RA: Conjunctival transplantation. Arch Ophthalmol 95:1425–1427, 1977

70. Thoft RA: Role of the ocular surface in destructive corneal disease. Trans Ophthal Soc UK 98:339–342, 1978

71. Thoft RA: Indications for conjunctival transplantation. Ophthalmology 89:335–339, 1982

72. Thoft RA: Keratoepithelioplasty. Am J Ophthalmol 97:1–6, 1984

73. Thoft RA, Dohlman CH: Chemical and thermal burns of the eye, in Freeman HM (ed): Ocular Trauma. New York, Appleton-Century-Crofts, 1979, pp 125–131

74. Thygeson P: Marginal corneal infiltrates and ulcers. Ophthalmology 51:198–207, 1947

75. Tseng SCG, Maumenee AE, Stark WJ, et al: Topical retinoid treatment for various dry-eye disorders. Ophthalmology 92:717–727, 1985

76. Webster RG Jr: Surgical adhesives in the treatment of corneal perforations. Perspectives in Ophthalmology 1:261–268, 1977

77. Webster RG, Slansky HH, Refojo MF, et al: The use of adhesive for the closure of corneal perforations; report of two cases. Arch Ophthalmol 80:705–709, 1968

78. Weiss JL, Williams P, Lindstrom RL, et al: The use of tissue adhesives in corneal perforations. Ophthalmology 90:610–615, 1983

79. Wilson FM II, Grayson M, Ellis FD: Treatment of peripheral corneal ulcers by limbal conjunctivectomy. Br J Ophthalmol 60:713–719, 1976

80. Womack LW, Liesegang TJ: Complications of herpes zoster ophthalmicus. Arch Ophthalmol 101:42–45, 1983

# 8

# Corneal Perforations Associated with Infectious Agents

## Sid Mandelbaum        Ira J. Udell

Medical and surgical approaches to perforations developing in noninfected corneas were discussed in Chapter 7. When the perforation results from infection of the cornea by a microbial agent, however, the goals of therapy must be modified. Sealing the perforation as rapidly as possible is no longer the primary goal. If the cornea is both infected and perforated, it is necessary to identify and eradicate the responsible organisms as well as to restore the integrity of the globe. Failure to do so may result in progressive ocular damage due to persistent infection. This additional constraint affects both the timing of intervention and the selection of the surgical procedure. It is often preferable to delay definitive treatment of the perforation until control of the infection is achieved.

The importance of suspecting a microbial etiology for any corneal perforation must again be stressed. Appropriately performed cultures of the cornea are required to make certain that bacteria, fungi, or Acanthamoeba are not causing or contributing to corneal ulceration. Even when dealing with diseases that may result in corneal perforation (e.g., neurotrophic keratitis) a high index of suspicion should be maintained, for these same diseases also predispose to microbial superinfection.

The variations in morphology and in presentation of infectious keratitis make it impossible to discuss all possible circumstances. Rather, we will present general guidelines for management of perforations or impending perforations in patients with corneal ulceration due to or associated with infectious agents. Unfortunately, there are few clinical studies and limited experimental data that address the optimum timing of intervention and the surgical techniques in these situations. These guidelines are therefore based primarily on clinical experience, much of it anecdotal, and reflect our approach to these problems. Since there are differences in the strategy of management depending on the class of organism involved, this chapter is divided into five sections discussing management of perforations developing in corneas

infected by bacteria, fungi, herpes simplex, herpes zoster, or Acanthamoeba. Details of the surgical techniques required were presented in Chapter 7.

## BACTERIA

Bacterial keratitis probably represents the most frequent cause of corneal perforation. Stromal necrosis results from lytic enzymes released by polymorphonuclear leukocytes chemotactically attracted to the area of infected cornea,[22,26,56] and by enzymes produced by some strains of bacteria (notably the proteases that characterize pseudomonas[25,55]). As the infection progresses, the ulceration may extend in diameter and involve deeper layers of the corneal stroma. Descemet's membrane presents a barrier to bacteria, and is relatively resistant to destruction by proteolytic enzymes.[10] This property of Descemet's membrane explains the development of a descemetocele in cases of rapidly destructive bacterial keratitis where the overlying stroma has been digested as a result of progressive ulceration. Descemet's membrane is not, however, indestructible; it may be damaged as a result of continued exposure to leukocyte-derived enzymes and/or mechanical forces, and may perforate.

Appropriate management of bacterial keratitis includes corneal cultures, prompt initiation of broad-spectrum fortified bactericidal antibiotics, and modification of the drug regimen depending on antibiotic sensitivies of the organisms isolated. Cultures obtained from the ulcer bed and margins with a Kimura or other type of spatula are best directly inoculated onto blood, chocolate, and Sabouraud's agar, and into thioglycolate broth. Special media are available to enhance growth of unusual pathogens. Directly inoculating culture media after scraping provides a much higher yield than placing a swab of the cornea into transport medium and relying on laboratory personnel to inoculate it. Gram and Giemsa-stained smears may assist in identification of the

SURGICAL INTERVENTION IN CORNEAL AND EXTERNAL DISEASES
ISBN 0-8089-1850-8

corneal pathogen. Caution is required in scraping an ulcer already thinned to the point of impending perforation. In this situation, the safest region to scrape is involved cornea peripheral to the area of maximal thinning. Detailed reviews of the diagnosis and treatment of bacterial corneal ulcers are available.[1,29]

There is uniform agreement as to the importance of frequently-administered, topical, fortified antibiotics in treating bacterial keratitis. Periocular administration of antibiotics may be a useful adjunct. The role of topical corticosteroids in this setting is controversial, however. Theoretically, suppressing the host immune response with steroids could decrease stromal necrosis.[26] Experimentally, however, corticosteroids also suppress the polymorphonuclear leukocytes's ability to kill phagocytosed bacteria.[34] Interfering with the cornea's natural response to bacterial infection thus may pose a double-edged sword. Liebowitz has recommended the concomitant administration of bactericidal antibiotics and topical steroids in cases of central or paracentral bacterial keratitis after the infecting organism has been identified and has been treated with antibiotics to which it is sensitive for 24–48 hours,[29] supporting this recommendation with experimental studies in rabbits.[31] A beneficial effect of a combined antibiotic-steroid regimen as compared to antibiotics alone for eyes with bacterial keratitis has **not** been documented clinically in man, however.

We feel that the risks of corticosteroids outweigh their potential benefits in this clinical setting, and only very rarely administer steroids to eyes with bacterial keratitis. If one chooses to use steroids, the risks involved must be recognized, and the patient should be carefully monitored. We have seen situations where the addition of topical steroids appears to have increased rather than diminished corneal stromal melting, or where apparently effectively treated bacteria were reactivated despite concomitant antibiotic therapy.

If the patient is already using topical corticosteroids when microbial keratitis develops, it is important not to abruptly discontinue them. Abrupt cessation of topical steroids, especially when they had been administered frequently and/or chronically, may result in severe rebound inflammatory corneal necrosis.[2] We prefer to initially decrease steroids to about half the former dosage while administering appropriate antibiotics. Over the next few days, we slowly taper and discontinue topical steroids.

If a descemetocele develops during treatment of a patient with bacterial keratitis, it is reasonable to attempt to minimize the pressure behind it by decreasing aqueous secretion with topical beta blockers and/or systemic carbonic anhydrase inhibitors. A therapeutic soft contact lens may stabilize the region of the descemetocele and possibly prevent corneal perforation.[30] If the surrounding corneal stroma is not necrotic, and the patient has already received several days of topical antibiotic therapy, cyanoacrylate adhesive may be applied to the descemetocele in an attempt to prevent perforation. Topical antibiotics are continued after application of a contact lens or of adhesive. Several cautions are in order if glue is used. Solid adjacent corneal tissue is needed for the glue to adhere to; if stromal necrosis has occurred over a large area, application of the glue is not likely to be useful. Excess adhesive or glue that is not adherent to firm corneal stroma may move with each blink, increasing the shearing forces on the descemetocele.

In a patient with bacterial keratitis who presents with a corneal perforation but retains a formed anterior chamber, we recommend both fortified topical antibiotics to treat the keratitis, and intravenous antibiotics as prophylaxis against bacterial endophthalmitis. Nursing personnel must be apprised of the situation so that they can be particularly careful not to apply pressure to the globe when drops are administered. A protective eye shield should be worn. If the chamber remains formed, there is no need to treat the perforation specifically prior to completing a full course of antibiotic therapy. Unfortunately, if there is a perforation the chamber usually shallows sufficiently to make the development of peripheral anterior synechiae (PAS) a concern. If the history or sequential examinations indicate that the perforation is recent, we prefer to administer topical antibiotics for 24–48 hours prior to sealing it. With a very small perforation, the application of a therapeutic soft contact lens may result in reformation of the chamber. If the perforation is less than 2 mm in size and the adjacent cornea is not necrotic, glue can be used to seal it. Antibiotic therapy is continued if the chamber reforms with these measures.

Perforations larger than 2 mm in diameter in eyes with bacterial keratitis generally occur in the setting of severe ulcers involving large portions of the cornea. The majority of these will require therapeutic penetrating grafts, as it is preferable to completely excise and replace the infected portions of cornea. We do not recommend lamellar patch grafts in this situation. The patch graft may cover cornea that is still infected, thus limiting antibiotic penetration to residual viable bacteria. Again, we usually prefer to treat for approximately 24–48 hours with intensive fortified topical antibiotics and intravenous antibiotics before undertaking the large penetrating keratoplasty usually required in this setting. The opposing considerations are the benefits of eradicating as many organisms as possible prior to surgery, versus the increasing likelihood of PAS the longer the chamber remains flat. Given the problems of either early or delayed surgery, we will sometimes apply adhesive to a perforation even larger than 2 mm, preparing for a penetrating keratoplasty in case the glue is not effective in sealing the leak and reforming the chamber.

Techniques for performing penetrating keratoplasty on an eye with a corneal perforation are described in Chapter 7. We routinely place portions of the excised host button directly on appropriate culture media to ascertain if viable bacteria are still present within the cornea. If an inflammatory membrane is removed from the surface of the iris, it too should be cultured; if one is not present, a sample of aqueous is plated instead. It is particularly important that several large iridectomies be fashioned, for the intense intraocular inflammation will frequently result in closure of smaller ones. The anterior chamber is irrigated with physiologic saline solution. We are more conservative regarding lens extraction when operating on infected compared to nonin-

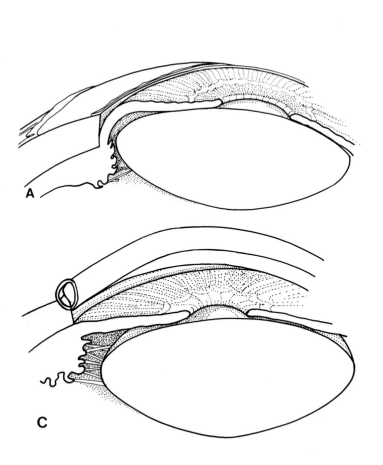

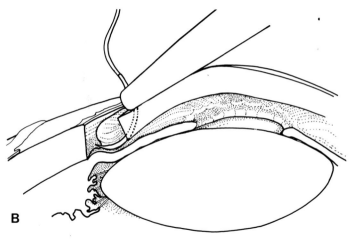

**Fig. 8-1.** (A) If the host cornea is removed to the limbus at the time of therapeutic keratoplasty for a corneal perforation, bulging of the lens-iris diaphragm may limit visualization of the full thickness of the scleral edge. (B) In order to obtain deep bites on the scleral side, the curved back portion of the needle (after it is passed through the donor cornea) is used to gently push the iris posteriorly, thus facilitating visualization of the posterior aspect of the host scleral edge. (C) Override of the donor cornea that results if sutures are not passed deeply into the host sclera.

fected corneas because the lens may act as a relative barrier to microbial spread from the anterior chamber to the vitreous, and because we prefer to minimize intraocular manipulation in these more inflamed, infected eyes.

When surgery is required for bacterial keratitis, involvement is often so extensive that resection of the cornea to the limbus in at least some areas is necessary. To facilitate placement of sutures into the sclera, it is best if a conjunctival peritomy is performed in the appropriate quadrants prior to removing the cornea. This usually causes extensive bleeding from engorged episcleral vessels; low suction applied through a glass dropper bottle tip is an effective way to obtain visualization despite the bleeding if the entire host cornea requires excision, a donor cornea 11–13 mm in diameter is usually necessary, depending on the size of the eye. In this range only nondisposable trephines are available in 1 mm increments; the donor is usually punched 1 mm larger than the trephine used to mark the host. Occasionally the host cornea is so ectatic that it cannot be marked at all with a trephine, and must be excised freehand at the corneoscleral junction. Measuring from limbus-to-limbus horizontally prior to removing the cornea will help in sizing the donor cornea.

In suturing donor grafts into the sclera, it is crucial to identify the full thickness of the host scleral margin. This may be difficult to do because the lens-iris diaphragm bulges forward, obscuring the scleral edge (Fig. 8-1A). After the suture needle is passed through the donor cornea, the curved back portion of the needle may be used to push the iris posteriorly, improving visualization of the posterior aspect of the host sclera (Fig. 8-1B). If this is not carefully done for each suture bite, the donor cornea may override the opening rather than nestle within it (Fig. 8-1C). In areas where the donor is being sewn into sclera, we prefer interrupted 9/0 nylon sutures; these larger diameter sutures better secure the graft into the sclera than does 10/0. Where donor and host cornea are being joined, 10/0 nylon sutures are preferable, so the knots can be buried. Suture bites through the host cornea should be relatively long to avoid subsequent cheesewiring through soft, edematous tissue. It is important that interrupted sutures be used because of differential rates of vascularization and suture loosening. Since the circumference of a therapeutic graft is often considerably larger than that of an optical penetrating keratoplasty and the donor–host match is not as precise, we usually find that at least 24 sutures are required. At the end of the procedure, we use a fluorescein strip to "paint" the donor–host junction and carefully inspect it with the cobalt blue filter of the microscope, making absolutely certain the wound is watertight. A wound leak resulting in a shallow chamber will aggravate the tendency to PAS formation in these inflamed eyes.

Postoperatively, there is usually severe inflammation;

frequently a large fibrin clot admixed with blood fills the anterior chamber. Since the inflammation increases the likelihood of PAS, and since the infected tissue has been excised, we utilize frequent topical steroids postoperatively. Administration of fortified topical antibiotics is resumed. Systemic antibiotics are discontinued after 2–3 days if there is no clinical evidence suggesting bacterial endophthalmitis, and if the membrane removed from the anterior chamber is culture-negative. Orally-administered antibiotics do not penetrate the eye well enough to be useful.

The proximity of these large grafts to the limbus and the inflammation usually present at the time they are placed, predispose to homograft reaction. In our experience, graft rejections in this situation often occur early, are intense, and are difficult to reverse. The goal in this situation is to sterilize and maintain the structural integrity of the globe; a central optical keratoplasty can subsequently be performed when the eye is quiet.

## Bacterial Scleritis

Since sclera is relatively resistant to bacterial infection, it is usually not necessary to excise sclera when operating for a perforated bacterial keratitis. Resecting sclera at the time of therapeutic keratoplasty damages the filtration angle and may increase the already substantial risk of glaucoma postoperatively. There are specific circumstances, however, in which bacterial scleritis is more likely. The causative organism is nearly always pseudomonas, usually involving sclera by spread from a contiguous keratitis.[11,45] Elderly patients or those with immunocompromised corneas are particularly susceptible.[8,11,45] Sudden increase in pain after initial improvement during treatment of bacterial keratitis should raise suspicion of this entity. Development of one or more subconjunctival abscesses peripheral to the limbus is virtually diagnostic of microbial scleritis.

In cases of extensive pseudomonas keratitis involving paralimbal cornea in a susceptible host, we usually administer intravenous and subconjunctival aminoglycosides in an attempt to prevent development of microbial scleritis, although there is no evidence to support this approach. Once bacterial scleritis has developed, it is difficult to treat. Cryotherapy to the involved sclera combined with penetrating keratoplasty has occasionally been useful.[11] Scleral resection can be attempted; unfortunately, the area of sclera infected is usually extensive. The prognosis if bacterial scleritis develops is poor; most eyes reported have lost useful vision, and many have required enucleation or evisceration.[8,45] Except for these uncommon cases where sclera has become infected, however, removal of the cornea to the limbus is usually sufficient to eliminate microbial keratitis.

## Peripheral Bacterial Perforations

Certain bacteria, including *Moraxella* and *Neisseria gonorrheae,* have a predilection for involving the peripheral cornea.[52] Gonococcal keratitis is particularly dangerous because it progresses so rapidly; a patient may present with a perfora-

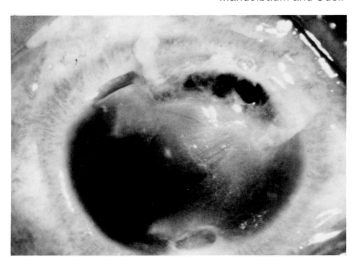

**Fig. 8-2.**   Superior peripheral corneal ulceration and large perforation in the left eye of a 20-year-old male with gonococcal keratitis and conjunctivitis. Ulcer rapidly progressed to perforation despite systemic and intensive topical antibiotic therapy. Iris is visible within the perforation superiorly; the chamber is flat. The central cornea is edematous but not involved with the ulceration. Another marginal ulcer (which did not perforate) is present inferiorly.

tion relatively soon after developing symptoms (Fig. 8-2). While large peripheral perforations in noninfected corneas are often best managed by a lamellar patch graft as described in Chapter 7, this procedure is not appropriate if the cornea is infected.

For a peripheral bacterial perforation too large to seal with glue, the principles regarding timing of surgical intervention discussed above apply. In the patient shown in Figure 8-2, a crescentic full-thickness penetrating keratoplasty extending to the limbus can be performed (Fig. 8-3). Should the graft subsequently become edematous, there would be

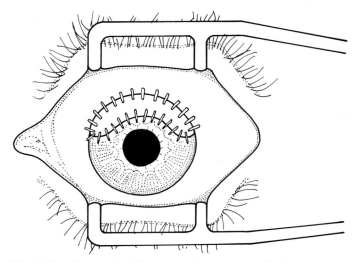

**Fig. 8-3.**   Crescentic full-thickness keratoplasty which can be performed for the large marginal perforation in Figure 8-2. Should it opacify, a graft of this shape would have less effect on visual acuity than a large circular keratoplasty that would involve the visual axis.

much less effect on visual acuity if the donor were crescentic than if the donor were circular, since a circular penetrating keratoplasty would need to be large enough to extend into the visual axis. A full-thickness crescentic donor button may be matched to the host defect using the techniques described in Chapter 7 for peripheral lamellar grafts.

## FUNGI

Although the appearance of a corneal infiltrate may suggest fungal keratitis (particularly infiltrates that are dry, gray, and slightly elevated with feathery edges and/or satellite lesions), and the clinical setting may suggest the possibility of a fungal etiology (particularly trauma with organic material or superinfection in eyes immunocompromised by chronic use of topical steroids), the cornerstone of diagnosis remains the laboratory. We have seen corneal ulcers "typically" fungal in appearance that have actually been caused by bacteria. Since it is impossible to determine the etiologic agent solely from the clinical appearance, and since bacterial keratitis generally progresses more rapidly than fungal keratitis, we recommend that corneal ulcers be treated as if they were bacterial unless laboratory evaluation provides evidence of fungal infection. Careful examination of Gram and Giemsa-stained scrapings from the ulcer bed are the most rapid diagnostic technique for determination of fungi. In a large series, experienced observers could identify fungal hyphae in approximately 80 percent of cases of culture-proven fungal keratitis.[33] Grocott's methenamine silver (GMS)-stained smears, if available, may be even more reliable.[18] If smears do not show hyphae, broad-spectrum fortified topical antibacterials should be frequently administered pending culture results. Fungi, if present, will usually grow in culture within 48 hours.[14] If fungi rather than bacteria are isolated, topical antifungals can be substituted. Because rapid deterioration may occur if bacterial keratitis "masquerading" as fungal is not appropriately treated, and because of the corneal toxicity of antifungals and the long course of therapy required once they are begun, we do not treat for fungal keratitis unless there is laboratory confirmation of fungal infection in the form of a smear showing hyphae or a positive culture. In smear and culture-negative cases strongly suspected of being fungal and clinically not responding to antibacterial agents, a small corneal biopsy can be obtained at the slit-lamp or in the minor operating room. Sometimes fungi cannot be isolated from superficial corneal scrapings, but can be cultured from or histopathologically located in deeper corneal stroma.[6,41] A corneal biopsy is generally preferable to anterior chamber paracentesis for diagnostic purposes in these cases.

Topical natamycin (Natacyn, Alcon, Ft. Worth, TX) is currently the drug of choice for fungal ulcerative keratitis. Natamycin is the only antifungal approved for topical ocular therapy by the Food and Drug Administration. Experience has shown it to be generally more effective and less toxic than amphotericin B. Forster and Rebell have found natamycin to be effective in approximately 85 percent of *Fusarium solani* infections, 60 percent of infections caused by other monilia-ceous (nonpigmented) fungi, 90 percent of keratitis caused by dematiaceous (brown-pigmented) fungi, and 75 percent of yeast infections of the cornea.[13] The imidazoles, including clotrimazole, miconazole, and ketaconozole, are another category of antifungals that may be useful. Of the filamentous fungi, Curvularia, Aspergillus, and Paecilomyces species are usually sensitive to the imidazoles, while Fusarium species are relatively insensitive.[13] Oral flucytosine may be helpful in certain yeast infections; it is best used in combination with amphotericin B, as resistance may rapidly develop when flucytosine is used as a single agent. Since all available drugs are fungistatic, the host immune response plays an important role in eliminating these infections. Principles of management and sensitivities to antifungal agents have been reviewed elsewhere.[13,23]

The availability of better antifungals has probably decreased the incidence of surgical intervention for fungal keratitis.[15,46] Nevertheless, in our experience surgery is more frequently required in the management of eyes with fungal keratitis than in cases of bacterial keratitis. From 1979 to 1985, approximately 30 percent of eyes treated for fungal keratitis at the Bascom Palmer Eye Institute required penetrating keratoplasty in the acute phase of their disease.* Other procedures besides penetrating keratoplasty that have been helpful in the management of fungal keratitis include debridement and, rarely, localized conjunctival flaps.

### Debridement

Fungi that have infected the cornea may grow in a more localized fashion than do bacteria. In these cases, debulking the lesion may be beneficial as an adjunct to topical antifungal agents. Vigorous scraping with a spatula or blade in the course of obtaining material for smears and culture may be sufficient. In certain cases where fungi are growing superficially in a "plaque-like" fashion, debriding the superficial cornea by lamellar keratectomy may be required to remove infected material and improve penetration of topical antimycotics to deeper corneal layers. An example of this growth pattern is shown in Figure 8-4A; removal of the fungal plaque combined with antifungal chemotherapy resulted in rapid resolution in this case of aspergillus keratitis (Fig. 8-4B).

### Penetrating Keratoplasty

If a fungal corneal ulcer is progressing despite treatment with antimycotics, penetrating keratoplasty is indicated. Keratoplasty allows removal of replicating organisms and/or antigenic material stimulating inflammation. With fungi particularly, in vitro sensitivity to drug does not necessarily correlate with a positive in vivo response. Other factors including the poor tissue penetration of most antifungal preparations, the host inflammatory response, and as yet undetermined host–fungal interactions may account for pro-

---

*Lee Klein, M. D., unpublished data.

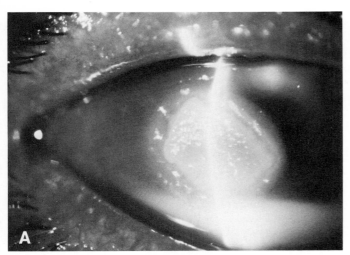 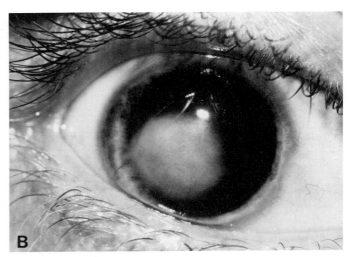

**Fig. 8-4.** (A) Twenty-eight-year-old male with ulcerative keratitis and a raised, firm, central corneal plaque. Note the large hypopyon. Cultures grew *Aspergillus* species. The patient had not responded to one month of topical antifungal therapy. Lamellar excision of the plaque was then performed. Histopathologically, the specimen was extensively infiltrated with hyphae. (B) Subsequent to lamellar keratectomy and antifungal therapy, the ulcer healed promptly. There is a residual corneal scar limiting visual acuity to 20/80.

gressive corneal ulceration despite treatment with an antifungal to which the organism is "sensitive."

Continued fungal replication despite appropriate topical therapy may particularly occur if fungi have been inoculated deeply into the corneal stroma (e.g. as a result of trauma), even if confined to a small area of cornea. Since unlike bacteria, fungi are capable of penetrating through intact Descemet's membrane,[41] it is preferable to excise the portion of cornea containing a deep, progressing fungal infection prior to development of fungal endophthalmitis. Topical antifungal therapy is generally worthwhile for at least several days to determine if it will control the infectious process.[16] If the ulcer continues to enlarge or extend more deeply into the cornea despite topical therapy, penetrating keratoplasty is indicated.

The difficulties that may be encountered if fungi are inoculated deeply in the cornea are demonstrated in the case shown in Figure 8-5. A 16-year-old male sustained an oblique injury to the left cornea with a tree branch; by slit-lamp examination, the cornea but not the anterior chamber was penetrated. There was no growth from corneal cultures. A deep stromal infiltrate and underlying endothelial plaque developed (Fig. 8-5A). Over the next month, the plaque enlarged to form a spherical mass despite treatment with antibacterials and natamycin. Anterior chamber paracentesis was performed, aspirating the mass attached to the endothelium (Fig. 8-5B). Although cultures of this were negative, pathologic examination revealed many hyphae within a dense coagulum of inflammatory cells and debris. Despite injection of intracameral amphotericin B, the mass recurred. A 2 mm penetrating keratoplasty was then performed, excising the cornea containing the deep infiltrate and adherent mass (Fig. 8-5C). Pathology showed many hyphae both in the deep corneal stroma and within the recurrent inflammatory ball.

In this patient, fungal organisms were sequestered in

the deep corneal stroma, a region where topical antimycotics penetrate poorly. Continued fungal replication resulted in recurrent formation of a "fungal ball" adherent to the endothelium. Aspiration of this mass did not solve the problem because viable fungi were still present in the deep stroma. The infection could only be eradicated by excising the deep cornea containing the fungi. As this case demonstrates, it can be difficult to clinically distinguish presumably sterile plaques from true extension of organisms through Descemet's membrane. Frequent careful slit-lamp observation with attention to the change in thickness of clear stroma between Descemet's membrane and the infiltrate may be helpful in making this determination.

Another group who may require penetrating keratoplasty are patients with fungal keratitis who develop impending or frank perforations. Many of these patients have been treated with corticosteroids during their course. Our personal experience certainly confirms reports in the literature indicating that steroids aggravate fungal keratitis, sometimes dramatically so.[6,24,41] Possible mechanisms include enhanced fungal replication, depression of host immune responses, or a combination of these. We strongly recommend avoiding the use of topical or subconjunctival steroids in the management of keratitis suspected or proven to be caused by fungi.

Lamellar keratoplasty is generally contraindicated in the management of fungal keratitis. Residual organisms (sometimes present deeper than the visible infiltrate) may replicate at the donor–host interface after lamellar keratoplasty. Penetration of topical antifungal drugs is likely to be inhibited by the donor lamellar button. If keratoplasty is required in a case of fungal keratitis, experimental evidence[51] and clinical experience[43,51] indicate that it should be a penetrating rather than a lamellar procedure.

Considerations in performing therapeutic penetrating keratoplasty for fungal keratitis are similar to those already discussed for bacterial infections. It is important to circum-

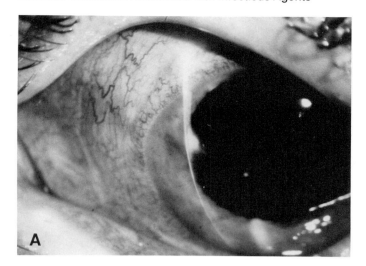

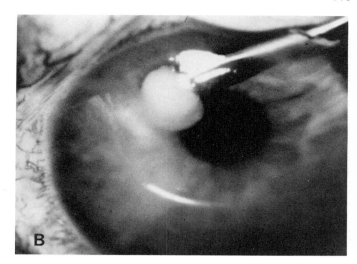

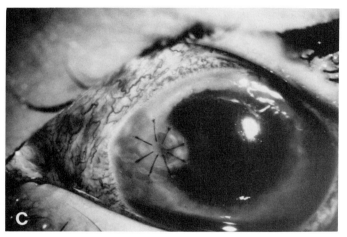

**Fig. 8-5.** (A) Deep, focal corneal infiltrate in the left eye of a 16-year-old male who sustained a glancing injury with a tree branch. The stroma anterior to the infiltrate is clear and the epithelium is intact. A small plaque is adherent to the endothelium directly under the infiltrate. (The patient's right eye had been enucleated 6 years previously as a result of a severe injury. (B) Intraoperative photograph approximately 1 month later. The previously small plaque has become a much larger mass. A needle has been introduced into the anterior chamber; the mass, which was quite adherent to the endothelium, was aspirated. Pathologic examination revealed many hyphae and inflammatory cells. (C) Because of recurrence of the mass adherent to the endothelium, a 2 mm penetrating keratoplasty was performed. The cornea containing the deep infiltrate and the adherent mass were excised. The eye has remained free of infection since (Courtesy of William Culbertson, M.D.).

scribe the area of cornea clinically involved. The graft should extend at least 1–2 mm peripheral to the corneal infiltrate. With peripheral ulcers or very large ulcers, this may require that the graft extend close to the limbus. In our experience, fungi are more likely to extend into the sclera than are bacteria. Sclera adjacent to involved paralimbal cornea should therefore be carefully inspected. If there is evidence of infection, the affected sclera must be excised and replaced along with the cornea. Fungi may also grow through peripheral cornea and into the chamber angle. If this occurs, the involved cornea, sclera, and iris should be removed en-bloc. Resecting all involved tissue is a key factor in successfully sterilizing the eye if the fungal infection has progressed to the point where surgery is necessary. We routinely culture a portion of the excised corneal button. Sections of the peripheral margins of the excised cornea can be examined histopathologically to ascertain completeness of resection, although the clinical course postoperatively rather than pathology results should be the primary factor determining the need for additional surgery (Fig. 8-6).

There is frequently a dense inflammatory plaque in the anterior chamber in cases of severe fungal keratitis, often adherent to the iris. This plaque should be removed at the time of keratoplasty to improve aqueous circulation and

decrease the risk of pupillary block postoperatively. Although the plaque is usually sterile, we recommend that it also be cultured and examined histopathologically. If progressive intraocular inflammation occurs after surgery, it will be important to know if organisms had extended into the anterior chamber. Even if fungi grow from the plaque, however, we would not inject intracameral antifungal drugs unless there was clinical evidence of intraocular infection. The eye may be capable of eliminating a small inoculum of fungi by its own immune mechanisms.[23,46] Fungal endophthalmitis developing as an extension from fungal keratitis is uncommon, although in our experience it occurs more frequently than does bacterial endophthalmitis as a result of bacterial keratitis. If fungal endophthalmitis develops, therapy should include resection of all clinically involved ocular tissues, and administration of appropriate intraocular antifungal drugs. The prognosis for salvaging the eye in this situation is reduced,[24,28,44,49] but appears better with an aggressive surgical approach.[44,48]

There is no concensus regarding the use of steroids after surgery for fungal keratitis. Although reduction of postoperative inflammation is a desirable effect of steroid administration, steroids may adversely affect the eye's limited ability to eliminate residual fungi. If keratoplasty is required for pro-

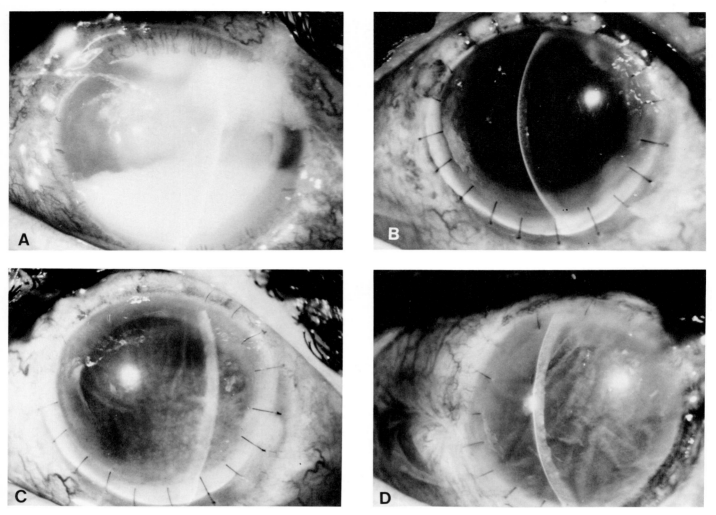

**Fig. 8-6.** (A) Left eye of a 40-year-old male with a 2 month history of a culture-negative corneal ulcer that developed after organic material accidentally fell into his eye. There had been progressive deterioration despite administration of multiple antibacterials and antifungals. There is a temporal arcuate ulceration from 2 to 5 o'clock, dense stromal infiltrates superiorly, and a 40 percent hypopyon. The temporal cornea perforated several days after this photograph was taken. (B) Same eye, 1 week after a 10 mm penetrating keratoplasty, cataract extraction, and anterior vitrectomy. The donor cornea has been sewn to host sclera superiorly and to a rim of host cornea inferiorly. Cultures of the excised cornea and the fibrin plaque removed from the anterior chamber at the time of surgery grew *Fusarium oxysporum*. (C) Ten days later, there has been development of a deep infiltrate of the host cornea at 3:30 o'clock, visible between two sutures. There was also a mass adherent to the iris in this region. The temporal cornea is edematous, and there are multiple small clumps on the endothelium. (D) Two weeks after total keratoplasty, and removal of iris and a 3 mm rim of sclera in the inferotemporal quadrant. A corresponding donor graft was fashioned from a whole globe. Intraocular amphotericin B was administered. Cultures of excised cornea and iris again grew fungus; there was no growth from the vitreous. The cornea is edematous. This patient is at high risk for recurrent intraocular infection, although there was no evidence of it when this photograph was taken. Unfortunately, the patient was lost to follow-up (Courtesy of Richard K. Forster, M.D.).

gressive, medically uncontrollable fungal keratitis, or there is evidence of fungal extension within the eye, we recommend avoiding use of steroids postoperatively. If keratoplasty is performed for an impending or actual perforation and the involved cornea appears completely circumscribed at surgery, the use of steroids should be considered on a case-by-case basis depending on the extent of inflammation, and the results of culture and histopathology of the excised cornea. If inflammation is so intense as to threaten survival of the eye, steroids are required despite their risks. In this situation, a short course of oral steroids may be

preferable in that they affect intraocular inflammation but do not achieve as high a concentration in the cornea as do topical steroids. There are no data as to when the use of steroids postoperatively are "safe" after penetrating keratoplasty for fungal keratitis; fungal infection recurring in the cornea or in the anterior chamber has been reported even months after surgery.[17] It is important to recognize that the primary goal of keratoplasty in these situations is to permanently eliminate the infecting fungi and to salvage the eye; maintaining a clear graft should be a subordinate consideration.

## Conjunctival Flap

Conjunctival flaps have only a very limited role in the treatment of fungal keratitis. Although occasional cases of central fungal keratitis may respond to debridement and a conjunctival flap, this approach is not as likely to be effective in eliminating the organisms as is a penetrating keratoplasty. Sanders reported that four of nine patients treated with conjunctival flaps for progressive fungal keratitis showed evidence of continued fungal replication despite presence of the flap, resulting in "abscess perforation through the flaps."[46]

More recently, Sanitato and coworkers have recommended excisional keratectomy and a localized conjunctival flap for peripheral fungal ulcers unresponsive to medical therapy.[47] Since the surrounding cornea and anterior chamber can still be monitored for signs of progressive infection after this procedure, a partial flap would seem to be a reasonable alternative in this situation. Should there be evidence of progressive infection despite the flap, full-thickness excision of the involved cornea would be warranted.

## HERPES SIMPLEX

The diagnosis of herpes simplex keratitis differs from bacterial or fungal keratitis in that it is usually made based on clinical appearance and course rather than by laboratory studies. Facilities for culturing herpes virus are not readily available, recovery of virus may not be possible even from cases that are clearly herpetic, and virus isolation takes sufficiently long as to significantly limit its clinical utility. Techniques for rapid detection of herpes antigens using monoclonal antibodies and DNA probes are now becoming more readily available, and may be helpful in difficult cases.[20] Laboratory studies are still best viewed as an adjunct, however.

The vast majority of patients with herpetic keratitis never require surgical intervention. Those who do, usually require penetrating keratoplasty to replace a scarred cornea. Patients may also require corneal grafting if they develop progressive stromal melting leading to a descemetocele or to corneal perforation—fortunately, a relatively uncommon sequence of events.

The pathogenesis of corneal stromal melting in herpetic keratitis is incompletely understood and appears to be multifactorial. Host factors including HLA type[37] and systemic immune status may be important. It has been generally accepted that herpetic stromal inflammatory disease is a consequence of nonviable viral components, soluble viral antigens, and virally altered keratocytes. Recently, however, Tullo and coworkers have isolated herpes virus from the stroma of human keratoplasty specimens.[54] Their work suggests that some cases of stromal keratitis may be caused by live virus, and supports the concept of empiric antiviral administration in cases treated with steroids. Although corticosteroids are beneficial in the management of stromal herpetic keratitis involving the visual axis, possible consequences of their use include steroid dependence, recurrent

herpes virus infection, bacterial or fungal superinfection, cataracts, and glaucoma. Occasionally, particularly in eyes with epithelial defects, chronic administration of topical steroids may contribute to progressive corneal stromal melting.

Management of a descemetocele or perforation occurring in a cornea with herpes simplex keratitis depends on its location, size, and the status of surrounding tissue. Cultures to rule out development of a secondary bacterial or fungal infection are important. These locally immunocompromised corneas are prone to secondary infection, which may develop without detectable change in the slit-lamp appearance of the eye.

If the perforation is peripheral to the visual axis, we prefer to use cyanoacrylate adhesive or to fashion a lamellar patch graft as described in Chapter 7. These modalities will often allow the cornea to heal; since scarring will be outside the visual axis, good visual acuity may be attained. Patients who develop a central perforation pose a more difficult management problem. Glue or a lamellar patch graft will cause visually significant scarring, thus necessitating a secondary optical keratoplasty. Proceeding directly to a central keratoplasty, however, may adversely affect the prognosis of the graft because of the substantial ocular inflammation present at the time of surgery.

There is disagreement in the literature regarding the prognosis when penetrating keratoplasty is performed at a time of active herpetic keratitis. Fine and Cignetti were unable to determine that the state of activity of the disease at the time of keratoplasty significantly influenced the final result.[12] Polack and Kaufman,[42] Cobo and coworkers,[7] Foster and Duncan,[19] and Beekhuis and associates[3] have disagreed, finding a worse prognosis in their patients when penetrating keratoplasty was performed at a time of active stromal necrosis. The difference in Foster's series in eyes with corneal perforations was particularly striking: none of the 16 eyes in which penetrating keratoplasty was performed for corneal perforation retained a clear graft for even 2 years. Perforations initially treated with a lamellar patch graft or cyanoacrylate adhesive, with optical keratoplasty deferred for 6–24 months until the eye was quiet, had a much better prognosis: 11 of 13 of these eyes maintained clear grafts. Based on these results, Foster has recommended either a patch graft or tissue adhesive and anti-inflammatory therapy to achieve and maintain a quiescent state prior to penetrating keratoplasty for corneal perforations in eyes with herpes simplex keratitis.[19] This is directly opposite to Cavanagh, who has maintained that immediate central keratoplasty is the most effective form of treatment for corneal perforation in these eyes.[5]

We consider the status of the surrounding cornea and the extent of ocular inflammation as the important parameters in determining the management for central perforations resulting from herpes simplex keratitis. If the adjacent tissue is healthy, adhesive or a small patch graft are likely to be effective in sealing the perforation. If the eye is then allowed to quiet, we believe the prognosis for subsequent central keratoplasty is improved. Should the perforation occur within a large area of corneal necrosis, however, a patch graft is technically very difficult to perform. An appropriate corneal bed may be impossible to fashion; the sutures have a tendency to cheesewire through the soft, thin host tissue, with possible recurrence of the leak. Similarly, a large area of corneal necrosis surrounding a perforation is a relative contraindication to the application of cyanoacrylate adhesive since there is nothing solid for the glue to adhere to. Therefore, given a central perforation developing within a large area of corneal stromal necrosis, we prefer penetrating keratoplasty, choosing the diameter of the graft to reach relatively normal cornea. If a corneal perforation that has been glued fails to heal after several months, penetrating keratoplasty is also indicated. Finally, if a central corneal perforation develops in an eye that is relatively quiet, at least by clinical criteria, we believe it is reasonable to proceed directly with central penetrating keratoplasty. Even eyes that appear clinically quiet, however, may develop substantial postoperative inflammation.

A major factor in improving the prognosis of penetrating keratoplasty for herpes simplex keratitis, especially in inflamed eyes, has been the use of corticosteroids in the postoperative period. It is generally agreed that topical corticosteroids should be given as necessary to control intraocular inflammation, as frequently as hourly if required. This reduces the likelihood of developing synechiae and corneal vascularization. Occasionally, systemic corticosteroids, which decrease intraocular inflammation but have less effect on the cornea than do topical steroids, may be warranted. Whenever frequent topical steroids are being used, we also empirically administer topical antivirals (usually four times per day) as prophylaxis against the development of epithelial herpes. Recurrent herpes is rarely a problem in the immediate postoperative period and poses less of a risk to long-term graft survival than does rejection.[7] Steroids are tapered based on ocular inflammation; we continue prophylactic topical antivirals until the eye requires the equivalent of 1 drop per day or less of 1 percent prednisolone acetate. Cobo and coworkers, however, do not recommend prophylactic antivirals (except if steroids are being intensively administered for graft rejection) for they did not find a higher recurrence rate without antiviral use.[7] Cycloplegics, dilating agents, beta blockers, and carbonic anhydrase inhibitors are administered as necessary postoperatively.

## HERPES ZOSTER

The cornea is frequently affected in patients with herpes zoster ophthalmicus. Sixty-five percent of patients reported by Liesegang had corneal involvement during their course, including early or late epithelial keratitis, anterior stromal infiltrates, disciform keratitis, sclerokeratitis, or neurotrophic keratopathy.[32] While necrotizing corneal stromal inflammation may occur months or years after the acute episode, and peripheral corneal ulcers have been reported,[38] it has been our experience that factors other than stromal necrosis directly caused by the zoster virus are usually associated with corneal perforation in this setting.

Chief among these factors is the marked diminution of corneal sensation that often accompanies even mild corneal involvement by the zoster virus. The hypesthesia that occurs with herpes zoster appears to be greater than would occur for a comparably severe episode of herpes simplex keratitis. This neurotrophic state predisposes to the development of epithelial defects, which heal poorly. There is frequently an element of exposure or incomplete blinking due to scarring of the lids, an added insult to the epithelium.[57] Topical steroids, which may have previously been administered for keratouveitis, are often inappropriately continued or even increased when an epithelial defect develops. The chronic administration of topical steroids to a neurotrophic, epithelium-deficient cornea will only hasten stromal melting and the development of a corneal perforation.

It is obviously best to treat epithelial defects or early stromal ulcers before they progress. We prefer lubricants and semi-pressure patching to a therapeutic contact lens in this setting. Neurotrophic corneas are prone to lens-related complications, especially bacterial infection. Caution is required even if a contact lens is applied only briefly; long-term contact lens use on a neurotrophic cornea is not advisable. Structural lid abnormalities limiting blinking or lid closure should be surgically repaired. A large lateral, or lateral and medial tarsorrhaphies are best performed before the cornea begins to melt. A culture-negative corneal infiltrate and a hypopyon may develop in a zoster-affected eye with a persistent epithelial defect; these generally resolve if a tarsorrhaphy is promptly placed. Should there be progressive melting despite these measures, a partial or complete conjunctival flap is often the best approach. We have not found cyanoacrylate adhesive to be as effective in encouraging stromal healing in these neurotrophic corneas as in corneas with more normal sensation.

When faced with a perforation in an anesthetic zoster cornea shown not to be secondarily infected, we prefer a lamellar patch graft to a large penetrating keratoplasty. Epithelial defects, poor healing along the donor-host junction, and recurrent stromal melting are complications more likely to develop after a large penetrating keratoplasty than after a lamellar patch graft. Strong consideration should be given to performing a tarsorrhaphy or a partial conjunctival flap at the time of the corneal surgery to provide the optimum environment for healing of the grafted tissue, and to prevent recurrence of epithelial defects.

## ACANTHAMOEBA

Acanthamoeba, a free-living protozoa, was first reported as a cause of keratitis in 1974.[40] An increasing number of cases of keratitis caused by these organisms are being reported.[4,9,21,39,53] Clinical features may include: (1) a history of relatively minor corneal trauma; (2) use of soft contact lenses; (3) pain, often beyond that expected for the degree of keratitis present; (4) a waxing and waning course, initially indolent but generally progressive; (5) epithelial defects that may heal and recur; and (6) stromal infiltrates, often in a partial or complete ring configuration.

Diagnosis of acanthamoeba keratitis requires a high

index of suspicion since clinical features may suggest herpes simplex keratitis, fungal keratitis, or low-grade bacterial keratitis (such as mycobacteria). The amoeba may be seen on Gram, Giemsa, Giemsa-Wright, trichrome, GMS, or periodic acid-Schiff (PAS)-stained smears, but familiarity with the double-walled, polygonal shape of the organisms is essential to avoid overlooking or misinterpreting them.[53] Acanthamoeba require special culture media for optimum growth, such as non-nutrient agar with an overlay of *E. coli*. Even appropriately cultured corneal scrapings may not yield growth of the organisms; if suspicion is high, a corneal biopsy for histopathologic examination is indicated. The variable clinical appearance and course, lack of familiarity with the organism, and its special culture requirements have been responsible for delayed diagnosis in many of the reported cases.

Unfortunately, even once the diagnosis is made, therapy for the condition is unsatisfactory. Acanthamoeba are rather resistant to chemotherapeutic agents. In cases that appear to have clinically responded to medical therapy, it is difficult to determine which of the many agents the patients had been treated with was helpful, and what proportion of the success can be attributed to therapy as opposed to unknown host factors. Results of in vitro sensitivity testing have not been uniform, possibly varying with the species, strain, and testing techniques.[21,53] The antibiotics that appear most useful at present include propamidine isethionate 0.1 percent drops and dibromopropamidine isethionate 0.15 percent ointment (both available commercially in England as Brolene, an over-the-counter preparation),[58] neomycin, miconazole, and systemic ketaconozole.[21,39,53] Caution must be exercised if systemic ketaconozole is used because of risks of anaphylaxis, liver damage, and drug interactions.[27] Topical steroids may have a role in the therapeutic regimen by decreasing corneal inflammation, though some have avoided their use for fear of depressing host defenses.[31] Cryotherapy will kill Acanthamoeba trophozoites in vitro, but its inability to eliminate the cyst form of the organism makes it unlikely to be a useful therapeutic modality.[36]

The role of penetrating keratoplasty in the management of Acanthamoeba keratitis is uncertain. Penetrating keratoplasty is required in patients who develop progressive stromal ulceration leading to descemetocele formation or perforation; 8 of 11 cases reviewed by Hirst and associates (10 of which had been previously reported) ultimately progressed to this stage.[21] Less clear, however, is the optimum timing for keratoplasty in patients diagnosed as having Acanthamoeba keratitis, but in whom there is no immediate danger of corneal perforation. Some contend that the difficulty in medically treating the infection argues for surgically replacing the involved cornea once the diagnosis is made, while the infection is presumably localized.[21,35] Some patients who have undergone relatively early keratoplasty, however, have had complicated postoperative courses.[39] Based on current experience, it would seem reasonable to attempt medical therapy with topical Brolene, neomycin, miconazole, and possibly oral ketaconozole in patients who have not progressed to the verge of perforation. Concomitant topical steroids may be required to limit progressive stromal and intraocular inflam-

mation. If this regimen is effective, it should probably be continued for many months before considering penetrating keratoplasty for visually significant corneal scarring. Should the keratitis progress despite this medical regimen, however, penetrating keratoplasty is the only other approach currently available. Lamellar patch grafts and conjunctival flaps do not appear to have any role in the treatment of this infection.

If penetrating keratoplasty is performed, the margin of resection should extend several millimeters peripheral to clinically involved cornea, even if this requires a very large graft. Unfortunately, encompassing the infiltrate does not assure removal of all organisms, as Acanthamoeba may be present in the cornea without inciting biomicroscopically visible inflammation.[4] It would therefore seem reasonable to prophylactically treat postoperatively with the antibiotic regimen described above. Histopathologic evidence of Acanthamoeba at the margins of the resected specimen is a poor prognostic sign, and should alert the ophthalmologist to be particularly vigilant for signs of recurrence in the host cornea postoperatively.

Despite the increasing reports of Acanthamoeba keratitis, therapy for this condition is likely to remain suboptimal until more effective chemotherapeutic agents are introduced.

## REFERENCES

1. Abbott RL, Abrams M: Bacterial corneal ulcers, in Duane TD (ed): Clinical Ophthalmology, Vol. IV. Philadelphia, Harper and Row, 1986, Chapter 18, pp 1–34
2. Aronson SB, Moore TE Jr: Corticosteroid therapy in central stromal keratitis. Am J Ophthalmol 67:873–896, 1969
3. Beekhuis WH, Renardel de Lavalette JGC, Van Rij G, et al: Therapeutic keratoplasty for active herpetic corneal disease: viral culture and prognosis. Documenta Ophthalmologica 55:31–35, 1983
4. Blackman HJ, Rao N, Lemp MA, et al: Acanthamoeba keratitis successfully treated with penetrating keratoplasty; suggested immunogenic mechanisms of action. Cornea 3:125–130, 1984
5. Cavanagh HD, Pihlaja DH: The management of corneal perforation in herpes simplex keratitis. Perspectives in Ophthalmology 1:269–273, 1977
6. Chin GN, Hyndiuk RA, Kwasny GP, et al: Keratomycosis in Wisconsin. Am J Ophthalmol 79:121–125, 1975
7. Cobo LM, Coster DJ, Rice NSC, et al: Prognosis and management of corneal transplantation for herpetic keratitis. Arch Ophthalmol 98:1755–1759, 1980
8. Codere F, Brownstein S, Jackson WB: *Pseudomonas aeruginosa* scleritis. Am J Ophthalmol 91:706–710, 1981
9. Cohen EJ, Buchanan HW, Laughrea PA, et al: Diagnosis and management of *Acanthamoeba* keratitis. Am J Ophthalmol 100:389–395, 1985
10. Dohlman CH, Balazs EA: Chemical studies on Descemet's membrane of the bovine cornea. Arch Biochem Biophys 57:445–457, 1955
11. Eiferman R: Cryotherapy of *Pseudomonas* keratitis and scleritis. Arch Ophthalmol 97:1637–1639, 1979
12. Fine M, Cignetti FE: Penetrating keratoplasty in herpes simplex keratitis; recurrence in grafts. Arch Ophthalmol 95:613–616, 1977
13. Forster RK: Fungal diseases, in Smolin G, Thoft RA (eds):

The Cornea; Scientific Foundations and Clinical Practice. Boston, Little, Brown and Company, 1983, pp 168–177

14. Forster RK, Rebell G: The diagnosis and management of keratomycoses. I. Cause and diagnosis. Arch Ophthalmol 93:975–978, 1975

15. Forster RK, Rebell G: The diagnosis and management of keratomycoses. II. Medical and surgical management. Arch Ophthalmol 93:1134–1136, 1975

16. Forster RK, Rebell G: Therapeutic surgery in failures of medical treatment for fungal keratitis. Brit J Ophthalmol 59:366–371, 1975

17. Forster RK, Rebell G, Stiles W: Recurrent keratitis due to *Acremonium potronii*. Am J Ophthalmol 79:126–128, 1975

18. Forster RK, Wirta MG, Solis M, et al: Methenamine-silver-stained corneal scrapings in keratomycosis. Am J Ophthalmol 82:261–265, 1976

19. Foster CS, Duncan J: Penetrating keratoplasty for herpes simplex keratitis. Am J Ophthalmol 92:336–343, 1981

20. Fung JC, Shaney J, Tilton RC: Comparison of the detection of herpes simplex virus in direct clinical specimens with herpes simplex virus-specific DNA probes and monoclonal antibodies. J Clin Microbiol 22:748–753, 1985

21. Hirst LW, Green WR, Merz W, et al: Management of Acanthamoeba keratitis; a case report and review of the literature. Ophthalmology 91:1105–1111, 1984

22. Hyndiuk RA: Experimental *Pseudomonas* keratitis. Trans Am Ophthalmol Soc 79:541–624, 1981

23. Jones BR: Principles in the management of oculomycosis. Am J Ophthalmol 79:719–751, 1975

24. Jones BR, Richards AB, Morgan G: Direct fungal infection of the eye in Britain. Trans Ophthalmol Soc UK 89:727–741, 1969

25. Kessler E, Kennah HE, Brown SI: *Pseudomonas* protease, purification, partial characterization, and its effect on collagen proteoglycan and rabbit corneas. Invest Ophthalmol Vis Sci 16:488–497, 1977

26. Kessler E, Mondino BJ, Brown SI: The corneal response to *Pseudomonas aeruginosa*: histopathological and enzymatic characterization. Invest Ophthalmol Vis Sci 16:116–125, 1977

27. Ketaconozole labeling revised. FDA Drug Bull 14:17–18, 1984

28. Kozarsky AM, Stulting RD, Waring GO III, et al: Penetrating keratoplasty for exogenous *Paecilomyces* keratitis followed by postoperative endophthalmitis. Am J Ophthalmol 98:552–557, 1984

29. Leibowitz HM: Bacterial keratitis, in Leibowitz HM (ed): Corneal Disorders; Clinical Diagnosis and Management. Philadelphia, W.B. Saunders Co, 1984, pp 353–386

30. Leibowitz HM, Berrospi AR: Initial treatment of descemetocele with hydrophilic contact lenses. Ann Ophthalmol 7:1161–1166, 1975

31. Leibowitz HM, Kupferman A: Topically administered corticosteroids; effect on antibiotic-treated bacterial keratitis. Arch Ophthalmol 98:1287–1290, 1980

32. Leisegang TJ: Corneal complications from herpes zoster ophthalmicus. Ophthalmology 92:316–324, 1985

33. Leisegang TJ, Forster RK: Spectrum of microbial keratitis in south Florida. Am J Ophthalmol 90:38–47, 1980

34. Mandell GL, Rubin W, Hook EW: The effect of an NADH oxidase inhibitor (hydrocortisone) on polymorphonuclear leukocyte bactericidal activity. J Clin Invest 49:1381–1388, 1970

35. Margo CE, Brinser JH, Groden L: Exfoliated cytopathology of *Acanthamoeba* keratitis (photo/essay). JAMA 255:2216, 1986

36. Meisler DM, Ludwig IH, Rutherford I, et al: Susceptibility of *Acanthamoeba* to cryotherapeutic method. Arch Ophthalmol 104:130–131, 1986

37. Meyers-Elliott RH, Elliott JH, Maxwell WA, et al: HLA antigens in recurrent stromal herpes simplex virus keratitis. Am J Ophthalmol 89:54–57, 1980

38. Mondino BJ, Brown SI, Mondzelewski JP: Peripheral corneal ulcers with herpes zoster ophthalmicus. Am J Ophthalmol 86:611–614, 1978

39. Moore MB, McCulley JP, Luckenbach M, et al: *Acanthamoeba* keratitis associated with soft contact lenses. Am J Ophthalmol 100:396–403, 1985

40. Nagington J, Watson PG, Playfair TJ, et al: Amoebic infection of the eye. Lancet 2:1537–1540, 1974

41. Naumann G, Green WR, Zimmerman LE: Mycotic keratitis; a histopathologic study of 73 cases. Am J Ophthalmol 64:668–682, 1967

42. Polack FM, Kaufman HE: Penetrating keratoplasty in herpetic keratitis. Am J Ophthalmol 73:908–913, 1972

43. Polack FM, Kaufman HE, Newmark E: Keratomycosis; medical and surgical treatment. Arch Ophthalmol 85:410–416, 1971

44. Pflugfelder SC, Zwickey TA, Forster RK, et al: Exogenous fungal endophthalmitis. Ophthalmology 93 (Suppl): 95, 1986

45. Raber IM, Laibson PR, Kurz GH, et al: *Pseudomonas* corneoscleral ulcers. Am J Ophthalmol 92:353–362, 1981

46. Sanders N: Penetrating keratoplasty in treatment of fungus keratitis. Am J Ophthalmol 70:24–30, 1970

47. Sanitato JJ, Kelley CG, Kaufman HE: Surgical management of peripheral fungal keratitis (keratomycosis). Arch Ophthalmol 102:1502–1509, 1984

48. Savir H: Anterior segment resection because of *Fusarium solani* keratitis and endophthalmitis. Arch Ophthalmol 102:824–825, 1984

49. Searl SS, Udell IJ, Sadun A, et al: Aspergillus keratitis with intraocular invasion. Ophthalmology 88:1244–1250, 1981

50. Singh G, Malik SRK: Therapeutic keratoplasty in fungal corneal ulcers. Br J Ophthalmol 56:41–45, 1972

51. Singh G, Malik SRK, Bhatnager PK: Therapeutic value of keratoplasty in keratomycosis; an experimental study. Arch Ophthalmol 92:48–50, 1974

52. Smokin G, Tabbaa K, Whitcher J: Infectious Diseases of the Eye. Baltimore, Williams & Wilkins, 1984, pp 96–101

53. Theodore FH, Jakobiec FA, Juechter KB, et al: The diagnostic value of a ring infiltrate in Acanthamoebic keratitis. Ophthalmology 92:1471–1479, 1985

54. Tullo AB, Easty DL, Shimeld C, et al: Isolation of herpes simplex virus from corneal discs of patients with chronic stromal keratitis. Trans Ophthalmol Soc UK 104:159–165, 1985

55. Twining SS, Davis SD, Hyndiuk RA: Proteases and descemetoceles in experimental pseudomonas keratitis. Invest Ophthalmol Vis Sci 27 (Suppl): 209, 1986

56. Van Horn DL, Davis SD, Hyndiuk RA, et al: Experimental *Pseudomonas* keratitis in the rabbit: bacteriologic, clinical, and microscopic observations. Invest Ophthalmol Vis Sci 20:213–221, 1981

57. Waring GO, Ekins MB: Corneal perforation in herpes zoster ophthalmicus caused by eyelid scarring with exposure keratitis, in Sundmacher R (ed): Herpetic Eye Diseases. Munchen, JF Bergmann, 1981, pp 469–478

58. Wright P, Warhurst D, Jones BR: Acanthamoeba keratitis successfully treated medically. Br J Ophthalmol 69:778–782, 1985

# 9

# Corneal and Bulbar Conjunctival Tumors

## Richard D. Grutzmacher      Frederick T. Fraunfelder

This chapter discusses the diagnosis and management of the major corneal and conjunctival tumors. It is divided into four main sections that encompass congenital lesions, epithelial tumors, melanotic tumors, and soft tissue tumors. The pertinent features regarding etiology, clinical manifestations, differential diagnosis, diagnostic approach, and finally surgical approach are discussed. Emphasis is placed on the more commonly encountered tumors.

We provide details of our management of conjunctival and corneal tumors. We acknowledge that other authors may have different approaches to these entities that are successful in their hands. Our intent is to provide a practical approach to conjunctival and corneal tumors that we have found most useful.

## CONGENITAL LESIONS

This section discusses the two most commonly encountered congenital epibulbar tumors, namely dermoids and dermolipomas. These choristomas are congenital, nonprogressive, and usually not associated with other ocular or systemic anomalies. Clinically and histopathologically dermoid tumors are quite distinct from dermolipomas.

Associated ocular or systemic anomalies can occur in up to 30 percent of epibulbar dermoids.[47] The ocular anomalies can include lid colobomas, mircophthalmos, Duane's retraction syndrome, and aniridia. The most notable systemic anomaly associated with dermoids or dermolipomas is Goldenhar's syndrome (oculoauriculo-vertebral dysplasia). Goldenhar's syndrome consists of pretragal appendages, preauricular fistulas, and epibulbar dermoids or dermolipomas. Epibulbar tumors are found in approximately two-thirds of Goldenhar's syndrome.[1] Other systemic conditions associated with epibulbar tumors include neurocutaneous syndrome, nevus flammeus, and neurofibromatosis.

## Dermoids

Dermoids are firm, whitish, nodular masses that arise most frequently at the inferotemporal limbus (Fig. 9-1). The size is quite variable ranging from 2 mm to, rarely, as large as 15 mm in size. These tumors usually are of cosmetic concern; however, if large, they can interfere with lid closure, create astigmatism, or potentially obstruct the visual axis. A corneal lipid deposition is commonly present, separated from the dermoid by a clear zone.

Histopathologically, dermoids consist of stratified squamous epithelium which may be keratinized with fine hairs present. The stroma consists of a dense, collagenous tissue with pilosebaceous units including hair follicles, sweat, and sebaceous glands. Less commonly these tumors can include cartilage, adipose tissue or lacrimal glandular elements.[15]

In most cases surgical excision should consist of a superficial scleral keratectomy (Fig. 9-2). This is generally the treatment of choice even if the dermoid involves deeper scleral layers. The exposed scleral portion should be covered with conjunctiva. If necessary, a unilateral conjunctival transplant can be performed to lessen the incidence of pseudopterygia formation. Deep excisions should be avoided as potential complications can include inadvertent perforation. If deep excision is necessary, a lamellar keratoplasty should be performed to provide adequate support and smooth contour.[9] This approach often is required if a cosmetic result is the primary goal.

## Dermolipomas

Dermolipomas are soft, yellowish, diffuse tumors that typically arise in the lateral canthal region and superotemporal fornix (Fig. 9-3). They are variable in size and can extend both anteriorly toward the cornea or posteriorly into the orbit.

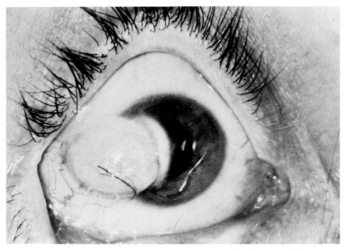

**Fig. 9-1.** Limbal dermoid with corneal lipid deposition.

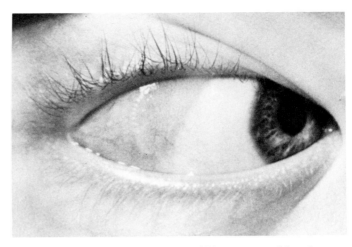

**Fig. 9-3.** Dermolipoma in 8-year-old boy managed by observation.

Histopathologically these choristomas consist of squamous epithelium covering a dense collagenous layer with excessive adipose tissue. Philosebaceous units are usually not present.

Management of dermolipomas varies with their size. Small dermolipomas, in general, should be observed to avoid operative complications. When excision is required partial removal of the anterior portion is recommended.[47] This can provide a good cosmetic result with minimal complications. Attempted complete excisions have resulted in significant ocular complications including keratoconjunctivitis sicca, excision of recti muscles, and excessive scarring.[9,13,47]

## EPITHELIAL LESIONS

### Papillomas

Conjunctival papillomas can be divided into two types: infectious and noninfectious. The noninfectious papillomas include an uncommon form termed "inverted papillomas," which are not discussed in this chapter.[57]

### Infectious Conjunctival Papillomas

*Infectious conjunctival papillomas* have clinical characteristics that are distinct from the noninfectious papillomas and there is rarely difficulty in the clinical diagnosis. Wilson and Ostler described the clinical features of infectious papillomas and how these differ from noninfectious causes (Table 9-1).[62] These benign tumors are usually asymptomatic in children or young adults, occurring most commonly in the inferior fornix. They may be multiple or bilateral in distribution. Although the inferior fornix and palpebral conjunctiva is the most common site, other areas of involvement include caruncle and, rarely, limbus. These tumors tend to be pedunculated, fleshy growths with little associated inflammatory reaction (Fig. 9-4).

Papovavirus has been implicated in the etiology of these papillomas.[38,39] Transmission to siblings from hand-to-eye contact is well documented.[62] These tumors rarely, if ever, undergo malignant transformation and generally show spontaneous resolution within a 2-year period.[62]

Treatment with the infectious form of conjunctival papillomas should be conservative. Multiple and extensive recurrences can occur following excision which can severely

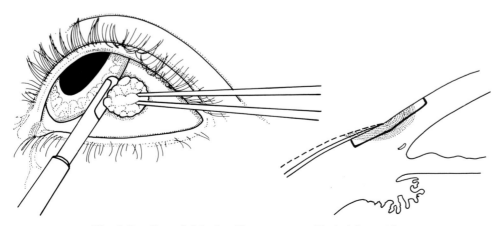

**Fig. 9-2.** Superficial scleral keratectomy of limbal dermoid.

**Table 9-1**
Clinical Characteristics of Conjunctival Papillomas*

| Infectious | Noninfectious |
|---|---|
| Usually in children or young adults | Usually in older adults |
| May be bilateral | Nearly always unilateral |
| May be multiple | Nearly always single |
| Usually on palpebral conjunctiva, fornix, or caruncle, especially below; less commonly at limbus | Usually on bulbar conjunctiva or at limbus |
| Pedunculated | Sessile or diffuse |
| Smooth surface | More surface irregularity and thickening |
| May occur with verrucae on eyelid or elsewhere | No such association |
| Multiple lesions may appear after excision of single lesion | Each recurrence usually single |
| Transmissible | Not transmissable |
| Usually little or no conjunctivitis; rarely moderate conjunctivitis | Occasionally marked conjunctivitis ("masquerade syndrome") |
| Occasionally fine ("toxic") epithelial keratitis | Cornea involved only by direct extension or mechanical factors |
| Rarely, if ever, malignant | Benign, dysplastic, or malignant |
| Spontaneous resolution common | Spontaneous resolution uncommon |

*Data from Wilson FM, Ostler HB: Conjunctival papilloma in siblings. Am J Ophthalmol 77:103–107, 1974. Published with permission from the American Journal of Ophthalmology. Copyright by The Ophthalmic Publishing Company.

aggravate this condition. In view of the common spontaneous resolution over a 2-year period, intervention should only be performed in the following circumstances: (1) if lid closure is not possible, (2) if it is cosmetically disfiguring, (3) following multiple extensive recurrences, or (4) if malignant transformation is suspected.

If treatment is indicated, we believe that surgical excision, combined with cryotherapy, is the management of

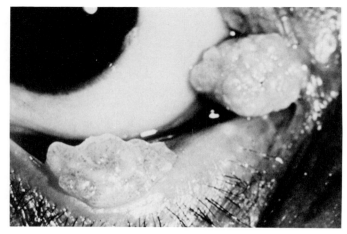

**Fig. 9-4.** Infectious conjunctival papillomas in 6-year-old managed by excision and cryotherapy.

choice.[20] These procedures are usually performed under general anesthesia due to the age group involved. Lid sutures may be advantageous for maximal exposure. Care must be taken to avoid seeding of uninvolved conjunctival areas. This may occur by grasping uninvolved tissue with forceps previously used in excision of an adjacent lesion. Because these lesions represent epithelial abnormalities, deep excisions are unnecessary. The surgical bed and immediate surgical margin should then be treated with a double freeze–thaw cryotherapy using a nitrous oxide cryoprobe. Contact should be made with a fully frozen cryoprobe tip for a 3-second interval. Contiguous areas of cryotherapy are applied to the entire bed. This is followed by a slow thaw and a reapplication of the cryotherapy. If liquid nitrogen cryogen is used with a 2–4 mm solid tip, the duration of contact should be 1 second. Irrigating solution should be available to release the probe from the tissues. If the probe is not completely frozen prior to contact it may adhere to the tissue. Postoperative treatment generally consists of topical antibiotics, corticosteroids, and cycloplegics.

Other treatment modalities have been described for particularly difficult cases with multiple recurrences. Included among these is carbon dioxide laser therapy immediately following excision of the main papilloma. This results in thermal ablation to the base and margins of the excision bed with reported good results.[53] Another treatment described includes the use of dinitro-clorobenzene (DCNB) together with surgical debulking of the papilloma.[5] This procedure consists of prior sensitization of the patient to DCNB utilizing skin contact. When hypersensitivity has been demonstrated surgical excision with application of DCNB to the surgical bed is performed. We feel these latter two modalities should be reserved for treatment failures utilizing excision plus cryotherapy.

### Noninfectious Papillomas

In contrast to infectious papillomas the *noninfectious papillomas* generally occur in older individuals at a single site that affects only one eye. The location is typically limbal or less commonly bulbar conjunctiva. They tend to be sessile in appearance and if large may have feeder vessels (Figs. 9-5 and 9-6). The clinical distinction between benign limbal papillomas and premalignant or malignant squamous epithelial neoplasms can be difficult. Noninfectious conjunctival papillomas should be treated in an identical fashion to precancerous and cancerous squamous epithelial lesions of the conjunctiva and limbus. This treatment consists of surgical excision combined with a double freeze–thaw therapy utilizing a nitrous oxide cryoprobe. This technique is described in detail under the precancerous and cancerous sections of epithelial lesions.

## Precancerous Lesions

### Conjunctival Intraepithelial Neoplasia

Pizzarello and Jakobiec initially coined the term "conjunctival intraepithelial neoplasia" (CIN) to describe nonpigmented in situ neoplasms of the epithelium.[48] This is a

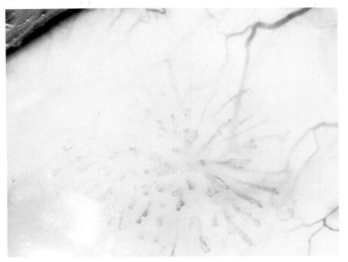

**Fig. 9-5.**   Limbal papilloma.

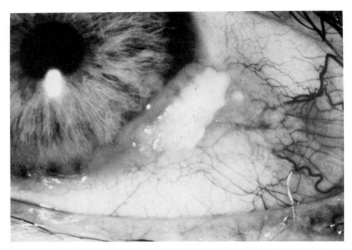

**Fig. 9-7.**   Conjunctival intraepithelial neoplasia-histopathology revealed carcinoma in situ.

useful designation because it encompasses a wide range of epithelial abnormalities from mild dysplasia to carcinoma in situ. Squamous cell carcinoma is diagnosed when this dysplastic process breaks through the epithelial basement membrane invading the substantia propria.

The clinical features of epithelial conjunctival tumors include the following. They occur in the elderly population usually in the sixth to seventh decade of life. There is a male predominance noted with a male:female ratio of approximately 5:1. They are typically located in the limbal area, most commonly in the interpalpebral portion of the limbus. These neoplasias typically form an exophytic thickening of the conjunctiva which is usually sessile in pattern and gelatinous in appearance (Fig. 9-7). A leukoplakic appearance is present in approximately 15 percent of these lesions.[48] *Leukoplakia* is a clinical, descriptive term referring to a whitish lesion on a mucous membrane. Although this term commonly is associated with hyperkeratosis or parakeratosis causing this whitish appearance, it is not a pathologic diag-

nosis. Local conjunctival inflammation is seen in approximately 50 percent of cases. These lesions are characteristically unifocal and slow growing with a low virulence. Large feeder vessels are frequently present if the lesion assumes a substantial size. Less commonly encountered are papillary forms, which are readily distinguished from the infectious conjunctival papillomas in children and young adults as described above.

The etiology of CIN and squamous cell carcinoma is felt by most to be a combination of two factors. The first is chronic actinic (ultraviolet) and general environmental exposure. The second factor is related to the characteristics of the limbal transition zone itself. Many believe this transition zone of conjunctiva to corneal epithelium predisposes this area to dysplastic processes analogous to cervical dysplasia of the uterus.

It is useful to review some basic histologic definitions when dealing with these lesions. Table 9-2 provides a basic definition of a variety of epithelial abnormalities and their histopathologic features including acanthosis, hyperkeratosis, parakeratosis, dysplasia, and squamous cell carcinoma. In CIN 90 percent of the cells are made up of dysplastic cells that appear as a "small, bland spindle cell."[48] The cytoplasm is typically eosinophilic with an ellipsoidal nucleus without prominent nucleoli. Approximately one-third of the lesions demonstrated mild dysplasia located in the basal one-third of the epithelium (Grade I dysplasia). The remaining 70 percent show more severe dysplasia with involvement up to full epithelial thickness which has been termed "Grade III dysplasia" or carcinoma in situ (Fig. 9-8).[48]

The differential diagnosis can include amelanocytic malignant melanomas, viral papillomas, actinic keratosis, and pseudoepitheliomatous hyperplasia. Pseudoepitheliomatous hyperplasia can occur anywhere on the conjunctiva. It is characterized by a rapid growth and can occur overlying an existing pterygium, pinguecula, or prior surgical excision site. It often has a whitish, inflamed, slightly elevated appearance which can cause confusion with CIN or

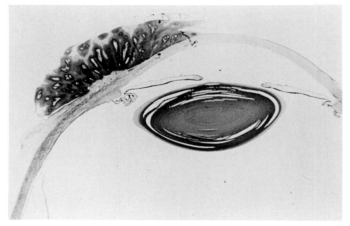

**Fig. 9-6.**   Histopathology-limbal papilloma (Courtesy of M. Reeh).

**Table 9-2**
Epithelial, Intraepithelial, and Subepithelial Lesions

| Histologic Diagnosis | Histopathologic Features | Clinical Appearance |
| --- | --- | --- |
| Acanthosis | Thickening of epithelium, particularly stratum spinosium | Clinical differentiation is difficult, but sometimes the larger and more hyperemic, elevated, and vascular are Grade III and squamous cell carcinoma |
| Hyperkeratosis | Surface keratinization of epithelium | |
| Parakeratosis | Same as above, but with cell nuclei persisting in keratin layer | |
| Dysplasia | Abnormal maturational sequence (disordered cellular polarity) from basal to surface layers of epithelium; usually implies some atypia (malignant appearance) of individual cells. Grade I only located in basal 1/3 and Grade III carcinoma in situ includes full thickness | |
| Squamous Cell Carcinoma | The dysplastic process has broken through the basement membrane | |

squamous cell carcinoma. Histologically, these lesions consist of a hyperplasia of a large epidermoid cell with surface parakaratosis and hyperkaratosis. The epidermoid cells themselves tend to show a low nuclear:cytoplasmic ratio without atypia. There is often a prominent inflammatory process at the base of this lesion and leukocytes frequently infiltrate the squamous proliferations.

*Diagnosis—CIN.* The clinical differentiation between various forms of dysplasias and squamous cell carcinomas can be difficult except with advanced lesions. Squamous cell carcinomas with invasion in the underlying sclera and fixation is a useful diagnostic point as is corneal invasion or any evidence of intraocular invasion. Certainly the latter would be rarely encountered. Leukoplakia is not a helpful clinical finding as this can be encountered in CIN, squamous cell carcinoma, papillomas, and a variety of conditions associated with hyperkeratosis. Often the extent of the epithelial lesion can be clinically underestimated. Rose bengal staining

as described by Wilson[61] is quite helpful in establishing the extent of involved conjunctiva. Retroillumination during slit lamp biomicroscopy can be of value to determine the extent of corneal involvement.

Other adjuncts to diagnosis can include exfoliative cytology. Scrapings performed in the office utilizing either Giemsa or Papanicolaou's smears can show atypical cytology.[25,44,56] These procedures are generally performed using a topical anesthetic and a platinum spatula. If multiple specimens are taken to outline a tumor area, individual #15 Bard-Parker blades are useful. The conjunctival scraping is placed on a glass slide and immediately fixed in 95% alcohol and submitted for the appropriate stains. We believe the main value of exfoliative cytology is in the early recognition of a recurrence of a previously treated lesion and in outlining the extent of dysplastic epithelium for surgical excision in cases with indistinct margins. This is especially true with large tumors (>180°) in order to identify and preserve normal conjunctiva.

If it is suspected that intraocular extension may have occurred and cells are present in the aqueous, then paracentesis for cytology can be of use in confirming intraocular invasion.[46] This is seldom necessary if gonioscopy shows no tumor invasion.

*Treatment—CIN and Squamous Cell Carcinoma.* Our current management for both CIN and squamous cell carcinoma consists of a combination of excision plus cryotherapy.[21,22] Prior studies utilizing excision alone for carcinoma in situ resulted in recurrence rates in the 30–40 percent range.[6,48,63] Freezing alone can be associated with a similar recurrence rate.[21,22] The combination of excision plus superficial cryotherapy has dramatically improved the results of treatment for these lesions.

The goals of cryotherapy are for a rapid freeze followed by a slow thaw. The best results are obtained using a double freeze–thaw technique to a temperature of approximately −25°C. This rapid freeze results in ice crystallization and

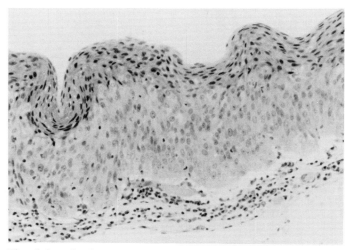

**Fig. 9-8.** Conjunctival dysplasia involving basal two-thirds of conjunctival epithelium.

**Table 9-3**
Cryogen Boiling Points

| Cryogen | Cryogen Boiling Points |
| --- | --- |
| Freon 12 | −29.8°C |
| Freon 22 | −41.0°C |
| Carbon dioxide | −38.5°C |
| Nitrous oxide | −89.5°C |
| Liquid nitrogen | −195.6°C |

mechanical injury to the involved cells, together with changes in electrolyte concentration and precipitation of proteins. Significant biochemical injuries occur during the thaw. At temperatures of 0°C smaller vessels constrict and can result in a localized ischemic necrosis of the involved tissue.[60] Table 9-3 lists the available cryogens and their corresponding boiling points. Liquid nitrogen has the lowest boiling point and thus greatest "heat sink." It remains the cryogen of

choice for treatment of skin and lid neoplasms. This generally is used with thermocouples to control the degree of freezing.

Initial reports on combination excision and cryotherapy for intraepithelial conjunctival tumors utilized liquid nitrogen cryogen.[21,22] Devine and Anderson have demonstrated, in a small series, that nitrous oxide cryoprobes are also highly effective although require slightly longer contact time.[10,11] The common availability and ease of use of nitrous oxide makes this attractive for most ophthalmologists.

Our procedure for management of these lesions is as follows (Fig. 9-9). We like to have two sets of instruments (scissors-forceps) available—one to be used solely in the tumor area and one to be used peripheral to this. Topical anesthesia is applied and the eye is prepped in the usual fashion. Rose bengal can be instilled if there is any question regarding the extent of involvement. Subconjunctival 1% lidocaine with epinephrine is next injected to elevate the

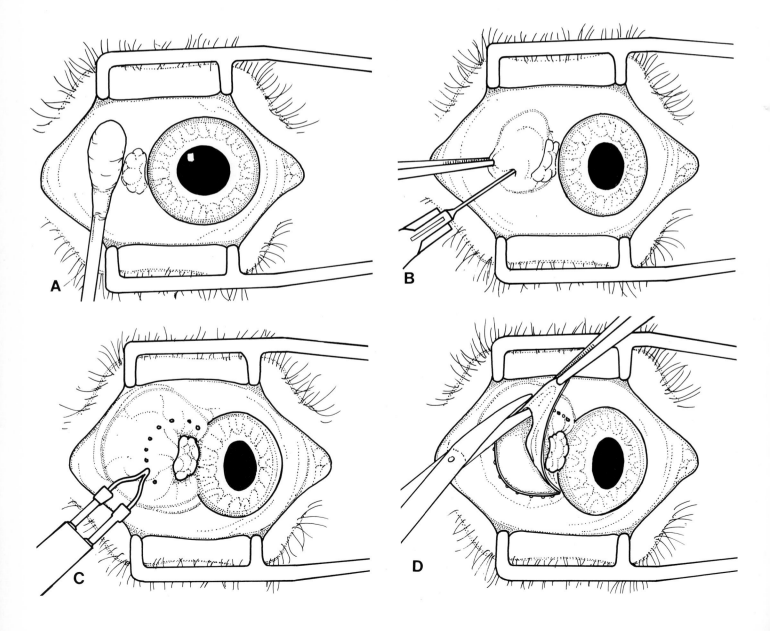

lesion from the underlying sclera. If the lesion does not elevate and there is no history of prior surgery, squamous cell carcinoma should be suspected with possible scleral invasion. Multiple drops of topical anesthetic are applied to the cornea to soften the epithelium. Cautery is next applied in normal conjunctiva 1.5 mm from the suspected edge of the lesion.

Westcot scissors are used to incise through the cautery marks down to bare sclera. If there is adherence of the lesion to the episcleral tissue a superficial sclerectomy is performed in the involved area. If the cornea is involved, slightly greater than 1 mm of normal corneal epithelium together with the involved epithelium is removed by gentle scraping toward

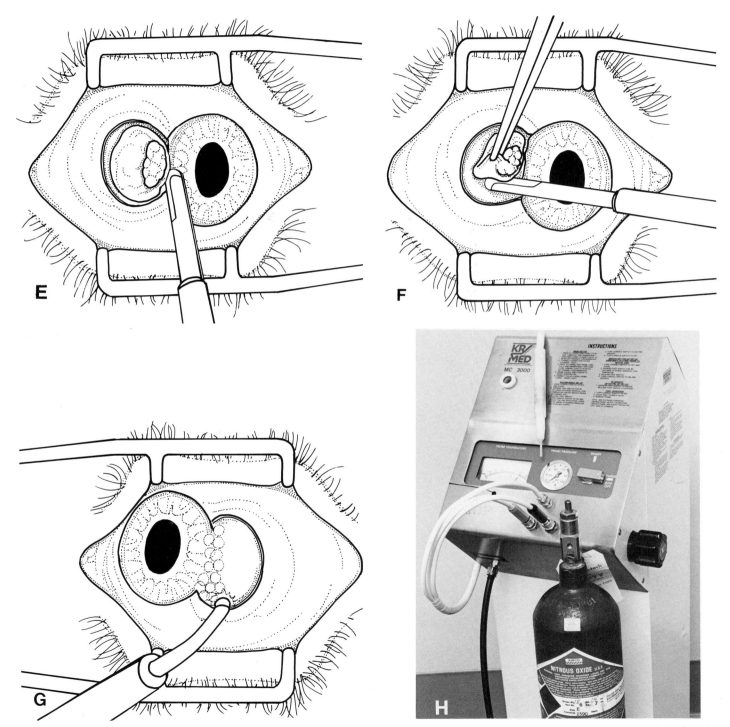

**Fig. 9-9.** Management of conjunctival intraepithelial neoplasia and squamous cell carcinoma: (A) cotton swab application of topical anesthetic; (B) subconjunctival injection of 1% lidocaine with epinephrine; (C) cautery applied 1.5 mm from lesion edge; (D) incision to bare sclera through cautery marks; (E) removal of adjacent corneal epithelium; (F) superficial sclerokeratectomy at limbus; (G) double freeze–thaw cryotherapy to involve limbus, areas of adhesions, and excision margins; (H) nitrous oxide cryounit.

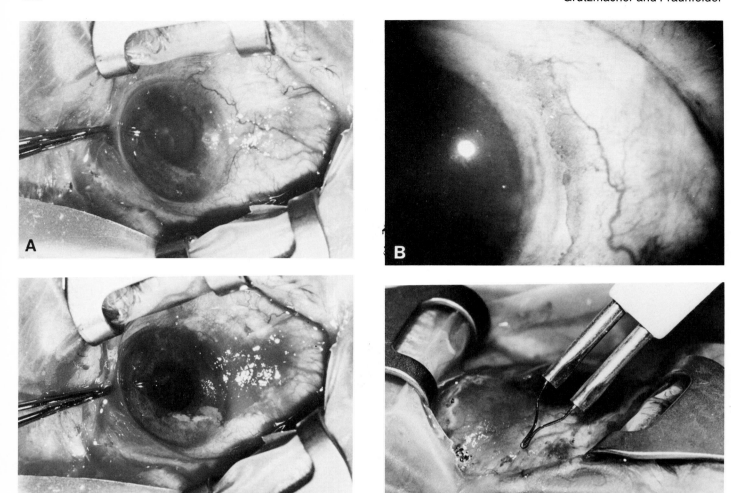

the limbus. If a suspected squamous cell carcinoma is present then a superficial keratectomy is performed in this area. Once both ends are freed a very superficial sclerokeratectomy can be performed at the limbus excising the mass as a whole. Instruments that are used on the tumor itself should not be used elsewhere during this procedure. Bleeding episcleral vessels can be lightly cauterized. The involved limbus, areas of adhesions, and excision margins are next frozen in a double freeze–thaw manner. Liquid nitrogen can be used through a 2–4 mm cryoprobe tip or nitrous oxide can be used utilizing a flat-tipped probe. The probe should be frozen entirely prior to contact with the tissues. If liquid nitrogen is the cryogen used then a 1-second application should be applied using overlapping imprints to cover the areas to be treated. This should then be allowed to thaw followed by a repeat treatment. If nitrous oxide is the cryogen chosen then the applications should be for a period of 3 seconds at each site. The most important area is the limbus as this is the most common site of recurrence. We do not allow freezing to extend greater than 1–1.5 mm onto the peripheral cornea. Finally, if the size of the defect permits, absorbable sutures can be used utilizing a different set of instruments to close

the conjunctival defect. It often, however, is unnecessary to close these defects and they will heal readily (Fig. 9-10).

Utilizing the above technique, a 92 percent cure was achieved with a minimum 3-year follow-up.[22] Complications are generally minimal using this superficial form of cryotherapy. Topical antibiotics are given postoperatively with a pressure dressing for 24 hours. Mild iritis is not uncommon. Corneal complications are usually minimal except for superficial scarring or pseudopterygia formation in areas of prior keratectomies. Because this can, early on, be confused with a recurrence it is important to perform only a very superficial "limbectomy" with little to no keratectomy. In the vast majority of cases removal of corneal epithelium without keratectomy is adequate.

Contraindications to this form of treatment include intraocular invasion or involvement of the fornix. Intraocular invasion requires enucleation. Deep corneal or scleral invasion requires lamellar grafting. Fornix involvement with squamous cell carcinomas often follow the globe posteriorly and the posterior extent of the lesion is unknown. Therefore, other modalities of treatment are required in these cases including possible exenteration.

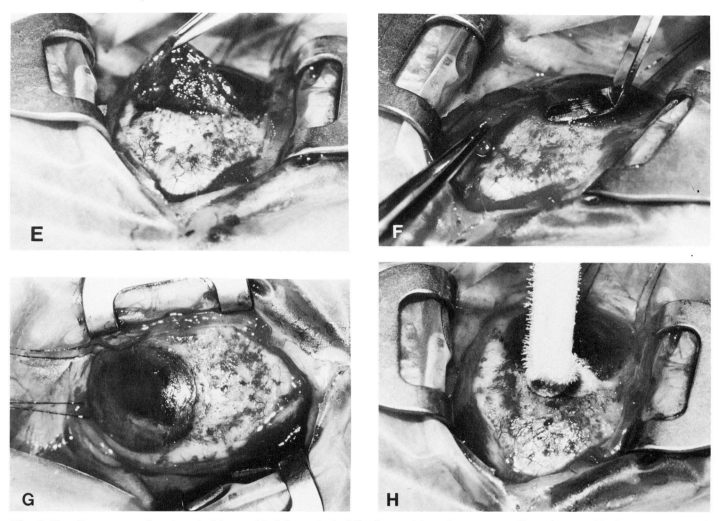

**Fig. 9-10.** Recurrence of conjunctival intraepithelial neoplasia following excision of squamous cell carcinoma of limbus: (A) dysplastic limbal and corneal conjunctiva; (B) 1% rose bengal outlining conjunctival epithelial involvement; (C) intraoperative rose bengal staining abnormal conjunctival and corneal epithelium; (D) cautery application surrounding involved lesion; (E) excision of lesion to bare sclera; (F) superficial scleral keratectomy of limbus; (G) bare scleral bed; (H) application of cryotherapy to limbus. (Fig. 9-8 is the corresponding histopathologic slide.)

The majority of recurrences occur within the first 6 months of treatment and nearly all recur within 2 years.[6,48] Recurrences are managed in an identical fashion to the above treatment.

### Corneal Intraepithelial Neoplasia

*Corneal intraepithelial neoplasia* consists of flat, gray plaques of epithelium extending from the limbal region onto the cornea. The central margin consists of fingerlike, fimbriated protrusions with abrupt transition from abnormal to normal epithelium. These corneal dysplasias typically arise adjacent to various limbal lesions (Fig. 9-11). Waring et al.'s report indicated the most common associated limbal lesion consisted of conjunctival intraepithelial neoplasia which ranged from dysplasia to carcinoma in situ.[58] Other limbal lesions can include squamous cell carcinoma, pinguecula, pterygium, and chronic conjunctival inflammation. These

lesions most commonly occur in men in the sixth to seventh decade. They are typically unilateral with a waxing and waning course if followed for months to years.

Histopathologically, these ground-glass sheets of epithelium demonstrate a hypercellular epithelium with pleomorphism and poor adhesion. The cell nuclei are pleomorphic and enlarged frequently with a course, hyperchromatic nucleoplasm. Mitotic figures are rarely encountered. Most cases represent a mild displasia. Waring et al. found no instance of corneal carcinoma in situ or invasion of Bowman's layer.[58]

The differential diagnosis can include a variety of entities that are usually readily distinguished from corneal intraepithelial neoplasia. These include squamous cell carcinoma invading the cornea, hereditary benign intraepithelial dyskeratosis,[50] corneal pannus, and epithelial basement membrane dystrophy.

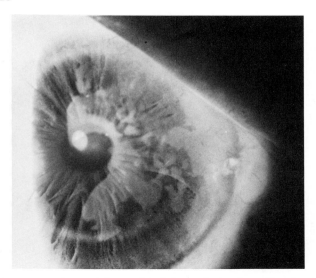

**Fig. 9-11.** Corneal intraepithelial neoplasia. Retroillumination demonstrates grey plaques of dysplastic epithelium.

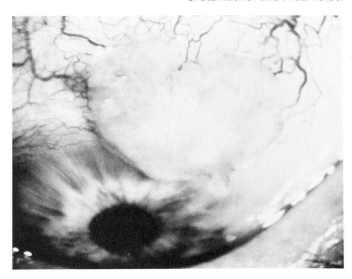

**Fig. 9-12.** Squamous cell carcinoma (Courtesy of R.E. Kalina).

Management of corneal intraepithelial neoplasia varies with the extent of the epithelial involvement and a nature of the associated limbal lesion. If a benign corneal dysplasia is associated with a pinguecula or pterygium with little suspicion of conjunctival intraepithelial neoplasia then observation is appropriate.

Surgical intervention is indicated when the visual axis is involved or if the associated limbal lesion is potentially premalignant or malignant. Anesthesia should consist of topical anesthetics for the corneal portion and subconjunctival injections of 1% lidocaine with epinephrine for excision of the associated limbal lesion. Instillation of 1% rose bengal facilitates recognition of the extent of the involved process. The corneal epithelium can be scraped using a #64 Beaver blade (Beaver, Belmont, MA) removing all the dysplastic epithelium toward the limbal area. Superficial keratectomy is not required. Limbal lesions can be excised as previously described. If there is suspicion of either conjunctival intraepithelial neoplasia involving the limbus or possibly squamous cell carcinoma then a double freeze–thaw cryotherapy should be applied to the limbal area. Cryotherapy of the limbus should not be associated with greater than 1–2 mm of corneal involvement and only with a superficial freeze.

## EPITHELIAL LESIONS

### Cancerous Lesions

#### Squamous Cell Carcinoma

As stated in the above section on CIN, a clinical differentiation between some forms of CIN and squamous cell carcinoma may not be possible. Fixation of the lesion to the underlying sclera, fixation of corneal epithelium to stroma, or ''iritis'' are features of invasive carcinomas. Certainly advanced, bulky lesions are more likely to represent carcino-

mas than intraepithelial neoplasias (Figs. 9-12–9-14). Often, however, histopathology is required to differentiate these lesions conclusively.

The etiology and management of squamous cell carcinoma is as described in the conjunctival intraepithelial neoplasia section. Evidence of intraocular invasion generally requires enucleation.[29,40,46,59] Extensive involvement into the fornices should not be treated by local excision and cryotherapy; rather, exenteration should be considered. Computerized tomography scans at the orbit and metastatic workup should be completed prior to consideration of exenteration. Orbit involvement with squamous cell carcinoma should be managed by exenteration.[43]

#### Mucoepidermoid Carcinoma

A rare form of carcinoma of the conjunctiva is a variant termed ''mucoepidermoid carcinoma.'' This tumor consists of epidermoid and mucus-producing cells. Mucoepidermoid carcinoma most commonly occurs in the salivary glands and

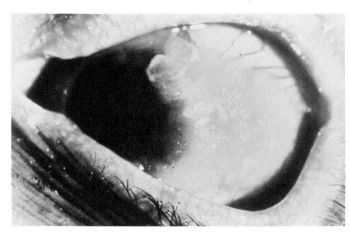

**Fig. 9-13.** Large, sessile squamous cell carcinoma.

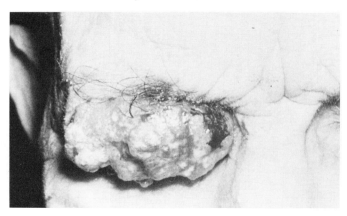

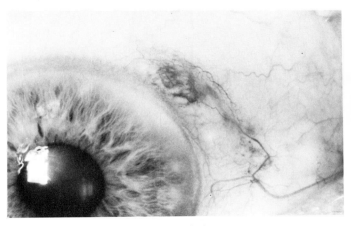

**Fig. 9-14.** Eighty-year-old man who refused surgery for limbal squamous cell carcinoma (courtesy of M. Reeh).

**Fig. 9-15.** Limbal nevus.

less commonly is found in the upper respiratory tract. Occurrence of the tumor in the conjunctiva is rare, but diagnosis is important in regards to its more aggressive tendencies.[3,23,49]

Clinically this tumor is indistinguishable from squamous cell carcinoma of the conjunctiva.[49] Histologically these tumors consist of epidermoid (squamous) cells together with clear or vacuolated cells which show positive staining for mucus. These stains include alcian blue, mucicarmine, and PAS. This form of carcinoma has a much more aggressive behavior and can result in both intraocular and orbital extension.

Initially treatment would be the same as for squamous cell carcinoma. Ocular invasion requires enucleation. Orbital invasion without evidence of metastasis should be managed by exenteration.

### Spindle-Cell Carcinoma

*Spindle-cell carcinoma* also resembles clinically squamous cell carcinoma. It is characterized by spindle-shaped cells in continuity with the overlying epithelium. Its tendency is for more aggressive behavior similar to the mucoepidermoid carcinoma. Initial management is the same as with squamous cell carcinoma.[8]

## MELANOTIC TUMORS

This section deals with conjunctival nevi, bilateral acquired melanosis, primary acquired melanosis, and malignant melanoma of the conjunctiva. Because ocular melanocytosis and oculodermal melanocytosis are not associated with conjunctival tumors, these entities are to be discussed.

### Conjunctival Nevi

Conjunctival nevi are felt to be congenital but only 50 percent are apparent during the first decade of life. These lesions are usually flat, sharply demarcated, and located near the limbus (Fig. 9-15), semilunar fold, or caruncle (Fig.

9-16). They can show variable pigmentation and can change in size and degree of pigmentation during childhood. This is especially true during puberty when they are commonly first noticed. Increased pigmentation does not equate with increased growth, and in addition to occurring during puberty can also be seen during pregnancy. Thirty percent may show no pigmentation or a very slight pigmentation at most.[26] Approximately half of conjunctival nevi have a cystic appearance.[64] These cysts are felt to develop from epithelial embryonic nests arising within the substantia propria. This is an important clinical finding as it strongly points to a diagnosis of conjunctival nevi.

There are three common histopathologic types of conjunctival nevi: (1) intraepithelial (junctional), which consists of nests of nevus cells confined to the basal epithelial area; (2) compound nevi, which consist of both an intraepithelial and subepithelial population of melanocytes; and (3) subepithelial nevi in which melanocytes are found only in the substantia propria with no intraepithelial presence. As with cutaneous nevi, conjunctival nevi tend to progress through these stages with age and can ultimately become involutional.

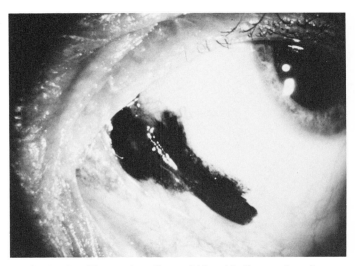

**Fig. 9-16.** Nevus of semilunar fold and bulbar conjunctiva.

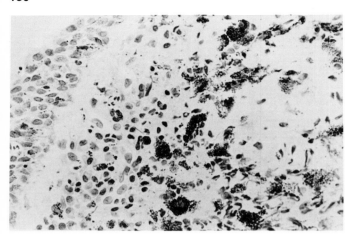

**Fig. 9-17.**　Compound nevus.

Intraepithelial (or junctional) nevi result in a flat, pigmented lesion. These are commonly seen in the first or early part of the second decade of life. The only significant confusion in differential diagnosis comes when a junctional nevus acquires pigmentation or becomes noticed past the second decade of life. This situation can cause confusion, both clinically and histopathologically, with early forms of primary acquired melanosis. Jakobiec has stated ". . . nevi invariably make their appearance within the first two decades of life."[32] The appearance of flat, new pigmentation past the second decade of life in whites should be considered possible primary acquired melanosis and managed appropriately for that condition.

Subepithelial and compound nevi constitute the majority of conjunctival nevi. These nevi may occasionally enlarge and even thicken in contrast to the intraepithelial nevus during puberty and pregnancy with the formation of epithelial cysts. These nevi seldom become inflamed or develop new blood vessels.

The histopathologic appearance of the nevus cell is a polyhedral cell with a round, oval nucleus and evenly distributed chromatin. The nuclei can occasionally assume a polygonal or a spindle-shaped appearance and can occasionally show nucleoli. The cytoplasm typically stains poorly with eosin, giving these cells a clear appearance on hematoxylin and eosin preparations. Approximately two-thirds of nevus cells, however, will demonstrate some pigment in the protoplasm (Fig. 9-17).[52]

The management of conjunctival nevi is general simple observation. If nevi are observed to grow significantly past puberty or are a cosmetic problem, simple excision is the treatment of choice. Acquired pigmented lesions past the second decade in patients not pregnant or on estrogen therapy should have simple excisions. Following topical anesthetic, a subconjunctival injection using 1% lidocaine with epinephrine is performed. A 1-2 mm margin of nonpigmented conjunctiva should be included in the excision as many nevi are only partially pigmented. Substantia propria is not excised and closure of the conjunctiva generally is not necessary. Topical antibiotics are used for 1 week.

Conjunctival nevi rarely give rise to malignant melanoma of the conjunctiva. This entity is discussed under "Malignant Melanomas."

## Bilateral Acquired Melanosis

*Bilateral acquired melanosis* can be racial, metabolic, or toxic.[66] The vast majority of cases are noted in blacks and other pigmented races. The characteristic location is in the limbal and perilimbal conjunctiva. In darkly pigmented individuals the conjunctival melanosis can rarely spread onto the cornea, resulting in a condition termed "striate melanokeratosis" (Fig. 9-18; see color insert following page 139). The racial form is characteristically nonprogressive past the second decade of life.[26] The histopathology is significant for increased melanin content in the basal epithelial cells with otherwise normal epithelial maturation and normal cytology. Bilateral acquired melanosis is a normal finding in pigmented races and does not predispose to the development of malignant melanoma. Its inclusion here is to point out differences between this form of melanosis and primary acquired melanosis.

## Primary Acquired Melanosis

*Primary acquired melanosis* (PAM) typically occurs as unilateral acquired pigmentation of the conjunctiva occurring in middle-aged whites. The earliest appearance is a flat, somewhat diffuse, lightly pigmented area of conjunctiva (Fig. 9-19; see color insert following page 139). Its clinical course is of slow progression with a waxing and waning pattern of growth. The most common location is at the limbus; however, the condition can be multifocal with involvement of the fornices, palpebral conjunctiva, semilunar fold, caruncle, and external lids (Fig. 9-20; see color insert following page 139). The use of ultraviolet light (Wood's lamp) can be helpful in determining the full extent of the conjunctival melanosis.[52] A histologic classification of primary acquired melanosis, modified from Spencer[55] and Folberg et al.[17] is clinically useful (Table 9-4).

Stage Ia-PAM without atypia histologically appears as a proliferation of typical-appearing melanocytes along the basal epithelial layer with increased pigmentation in the surrounding epithelial cells (Fig. 9-21). Stage Ib-PAM with atypical melanocytic hyperplasia occurs in varying types of patterns and degree of severity (Fig. 9-22):[18]

1. Basilar hyperplasia: proliferation of melanocytes confined to the basilar layer of the epithelium.
2. Basilar nests: cluster of melanocytes at the basilar level "pushing" the overlying epithelium upward.
3. Intraepithelial nests: cluster of melanocytes within epithelium.
4. Pagetoid involvement: individual melanocytes present within suprabasilar layers of epithelium.
5. In situ-like: full thickness of epithelium replaced by atypical melanocytes.

**Table 9-4**
Histologic Classification of Primary Acquired Melanosis and
Malignant Melanoma Associated with PAM*

I. Stage I—Primary Acquired Melanosis
   a. Without atypia
   b. With atypical melanocytic hyperplasia
      1. mild atypia—basilar hyperplasia
      2. moderate to severe dysplasia
II. Stage II—Malignant Melanoma Associated with PAM
   a. With superficially invasive melanoma (tumor thickness < 0.8 mm)
   b. With more deeply invasive melanoma (tumor thickness > 0.8 mm)

*Adapted from:

Spencer WH, Zimmerman LE: Conjunctiva. Neoplasms and related conditions, in Spencer WH (ed): Ophthalmic Pathology. An Atlas and Textbook. Philadelphia, WB Saunders Co., 1985, pp 177–122

Folberg R, McLean IW, Zimmerman LE: Malignant melanoma of the conjunctiva. Hum Path 16:136–143, 1985

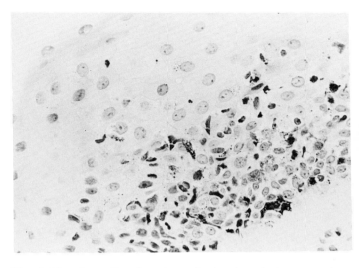

**Fig. 9-22.** Stage Ib-primary acquired melanosis demonstrating atypical melanocytic hyperplasia.

Recent work by Folberg, McLean, and Zimmerman[16,18] has shown that certain forms of atypical melanosis lead to a higher incidence of progression to malignant melanoma. They define two risk factors that show a significantly higher association of progression to melanoma: (1) a predominant pattern other than basilar hyperplasia (90 percent progression to malignant melanoma); and (2) any epitheloid cells present within the epithelium (75 percent progression to malignant melanoma) (Fig. 9-23).

Reese initially reported a 17 percent incidence of malignant melanomas arising from primary acquired melanosis.[51] This incidence occurred in lesions followed for a 5- to 10-year period. More recently Folberg et al. reported a 32 percent incidence of progression to malignant melanoma.[16,19] Of note was that primary acquired melanosis without atypia (Stage Ia) showed no progression to malignant melanoma in 13 cases. In contrast, primary acquired melanosis with atypia showed a 46 percent incidence of progression to malignant melanoma.

The distinction between primary acquired melanosis with and without atypia is a pathologic, not a clinical, distinction. Therefore acquired, unilateral, idiopathic, conjunctival pigmentations in whites that occur past the age of 20 years should be biopsied.

If the lesion is small, excisional biopsy as described under "Conjunctival Nevi" is adequate. If the biopsy is consistent with primary acquired melanosis without atypia and the margins show complete excision, further therapy is not necessary. If PAM with atypia is present, then excision, cryotherapy, or excision with cryotherapy should be performed.

Melanocytes are known to be sensitive to cryotherapy.[34,60] It is well established that a double freeze–thaw appli-

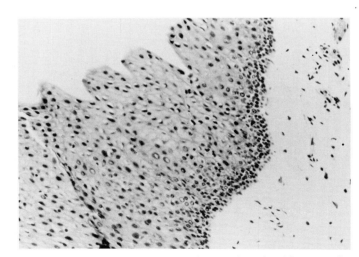

**Fig. 9-21.** Stage Ia-primary acquired melanosis without atypia. Typical-appearing melanocytic hyperplasia involving basal epithelium (histopathology slide of Fig. 9-19).

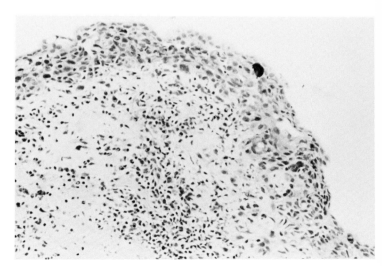

**Fig. 9-23.** Stage IIa superficially invasive malignant melanoma associated with primary acquired melanosis.

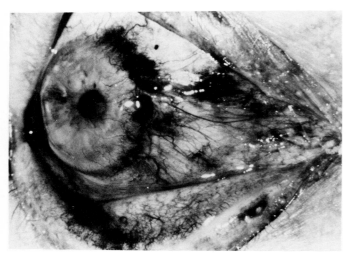

**Fig. 9-24.** Primary acquired melanosis with limbal melanomas.

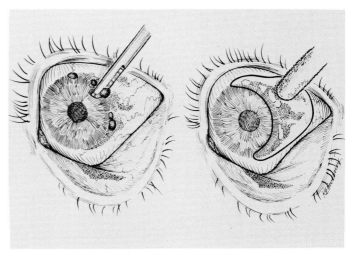

**Fig. 9-25.** Excision of all nodular lesions followed by application of cryotherapy to the surgical beds and contiguous areas of conjunctival pigmentation.

cation of cryotherapy is most efficacious. The intent is for a rapid freeze to $-20°C$ or lower together with a slow thaw. By definition PAM is an intraepithelial lesion. Therefore, nitrous oxide is a satisfactory cryogen for this condition.

Our management of primary acquired melanosis with atypia is as follows (Figs. 9-24 and 9-25). A topical anesthetic is applied followed by insertion of a speculum. One percent lidocaine with epinephrine is injected into the subconjunctival space ballooning the involved bulbar conjunctiva. A nitrous oxide cryoprobe is used with a flat tip. The cryoprobe is activated and "fully" frozen prior to touching the surgical bed. Contiguous applications of cryotherapy are applied for three seconds at each site.

Irrigating solutions should be available to release the probe from the tissue if necessary. A maximum of one-half of the bulbar conjunctiva can be treated at a single setting; however, it is safer to treat one quadrant per session.

Following completion of the initial cryo application, a second (double freeze–thaw) application is performed. Thermocouples are not used in the treatment of primary acquired melanosis involving the bulbar conjunctiva alone. The extent of cryotherapy should extend approximately 2 mm beyond the clinically apparent involved tissue. If flat corneal involvement is present the epithelium should be surgically removed using multiple surgical blades. In general no blade should be used for more than one scraping and multiple "clean" forceps should be available to avoid implantation of atypical melanocytes in uninvolved areas. Opposing palpebral and conjunctival areas of PAM should be treated on separate sessions to avoid symblepharon formation.

Postoperatively the treated area may show a sluffing of the conjunctiva with minimal disturbance in the underlying substantia propria. This allows for a healing of the conjunctiva from contiguous epithelium over a few weeks. Postoperative treatment consists of topical antibiotics and, if necessary, cycloplegics and corticosteroids. Patients should be seen frequently during the first few weeks to identify and lyse

symblepharon formation. In some patients daily lysis of symblepharon using a glass rod is required during the first week. Advanced cases are associated with a higher recurrence rate, undoubtedly due to migration of atypical melanocytes during the early stage healing.[32]

Fornix and palpebral conjunctiva can be treated in a similar fashion. If there is lid margin or external cutaneous involvement, liquid nitrogen spray utilizing a thermocouple may be the treatment of choice. The technique for liquid nitrogen spray cryotherapy for this and bulbar conjunctival lesions is well described.[19,60]

Recurrences are to be expected in primary acquired melanosis with atypia. Folberg reported a 61 percent incidence of recurrences in their 41 patients.[18] Factors associated with an increased incidence of recurrence include diffuse involvement, corneal involvement, and severity of atypia. Recurrences of conjunctival pigmentation should be biopsied prior to repeat treatment. Mild recurrences can result from melanin accumulation and macrophages (melanophages) in the substantia propria. Therefore recurrence of conjunctival pigmentation does not necessarily equate with recurrence of PAM. Recurrent pigmentation associated with increased thickening, however, should be managed by excisional biopsy with cryotherapy.

Complications of cryotherapy include early pain, erythema, and lid edema. Loss of lashes, depigmentation, and eyelid notching are potential complications when external lid or lid margins are treated. Extensive bulbar treatment has been reported to result in hypotony, corneal vascularization, iritis, and even cataract formation.[4] The severe complications generally occur, however, after using either liquid nitrogen cryogen or longer durations of treatment with a nitrous oxide cryoprobe. We have not encountered these severe intraocular complications utilizing the method described above.

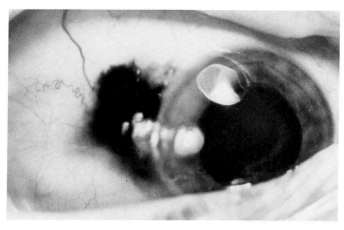

**Fig. 9-26.** Limbal malignant melanoma from conjunctival nevus.

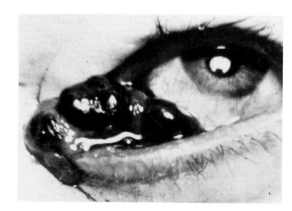

**Fig. 9-27.** Nodular melanoma involving medial fornix (Courtesy of M. Reeh).

## Malignant Melanoma

*Conjunctival malignant melanomas* are uncommon ocular tumors. The ratio of conjunctival to uveal malignant melanomas in major eye pathology laboratories is in the range of 1:20 to 1:30.[26] Malignant melanomas of the conjunctiva can arise from primary acquired melanosis, conjunctival nevi, and de novo. The exact incidence of these forms of melanoma is unclear because previous reports have varied greatly. Reese reported that 50 percent of conjunctival melanomas arise from PAM, 25 percent from nevi, and that 25 percent were de novo.[52] Previously, Zimmerman had reported that 50 percent of conjunctival melanomas arose de novo, 30 percent from primary acquired melanosis, and the remainder from nevi.[65] More recently, Folberg[17] reported a 70–75 percent association of conjunctival malignant melanomas with PAM.

Clinically these lesions appear as discrete, variably pigmented masses, most commonly encountered in the limbal or perilimbal areas (Fig. 9-26). They can occur anywhere on the bulbar or palpebral conjunctiva, semilunar fold, caruncle, or lid margins (Fig. 9-27). The degree of pigmentation does not equate in any way with the degree of malignancy,[26] nor is the location on the globe of particular prognostic significance.

It has been previously taught that the cytologic characteristics of conjunctival malignant melanoma do not give prognostic information regarding these tumors. This is in distinction to the prognostic information provided by the histology of uveal melanomas. Recently Folberg et al. reported the following histologic factors to be of prognostic significance in conjunctival melanomas associated with PAM:[16,17]

1. Palpebral conjunctival or caruncle involvement
2. Tumor thickness greater than 0.8 mm
3. Pagetoid or in situ growth
4. Moderate to severe atypia
5. Greater than or equal to five mitotic figures per high-powered field

They were, however, unable to identify any histologic prognostic factors in malignant melanoma unassociated with PAM. Amelanotic malignant melanomas of the conjunctiva occur in less than 10 percent of cases. The use of antimelanoma monoclonal antibodies can aid in their histopathologic diagnosis (Fig. 9-28).[19]

Yanoff and Fine state in their textbook that the incidence of mortality from conjunctival melanomas varies with the etiology and stated that melanomas arising from nevi are associated with a lower mortality.[64] The recent report of Folberg showed no difference in mortality in melanomas associated or unassociated with PAM. Their overall mortality rate was 26 percent; however, they allowed for follow-up as short as 1 year. Previous reports have given a 5-year survival figure of approximately 40 percent.[51] Jay's report in 1964 gave a more favorable prognosis to both localized and widespread forms of conjunctival melanoma. This study reported a 5- and 10-year survival for localized forms of 80 percent and a 10-year survival for the widespread form of conjunctival melanoma to be 50 percent.[35,36]

Tumor thickness has been shown to be of prognostic importance in various reports. Silvers reported in 1978 that a tumor thickness of less than 1.5 mm was associated with a favorable prognosis whereas tumors greater than or equal to 1.8 mm resulted in a high mortality.[54] The report by Folberg et al. also demonstrated that tumor thickness is significant; however, they found a cutoff of 0.8 mm maximal thickness to be more reliable prognostically.[17]

Management of conjunctival malignant melanomas should employ a combination of surgical excision plus cryotherapy. This combined approach toward malignant melanomas has risen due to the high recurrence rate noted following excision alone. Liesegang[42] noted a 60 percent recurrence rate following excision of localized (nodular) malignant melanoma of the conjunctiva. Jakobiec and others have reported improved results with combination surgery and cryotherapy.[12,31–33]

Our approach in the management of conjunctival malignant melanomas is as follows (Fig. 9-28). We believe two sets of instruments are helpful to avoid inadvertent

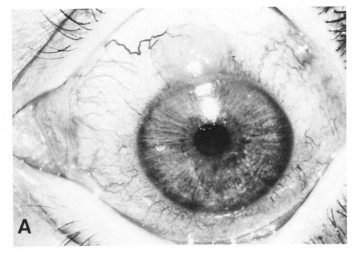

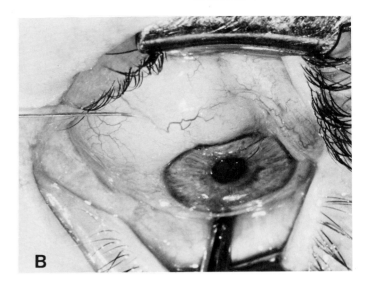

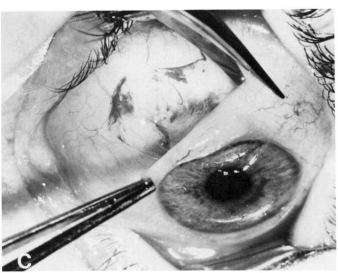

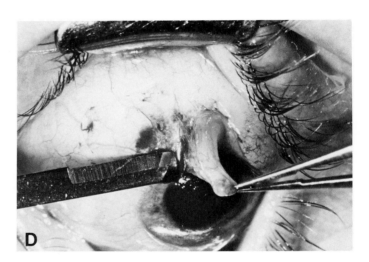

implantation of melanoma cells to uninvolved sites. Instruments involved with the handling of the suspected melanoma itself should not be used in other ocular sites. Following topical anesthetic, lid preparation, and insertion of a lid speculum, a subconjunctival injection of lidocaine with epinephrine is injected into the involved quadrants. Any tumor not readily elevated by this injection should be suspected of potential scleral invasion. All nodules should be excised including a wide, clinically uninvolved rim of conjunctiva. This "tumor-free" rim should measure approximately 2–3 mm in width.

Following excision of the tumor nodule cryotherapy is applied in the double freeze–thaw manner. This therapy is applied to the base and margins of the surgical excision and to any areas of surrounding flat pigmentation. Diffuse malignant melanomas may require multiple treatment sessions to avoid significant complications of cryotherapy. A nitrous oxide cryoprobe is sufficient for bulbar conjunctival treatment. The cryoprobe should be activated and completely

frozen prior to application to the involved bed. Contiguous areas of cryotherapy are applied to the surgical base and surgical margin maintaining contact for a minimum of three seconds. The area of cryotherapy should extend beyond visible pigmentation by approximately 2 mm. Following thawing of the treated area, the procedure is again repeated. If more than 50 percent of the conjunctiva is involved in acquired melanosis, multiple treatment sessions are generally required. We generally do not use the thermocouple in treating areas involving bulbar conjunctiva.

Treatment of malignant melanoma involving the palpebral conjunctiva generally is performed in two stages. Initially a full-thickness excisional lid biopsy is performed. These wedge-shaped or pentagonal defects are repaired in a typical fashion; however, conjunctival sutures are not placed in an attempt to avoid deep tumor implantation. The second stage of cryotherapy generally is applied 3–5 weeks following the initial excision to allow for early wound repair. If the biopsy shows complete excision with residual PAM then

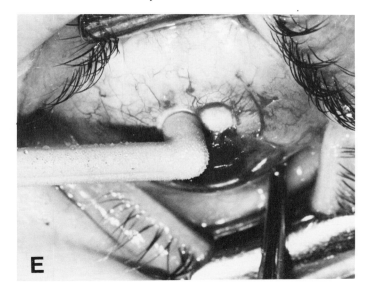

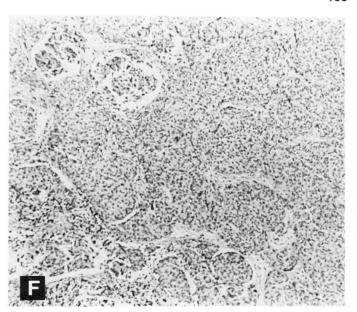

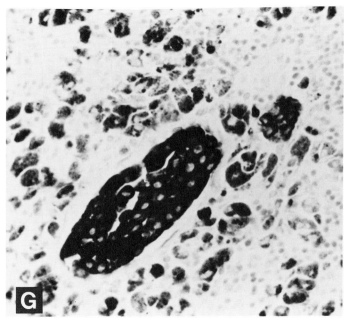

**Fig. 9-28.** Management of malignant melanoma. (A) Amelanotic malignant melanoma of limbus; (B) subconjunctival injection of 1% lidocaine with epinephrine; (C) incision 2–3 mm from lesion to bare sclera; (D) superficial scleral keratectomy at limbus; (E) double freeze–thaw nitrous oxide cryotherapy to entire surgical bed; (F) amelanotic melanoma; (G) positive monoclonal antimelanoma antibody stain (Courtesy of P. Kramer, J.C. Orcutt).

nitrous oxide is a suitable cryogen. Double freeze–thaw applications can be applied to the involved area after local injection of a combination of lidocaine and bupivacaine as described previously for PAM.

If the biopsy shows incomplete horizontal margins such as occurring with Stage IIa (residual malignant melanoma associated with PAM), then the cryogen of choice should be liquid nitrogen. Local infiltration should consist of combination lidocaine and bupivacaine. Thermocouples would be placed at the margin of the involved treated areas as cryotherapy of lid lesions to −25° will automatically be full thickness. Often two or more thermocouples are required to adequately monitor the cryotherapy. The thermocouple should be introduced into the skin at least 5 mm outside the treated area. Topical anesthetic should be applied and globe protec-

tors should be used consisting of either an appropriately cut styrofoam cup or a Yager plastic retractor. For this type of lesion a 20-gauge needle ("D" tip) is generally preferred to minimize liquid nitrogen "run-off." The tip is held 4–5 mm from the treated area starting at the center of the treatment area and perpendicular to the surface. The initial freeze is continued to a temperature of −25°C at the base and tumor margins. The thaw is allowed to occur to at least +2°C. The process is then repeated to −25°C to complete a double freeze–thaw application.

Postoperatively, significant erythema and lid edema is to be expected. Postoperative treatment should include topical corticosteroids, antibiotics, and cycloplegics. Systemic corticosteroids may be required to control the inflammatory reaction.

Management of ocular invasive malignant melanomas of the conjunctiva is a more difficult situation. Dutton has reported successful treatment of a superficially invasive melanoma involving the sclera with local excision and cryotherapy.[12] If there is clinical evidence of superficial scleral or corneal invasion we believe the superficial sclerectomy, and/ or keratectomy, is advisable followed by double freeze–thaw cryotherapy. We generally would use nitrous oxide as the cryogen for this condition; however we would maintain contact for 3–4 seconds to the surgical bed. Deep scleral or intraocular invasion requires enucleation.

Malignant melanoma involving the fornix is treated in a similar fashion with excision followed by a double application of freeze–thaw cryotherapy. If the pathologic report shows an incomplete deep excision with residual melanoma involving the fornix, exenteration may be advisable. In this situation we recommend obtaining a computed tomography (CT) scan to rule out subclinical orbital involvement in addition to a metastatic workup. Orbital invasion is associated with a 90 percent incidence of metastasis following exenteration.[16] If there is evidence of orbital invasion the value of exenteration is strongly in doubt. If there is no evidence of orbital invasion the options are (1) exenteration, or (2) cryotherapy utilizing liquid nitrogen spray together with thermocouples obtaining a double freeze–thaw to a value of −40°C or lower. The incidence of metastasis following exenteration without orbital invasion is 42 percent and it is unclear whether this is a preferred mode of treatment to cryotherapy. Nonetheless, if excision of a forniceal melanoma showed incomplete deep excision and subsequent CT scan showed no evidence of orbital invasion, we would recommend exenteration. If the patient refused this therapy, then cryotherapy would be performed utilizing multiple thermocouples and a liquid nitrogen spray to the forniceal area.

Recurrences following surgery and cryotherapy for malignant melanoma of the conjunctiva are common. Folberg reported a 41 percent incidence of recurrence in melanomas associated with PAM and a 21 percent recurrence rate in melanomas not associated with PAM.[16] Recurrent melanomas are handled in an identical fashion as described above. Their presence, however, is of prognostic importance as these patients do have a higher overall mortality rate than patients without recurrence.

## SOFT-TISSUE TUMORS

### Lymphoid Hyperplasia and Lymphoma

Benign and malignant lymphoid tumors of the conjunctiva can be difficult to distinguish, both clinically and histopathologically.[45] Jakobiec and Siegelman reported on 40 such patients with a median follow-up of more than 6 years.[30] They felt they could distinguish the benign versus the malignant group based on histopathologic criteria. Eighty-two percent of their patients demonstrated benign features and were therefore classified as pseudolymphomas (lymphoid hyperplasia). The remaining 18 percent represented malignant lymphomas.

### Lymphoid Hyperplasia

*Lymphoid hyperplasia* ( *pseudolymphoma*) appears as a pink, often fleshy-appearing mass usually arising in the inferior fornix (Fig. 9-29; see color insert following page 139). The soft masses are often sausage-shaped and of variable size. Less commonly, superior fornix or canthal areas are involved. The average age in Jakobiec and Siegelman's study was 55 years (a 9- to 78-years-old range) with equal male and female distribution.[30] The majority presented with unilateral involvement; however, 15 percent showed bilateral manifestations on presentation. Of the unilateral cases 7 percent went on to develop contralateral involvement. Approximately 20 percent of their cases had associated cervical adenopathy which on biopsy demonstrated a "benign lymphoid hyperplasia."

There are two clinical features that can be useful in helping to distinguish benign versus malignant lymphoid tumors. The first is a multifocal occurrence of subconjunctival masses. The second is a "pebbly" follicular appearance on the surface or leading edge of the subconjunctival mass. When either of these two features were present clinically they were associated with benign histopathologic diagnosis.

Pathologically, these benign lesions can be divided into two groups consisting of (1) benign follicular lymphoid hyperplasia, and (2) diffuse reactive lymphoid hyperplasia. The follicular group corresponds with the clinical follicular appearance and accounts for approximately 40 percent of benign cases.[30] These follicles consist of lymphoid elements with germinal centers. The diffuse or patternless group accounts for the remaining sixty percent and consists of infiltrations of mature lymphocytes. In both these groups the typical histopathologic features were masses of mature lymphocytes together without evidence of significant cytologic atypia.

Immunocytochemical staining greatly enhances histopathologic distinction between lymphoid hyperplasia and lymphoma.[14,24,37] Although exceptions exist, lymphoid hyperplasia is characterized by a polyclonal proliferation of lymphocytes. In contrast, lymphomas demonstrate a monoclonal proliferation of lymphocytes.

### Malignant Lymphomas

*Malignant lymphomas* involving the conjunctiva typically occur in the elderly population group with an equal sex distribution. Clinically these lesions are smooth, fleshy masses most commonly encountered in the inferior fornix. They are, in general, larger and more elevated than lymphoid hyperplasia (Fig. 9-30; see color insert following page 139). Roughly half of the lesions may show evidence of orbital involvement with either proptosis, globe displacement, or motility disturbances.

Histopathologically these tumors show diffuse lymphocytic proliferation with cytologic atypia. There can be a high mitotic activity (1–2 mitoses per high-power field) together with large nuclei and prominent nucleoli. Cell marker analysis demonstrates a monoclonal cell origin.[37]

*Treatment of lymphoid hyperplasia and conjunctival lymphoma.* The initial management of both lymphoid hyperplasia and conjunctival lymphomas is usually excision plus irradiation. The preoperative evaluation should include a general physical examination by an internist with attention directed toward possible hepatosplenomegaly and lymphadenopathy. In addition, noninvasive diagnostic tests should include chest x-ray, complete blood count, serum protein electrophoresis, and liver function tests. Any clinical evidence of orbital involvement mandates an orbital CT scan.

Surgical excision can be performed under local or general anesthesia. Following conjunctival incision, an excisional biopsy is performed when feasible. The surgeon should avoid deep forniceal excisions entering the orbit except for biopsy purposes. Fresh (nonfixed) specimens should be submitted for immunocytochemical analysis in addition to fixed specimens for routine histopathology.

Postoperative irradiation in lymphoid hyperplasia consists of 1500 rads of orthovoltage or beta-radiation.[7] Jakobiec and Siegelman used a higher dose of 3000 rads irradiation for their benign lesions in daily doses of 300 rads.[30] This group showed local recurrences in approximately 20 percent of their patients utilizing excision plus irradiation.

Cryotherapy is an acceptable alternative to irradiation in the initial management of lymphoid hyperplasia. This may be particularly true in the treatment of young patients. Following biopsy confirmation of lymphoid hyperplasia, 1% lidocaine with epinephrine should be injected deep into the conjunctival mass ballooning it forward. Thermocouples can be used to monitor a double freeze–thaw therapy to −25°C. For relatively thin lesions nitrous oxide cryogen is probably adequate provided the desired temperature of −25°C is established at the base.

If the histopathology following excisions demonstrates a malignant lymphoma, then higher doses of irradiation are generally employed. Often the malignant infiltrations will respond to doses as low as 1500 rads; however, some authors choose to go to larger doses with ranges up to 5000–6000 rads.[7,30] Patients demonstrating malignant conjunctival lymphomas require extensive systemic evaluation by an oncologist. Recurrences in the malignant group are interestingly less common than in the benign group.[30]

Management of recurrences in lymphoid hyperplasia following radiation treatment should consist of repeat biopsy followed by cryotherapy. Complete regression in five of eight cases treated in this fashion has been reported.[20] Two of eight showed significant improvement without need for further treatment. Only one of eight cases showed no improvement utilizing cryotherapy.

## Rhabdomyosarcoma and Kaposi's Sarcoma

*Rhabdomyosarcoma* rarely presents as a subconjunctival tumor in a child. In the absence of other findings this would not be the initial suspected diagnosis. Following excisional or incisional biopsy treatment would consist of thorough patient evaluation followed by irradiation treatment.

*Kaposi's sarcoma* is a rare vascular tumor which is believed to originate from pleuripotential vascular cells. Awareness of this rare tumor is important because of its association with immunocompromised states, in particular with acquired immunodeficiency syndrome (AIDS).[27] This tumor is often multicentric in origin, presenting as bluish-red maculas or nodules on the lower extremities. Subconjunctival involvement normally occurs following the development of nodules on the lower extremities, however, it can be the presenting feature of this disorder.[28,41] There is also a report of Kaposi's sarcoma in association with myasthenia following prolonged systemic corticosteroids.[2] The conjunctival involvement is characterized by bluish-red or hemorrhagic nodules involving the bulbar conjunctival or fornices. These vascular tumors can spontaneously hemorrhage, potentially complicating their clinical appearance. Ocular treatment consists of local excision of subconjunctival or forniceal nodules followed by radiotherapy.

## ACKNOWLEDGMENTS

Supported in part by an unrestricted award from Research to Prevent Blindness, Incorporated.

## REFERENCES

1. Baum JL, Feingold M: Ocular aspects of Goldenhar's syndrome. Am J Ophthalmol 75:250–257, 1973
2. Bedrick JJ, Savino PJ, Schatz NJ: Conjunctival Kaposi's sarcoma in a patient with myasthenia gravis. Arch Ophthalmol 99:1607–1609, 1981
3. Brownstein S: Mucoepidermoid carcinoma of the conjunctiva with intraocular invasion. Ophthalmology 88:1126–1230, 1981
4. Brownstein S, Jakobiec FA, Wilkenson RD, et al.: Cryotherapy for precancerous melanosis (atypical melanocytic hyperplasia) of the conjunctiva. Arch Ophthalmol 99:1224–1231, 1981
5. Burns RP, Wankum G, Grangiacomo J, et al.: Dinitrochlorolanzene and debulking therapy of conjunctival papilloma. J Pediatr Ophthalmol Strabismus 20:221–226, 1983
6. Caroll JM, Kuwabara T: A classification of limbal epitheliomas. Arch Ophthalmol 73:545–551, 1965
7. Char DH: The management of lid and conjunctival malignancies. Surv Ophthalmol 24:679–689, 1980
8. Cohen BN, Green WR, Iliff NT, et al.: Spindle cell carcinoma of the conjunctiva. Arch Ophthalmol 98:1809–1813, 1980
9. Daily EG, Lubowitz RM: Dermoids of limbus and cornea. Am J Ophthalmol 53:661–665, 1962
10. Devine RD, Anderson RL: Nitrous oxide cryosurgery for intraepithelial epithelioma and its implications. Presented at the American Society of Ophthalmic Plastic and Reconstructive Surgery, Atlanta, November 6, 1981
11. Devine RD, Anderson RL: Nitrous oxide cryotherapy for intraepithelial epithelioma of the conjunctiva. Arch Ophthalmol 101:782–786, 1983
12. Dutton JJ, Anderson RL, Tse DT: Combined surgery and cryotherapy for scleral invasion of epithelial malignancies. Ophthalmic Surg 15:289–294, 1984
13. Economidis I, Tragalais M, Mangouritsas N, et al.: Keratoconjunctivitis sicca following excision of dermolipoma of the lacrimal gland. Ann Ophthalmol 10:1973, 1978

14. Ellis JH, Banks PM, Campbell RJ, et al.: Lymphoid tumors of the ocular adnexa: Clinical correlation with the working formulation classification and immunoperoxidase staining of paraffin sections. Ophthalmology 92:1311–1324, 1985

15. Elsas FJ and Green WR: Epibulbar tumors in children. Am J Ophthalmol 79:1001–1007, 1975

16. Folberg R, McLean IW, Zimmerman LE: Conjunctival melanosis and melanoma. Ophthalmology 91:673–678, 1984

17. Folberg R, McLean IW, Zimmerman LE: Malignant melanoma of the conjunctiva. Hum Pathol 16:136–143, 1985

18. Folberg R, McLean IW, Zimmerman LE: Primary acquired melanosis of the conjunctiva. Hum Pathol 16:129–135, 1985

19. Folberg R, Donoso LA, Atkinson BF, et al.: An antimelanoma antibody and the histopathology of uveal melanomas. Arch Ophthalmol 103:275–279, 1985

20. Fraunfelder FT, Wallace TR, Farris HE, et al.: The role of cryosurgery in external ocular and periocular disease. Trans Am Acad Ophthalmol Otolaryngol 83:713–724, 1977

21. Fraunfelder FT, Wingfield D: Therapy of intraepithelial epitheliomas and squamous cell carcinoma of the limbus. Trans Am Opthalmol Soc 78:290–300, 1980

22. Fraunfelder FT, Wingfield D: Management of intraepithelial conjunctival tumors and squamous cell carcinomas. Am J Ophthalmol 95:359–363, 1983

23. Gamel JW, Eiferman RA, Guibor P: Mucoepidermoid carcinoma of the conjunctiva. Arch Ophthalmol 102:730–734, 1984

24. Garner A, Rahi AHS, Wright JE: Lymphoproliferative disorders of the orbit: An immunological approach to diagnosis and pathogenesis. Br J Ophthalmol 67:561–569, 1983

25. Gelender H, Forster RK: Papaniculaou cytology in the diagnosis and management of external ocular tumors. Arch Ophthalmol 98:909–912, 1980

26. Henkind P: Conjunctival melanocytic lesions: Natural history, in Jakobiec FA (ed): Ocular and Adnexal Tumors. Aesculapius, Birmingham, AL, 1978, pp 572–582

27. Holland GN, Gottlieb MS, Yee RD, et al.: Ocular disorders associated with a new severe cellular immunodeficiency syndrome. Am J Ophthalmol 93:393–402, 1982

28. Howard GM, Jakobiec FA, DeVoe AG: Kaposi's sarcoma of the conjunctiva. Am J Ophthalmol 79:420–423, 1975

29. Iliff WJ, Marbark R, Green WR: Invasive squamous cell carcinoma of the conjunctiva. Arch Ophthalmol 93:119–122, 1975

30. Jakobiec FA, Sigelman J: Lymphoma and pseudolymphoma of the conjunctiva, in Jakobiec FA (ed): Ocular and Adnexal Tumors. Aesculapius, Birmingham, AL, 1978, pp 532–552

31. Jakobiec FA, Brownstein S, Wilkinson RD, et al.: Combined surgery and cryotherapy for diffuse malignant melanoma of the conjunctiva. Arch Ophthalmol 98:1390–1396, 1980

32. Jakobiec FA, Brownstein S, Albert W, et al.: The role of cryotherapy in the management of conjunctival melanoma. Ophthalmology 89:502–515, 1982

33. Jakobiec FA, Brownstein S, Wilkinson RD, et al.: Adjuvant cryotherapy for focal nodular melanoma of the conjunctiva. Arch Ophthalmol 100:115–118, 1982

34. Jakobiec FA, Iwamoto T: Cryotherapy for intraepithelial conjunctival melanocytic proliferations. Ultrastructural effects. Arch Ophthalmol 101:940–942, 1983

35. Jay BS: Naevi and melanomata of the conjunctiva. M.D. thesis, University of Cambridge, 1964

36. Jay B: Naevi and melanomata of the conjunctiva. Br J Ophthalmol 49:169, 1964

37. Knowles DM, Jakobiec FA: Ocular adnexal lymphoid neoplasms: Clinical, histopathologic, electron microscopic, and immunologic characteristics. Hum Pathol 13:148–162, 1982

38. Lass JH, Grove AS, Papale JJ, et al.: Papillomavirus in human conjunctival papillomas. Am J Ophthalmol 95:364–368, 1983

39. Lass JH, Grove AS, Papale JJ, et al.: Detection of human papillomavirus—DNA sequences in conjunctival papilloma. Am J Ophthalmol 96:670–674, 1983

40. Li WW, Pettit TH, Zakka KA: Intraocular invasion by papillary squamous cell carcinoma of the conjunctiva. Am J Ophthalmol 90:697–701, 1980

41. Lieberman P, Lovera I: Kaposi's sarcoma of the bulbar conjunctiva. Arch Ophthalmol 88:44–45, 1972

42. Liesegang TS, Campbell RJ: Mayo Clinic experience with conjunctival melanomas. Arch Ophthalmol 98:1385–1389, 1980

43. Linberg JV, Orcutt JC, Van Dyk HJL: Orbital surgery, in Duane TD, Jaeger EA (eds): Clinical Ophthalmology, vol. 5. Philadelphia, Harper and Row, pp 1–46, 1985

44. Lopez Cardozo P, Oosterhuis JA, deWolff-Rouondaa PD: Exfoliative cytology in the diagnosis of conjunctival tumors. Ophthalmologica 182:157–164, 1981

45. Morgan G, Halby J: Lymphocytic tumors of indeterminate nature. A 5-year followup of 98 conjunctival and orbital lesions. Br J Ophthalmol 62:381–383, 1978

46. Nicholson DH, Herschler J: Intraocular extension of squamous cell carcinoma of the conjunctiva. Arch Ophthalmol 95:843–846, 1977

47. Nicholson DH, Green WR: Congenital epibulbar choristomas and hamartomas, in Nicholson DH, Green WR, (eds): Pediatric Ocular Tumors. New York, Masson, 1981, pp 131–138

48. Pizzarello LD, Jakobiec FA: Bowen's disease of the conjunctiva: A misnomer, in Jakobiec FA (ed): Ocular and Adnexal Tumors. Birmingham, AL, Aesculapius, 1978, pp 553–571

49. Rao NA, Font RL: Mucoepidermoid carcinoma of the conjunctiva. Cancer 38:1699–1709, 1976

50. Reed JW, Cashwell F, Klintworth GK: Corneal manifestations of hereditary benign intraepithelial dyskeratosis. Arch Ophthalmol 97:297–300, 1979

51. Reese AB: Precancerous and cancerous melanosis. Am J Ophthalmol 61:1272–1277, 1966

52. Reese AB, Tumors of the Eye. Hagerstown, MD, Harper and Row, 1976, pp 249–257

53. Schachat A, Iliff WJ, Kashima HK: Carbon dioxide laser treatment of recurrent squamous papilloma of the conjunctiva. Ophthalmic Surg 13:916–918, 1982

54. Silvers D, Jakobiec FA, Freeman T, et al.: Melanoma of the conjunctiva: A clinicopathologic study, in Jakobiec FA (ed): Ocular and Adnexal Tumors. Birmingham, AL, Aesculapius, 1978, pp 583–599

55. Spencer WH, Zimmerman LE: Conjunctiva. Neoplasms and related conditions, in Spencer WH (ed): Ophthalmic Pathology. An Atlas and Textbook. Philadelphia, Saunders, 1985, pp 177–222

56. Spinek M, Friedman AH: Squamous cell carcinoma of the conjunctiva. Value of exfoliative cytology in diagnosis. Surv Ophthalmol 21:351–355, 1977

57. Streeten BW, Carillo R, Jamison R, et al.: Inverted papilloma of the conjunctiva. Am J Ophthalmol 88:1062–1066, 1979

58. Waring GO III, Rother AM, Ekins MB: Clinical and patho-

logic description of 17 cases of corneal intraepithelial neoplasia. Am J Ophthalmol 97:547–559, 1984

59. Wexler SA, Wallow IHL: Squamous cell carcinoma of the conjunctiva presenting with intraocular extension. Arch Ophthalmol 103:1175–1177, 1985

60. Wilkes TD, Fraunfelder FT: Principles of cryosurgery. 10(8):21–30, 1979

61. Wilson FM: Rose bengal staining of epibulbar squamous neoplasms. Ophthalmic Surg 7(2):21–23, 1976

62. Wilson FM, Ostler HB: Conjunctival papilloma in siblings. Am J Ophthalmol 77:103–107, 1974

63. Winter F, Kleh T: Precancerous epithelioma of the limbus. Arch Ophthalmol 64:208–215, 1960

64. Yanoff M, Fine BS (eds): Ocular Pathology. A Text and Atlas. Philadelphia, Harper & Row, 1982, pp 796–805

65. Zimmerman LE: Squamous cell carcinoma and related lesions of the bulbar conjunctiva, in Bonick M (ed): Ocular and Adnexal Tumors; New and Controversial Aspects. St. Louis: Mosby, 1964, pp 49–74

66. Zimmerman LE: Melanocytic tumors of interest to the ophthalmologist. Ophthalmology 87:497–502, 1980

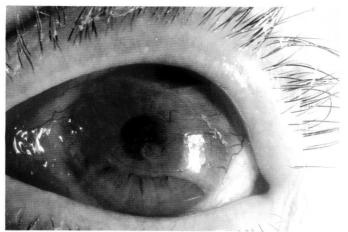

**Fig. 6-28.** Clinical appearance 2 months after conjunctival flap surgery. Graft has retracted slightly, but note its thinness.

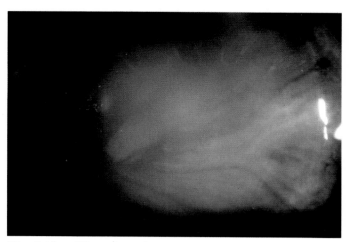

**Fig. 9-18.** Bilateral acquired melanosis with striate melanokeratosis.

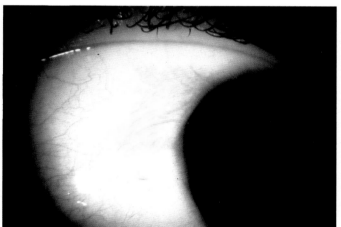

**Fig. 9-19.** Probable primary acquired melanosis of 1-year duration in 35-year-old Caucasian. Note: The earliest manifestation of PAM can be clinically and histopathologically identical to a junctional nevus. The age of onset, extent of involvement, and progression over time allow distinction between these entities.

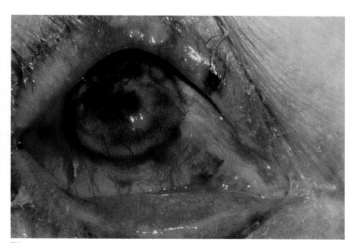

**Fig. 9-20.** Primary acquired melanosis with a history of multiple malignant melanomas.

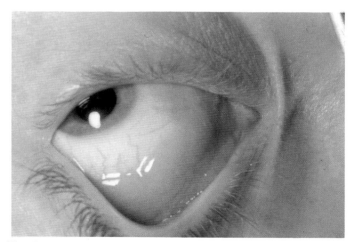

**Fig. 9-29.** Lymphoid hyperplasia in 35-year-old female demonstrating surface follicles.

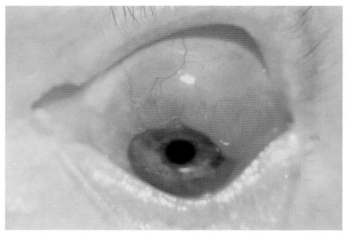

**Fig. 9-30.** Malignant lymphoma of conjunctiva in 60-year-old female treated with irradiation.

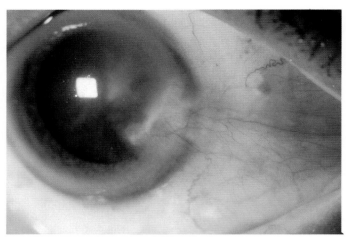

**Fig. 10-2.** A thin, large, noninflamed primary pterygium in a 40-year-old male signifying a good prognosis (Courtesy of Richard L. Abbott, M.D.).

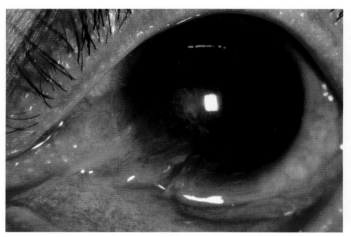

**Fig. 10-6.** An inflamed aggressive recurrent pterygium in a 35-year-old male signifying a poor prognosis.

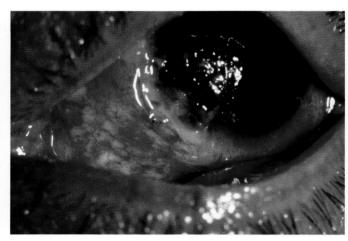

**Fig. 10-8.** Postoperative appearance of the aggressive pterygium seen in Figure 10-6, 1 week postexcision with conjunctival free transplant graft.

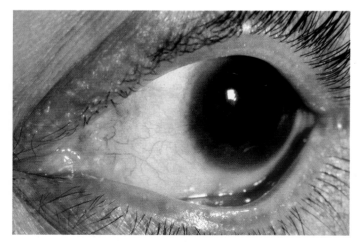

**Fig. 10-9.** Healed appearance of the same eye pictured in Figure 10-8 eight months after free conjunctival graft. Note the clear, smooth cornea and quiet cosmetic conjunctiva.

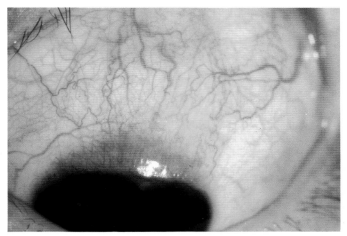

**Fig. 11-1.** A 31-year-old man with typical appearance of SLK. There is inflammation and hyperemia of the superior bulbar conjunctiva as well as proliferation of the superior limbal conjunctival epithelium. The area stains brightly with rose bengal dye (Courtesy of Richard L. Abbott, M.D.).

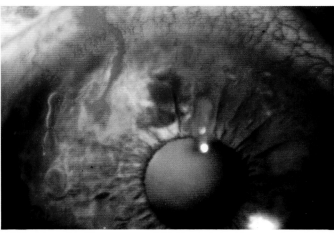

**Fig. 11-2.** A 42-year-old woman with SLK and filamentary keratitis involving the superior limbal area and cornea. The filaments are stained with rose bengal dye (Courtesy of Richard L. Abbott, M.D.).

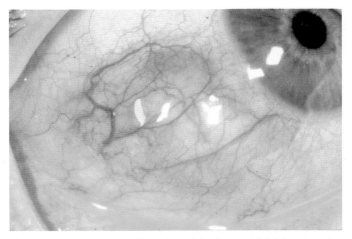

**Fig. 13-1.** Region of mild scleral thinning and bluish coloration in a patient with Crohn's colitis.

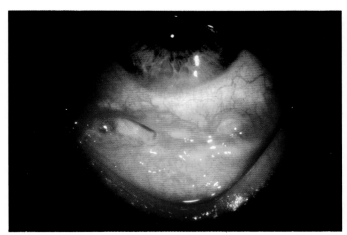

**Fig. 13-2.** Two areas of inferior epibulbar conjunctival and episcleral ulceration in an aphakic elderly female with rheumatoid arthritis.

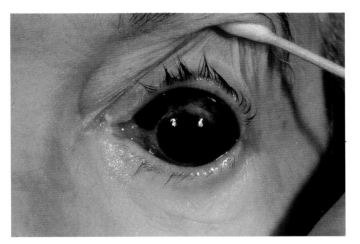

**Fig. 13-7.** Advanced scleral thinning and bluing in an elderly female with rheumatoid arthritis and sclerouveitis. There was no perforation.

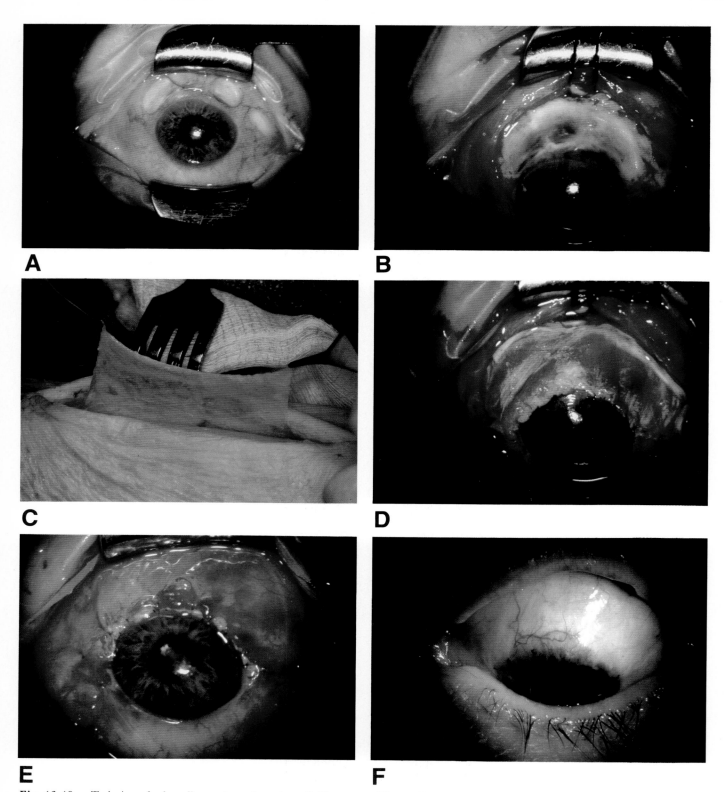

**Fig. 13-19.** Technique for lamellar periosteal patch graft (Courtesy of Steven B. Koenig, M.D.) (A) Multiple areas of conjunctival and scleral necrosis in a patient with scleromalacia perforans. (B) Completion of a fornix-based conjunctival flap with dissection of a large scleral bed and peripheral lamellar keratectomy. (C) Harvesting of pretibial periosteum. (D) Periosteum trimmed and sutured into lamellar scleral bed with interrupted 9-0 nylon suture. (E) Conjunctival flap covering periosteum and sutured to peripheral cornea with interrupted nylon or vicryl sutures. (F) Postoperative appearance at 6 months.

## 10

# Pterygium

## David R. Demartini    David W. Vastine

A *pterygium* (G. winglike) is a triangular patch of conjunctiva and hypertrophied subconjunctival connective tissue extending onto the cornea apex toward the pupil. The first 1–2 mm of the apex are often called the "head" of the pterygium (Fig. 10-1). The "neck" lies between the head and the limbus. The conjunctival "body" of a pterygium extends from the neck to the conjunctival fornix. The "cap" is the gray, subepithelial, fibrous tissue (Ilots de Fuch's, Fuch's Islands)[6] at the leading edge of the head. Very commonly a corneal epithelial iron line (Stocker's line) forms axial to and circumscribing the head of the pterygium. Nasal pterygiums are more common than lateral pterygiums. Occasionally both are seen in the same patient.

In its initial stages a pterygium is mostly a cosmetic problem of inflamation and redness. Although frequently assymptomatic it may produce burning, foreign body sensation, or mild photophbia. With progression, the pterygium may extend across the cornea, obscuring vision and inducing astigmatism (positive cylinder axis perpendicular to the pterygium apex) and/or extraocular motion limitation or diplopia. Many pterygiums stop progressing and become thin, white, uninflamed, and assymtomatic. (Fig. 10-2; see color insert following page 139). Despite the common occurrence of pterygium, there is much controversy regarding its etiology, pathogenesis, and surgery.

### DEFINITIONS

Elastotic degeneration is a fundamental characteristic of pterygium and pingueculum pathology. It is characterized by abnormal subepithelial connective tissue, which is a complex mixture of degenerating collagen, ground substance, normal and abnormal elastic tissue, and abnormal fibroblast activity. Normal elastic tissue will stain with elastic tissue stains and lyse with nonproteolytic elastase. Pterygium subepithelial connective tissue will stain with elastic tissue stains but will not lyse with nonproteolytic elastase, thus it is

termed "elastoid tissue" or "elastotic degeneration" of collagen.[45] Histologically, this tissue degeneration is thought to be identical to that seen in wrinkles of the skin. Current theories[40] of pathogenesis implicate ultraviolet light damage after long exposure times before elastoid tissue is seen. Hence a "recurrent pterygium," which regrows in a few months, will not have had enough time for elastotic degeneration to develop. However, elderly patients with conjunctival carcinomas may have coincidental elastoid tissue in addition to their carcinoma due to the many years of ultraviolet exposure before the carcinoma developed. Elastoid tissue fluoresces under ultraviolet light. This phenomenon should be considered when trying to differentiate this tissue from others.

Pterygium may be subdivided into three types based on clinical exam characteristics, pathology, and suspected pathogenesis: true pterygium, pseudopterygium, and "recurrent pterygium" (Table 10-1).

A true pterygium lies in the interpalpebral aperture and is firmly attached to the corneal stroma throughout its entire length. Histopathologically, the true pterygium shows elastotic degeneration of the subconjunctival connective tissue, invasion and firm adherence to corneal stroma with break-up of Bowman's layer, Fuch's islands, degeneration or proliferation of the overlying conjunctival epithelium (which causes fluorescein or rose bengal staining), vascular proliferation, engorgement, and inflammatory cell infiltration in subepithelial tissue. Rarely will a true pterygium transform into an epithelial carcinoma.

A pseudopterygium is similar to a true pterygium in appearance but is differentiated by either: (1) lying outside the palpebral aperture or (2) its very loose or absent adherence to the corneal limbus such that a small muscle hook or canalicular probe may be passed under the body without resistance. A pseudopterygium is thought to be caused by corneal irritation with secondary conjunctival fibrovascular response with extension onto the cornea. Progression across the cornea may continue as long as the corneal inflammation

SURGICAL INTERVENTION IN CORNEAL AND EXTERNAL DISEASES
ISBN 0-8089-1850-8

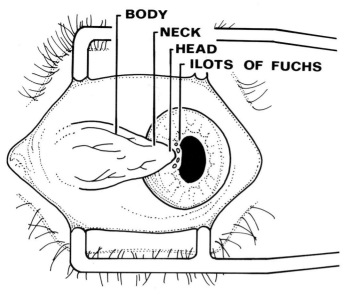

**Fig. 10-1.** Pterygium nomenclature.

persists. The degenerative elastoid histopathology may be present depending on the duration, anatomical location of the lesion, and its chance for exposure to ultraviolet light. Trauma, burns, infections, inflammations,[6] and corneal degenerations[18] have been implicated in the genesis of pseudopterygium. Carcinoma should always be suspected in any atypical pterygium.

A "recurrent pterygium" is a secondary fibrovascular growth[45] across the cornea from the corneoscleral defect of a previously excised pterygium or pseudopterygium. Its location should be similar to the pterygium excised and it should be strongly adherent to the underlying corneoscleral tissues. Usually a recurrent pterygium is reexcised before an elastoid degeneration can occur. Its formation is often rapid, relentless, and generally more aggressive than the original lesion. Recurrence following excision is more likely in younger patients with thick aggressive primary pterygiums, patients with an aggressive postoperative inflammatory reaction, and patients reexposed to an endemic area high in pterygium

etiologic factors (e.g., ultraviolet light, wind, etc.). Surgical prognosis is more cautious following a recurrence.

Pingueculum (fr. pinguiculus, fattish) describes a "fatty" appearing lesion, which histigically is elastoid tissue located in the interpalpebral conjunctiva but without corneal invasion. Histopathologically, it has all of the characteristics of the true pterygium except for its corneal invasion. It may also degenerate into a carcinoma. Its elastoid tissue fluoresces under ultraviolet light. Generally, a pingueculum appears before a pterygium; however, many authors disagree[6,33] with Fuch's dictum that every pterygium develops from a pingueculum.

Conjunctival carcinoma should always be considered whenever an atypical pterygium is encountered. This tumor usually develops at the limbus, with associated inflamation, reactive vasculature, and ulcerated epithelium which causes fluorescein or rose bengal staining. Noninvasive carcinoma in situ (intraepithelial) tumors are very weakly adherent to the underlying tissues and can be easily scraped off during surgery. Invasive squamous carcinomas are more firmly adherent and resist scraping similar to pterygium. Conjunctival carcinomas do not develop elastotic degeneration but may contain some degeneration if located near a previous pingueculum or pterygium. Carcinomas do not demonstrate fluorescence under ultraviolet light. The etiology of a conjunctival carcinoma is not known but intense ultraviolet exposure has been implicated.

## HISTORY

Pterygium was described as early as 1000 B.C. by the Indian physician Susruta.[6] Roman physicians recognized this lesion in the first century A.D. and described it as the "unguis of celsus." British ophthalmologists have referred to it as the "web of old English surgeons."[41]

Fuchs wrote the classic treatise in 1892, which dominated ophthalmologists' understanding for 50 years. He first popularized the differentiation of pterygium into either: (1) the thick, vascular, progressive type or (2) the thin, white, nonprogressive type. He felt that a temporal pterygium is

Table 10-1
Differential Diagnosis of Pterygium

|  | True Pterygium | Pseudopterygium | Pingueculum | Recurrent Pterygium | Conjunctival Carcinoma |
|---|---|---|---|---|---|
| Incidence: | Common | Uncommon | Common | Variable | Uncommon |
| Onset (decade): | 3rd, 4th | Variable | 2nd, 3rd | Postsurgery | 6th, 7th |
| Histopathology: | Elastotic degeneration | Fibrovasular | Elastotic degeneration | Fibrovascular | Carcinoma |
| Limbal adherence | Strong | None | Conjunctiva only | Strong | Weak |
| UV Fluorescence | Yes | No | Yes | No | No |
| Interpalpebral | Yes | Occasionally | Yes | Yes | Variable |
| Eiology | UV light, chronic keratitis | Keratitis, secondary fibrovasular in-growth | UV light | Pterygium excision | Age, dysplasia, UV light |

never seen without a medial pterygium. Finally, he believed that a pterygium always originates from a pingueculum. Others[6,33] disagree with these conclusions. Cameron's book, *Pterygium Throughout The World,* is a more recent summary of pterygium and its management.

## GEOGRAPHIC DISTRIBUTION

Pterygium is seen in all parts of the world but is more common near the equator. Cameron[6] has mapped worldwide distribution and finds it most prevalent inside the 30th latitude parallels and very rare north or south of the 40th parallels. Hence, a relative "pterygium belt" straddles the equator. Dimitry[13] has shown a similar geographic prevalence in the United States where pterygium is most common in southern cities. In Darrel and Bachrach's United States study,[9] a higher incidence of pterygium is seen in veterans living south of the 37th lattitude compared to those living in the north. Cameron noted a dramatic rise in pterygium incidence in similar genetic populations (e.g., British) who have migrated to more equatorial climates (e.g., Australia). McGavic[29] noted a sudden increase in pterygium in his veteran patients who served during World War II. This phenomenon of increased pterygium prevalence in the geographic "pterygium belt" has inspired or supported many of the theories of pterygium genesis.

## PREVALENCE

The prevalence of pterygium is documented in various studies (Table 10-2). Interpretation of this data requires analysis of the populations studied, geographic location, and sampling techniques. Some populations are very high or low risk for pterygium. Intrapopulation study groups also demonstrate a different risk for pterygium in accordance with cultural lifestyles, customs, or employment. Moran and Hollows[34] found aboriginal and nonaboriginal Australian women to have a lower prevalence of pterygium than their male counterparts, which they explain by the local custom that the females spend more time indoors, thus avoiding local pterygium etiologic factors (e.g., ultraviolet light). Detels and Dhir[12] found a higher prevalence of pterygium in indoor sawmill workers of British Columbia when compared

to outdoor farmers of the Indian Punjab region. Hence, numerous etiologic factors may be responsible for pterygium, not just geographic location or ultraviolet light exposure.

Prevalence of pterygium and pingueculum also depends on the age of the patient.[6,34,36] Generally, people between the ages of 20–50 years are more prone to pingueculum and pterygium, with diminishing incidence before and following this period. Zauberman[5] found that the highly aggressive and recurrent pterygiums were seen in younger patients. Hence a study of general pterygium prevalence or management may be affected by the age of the patients.

## ETIOLOGY

Despite the commonality of pterygium, little is truly known about its etiology. Many theories have been developed based on incidence observations, geographic distribution, histopathology, methods of treatment, and some speculation. There is probably no single explanation for every pterygium. It is more likely to be a degenerative response to a number of different stimuli.

Radiation damage by ultraviolet (UV) energy is the most widely accepted theory for pterygium formation. The following findings support this view. First, geographic distribution of pterygium prevalence generally parallels local atmospheric UV energy intensity.[6,34] Second, dermatologists[40] have experimentally produced dermal elastoid degeneration by intense UV irradiation in animals. Third, a large amount of UV energy is absorbed in the superficial layers of the conjunctiva and cornea explaining the location of elastoid degeneration and pterygium.[28] Fourth, retrospective studies of different methods of screening UV energy (spectacle,[6] or closing the nondominant eye [22]) cause a decrease in pterygium prevalence. Fifth, employment exposures (welders) has led to increased pterygium occurrence.[25] And sixth, uniform genetic populations that have low pterygium incidence in their low ambient UV homeland, experience higher incidence of pterygium when relocated to higher UV location.[6] Conversely, however, another study[12] demonstrated a higher incidence of pterygium among indoor lumbermill workers in Canada than in Punjab Indian farmers. Hence ultraviolet irradiation cannot be the complete explanation for pterygium genesis.

Table 10-2
Pterygium Prevalence

| Author (year) | Prevalence (%) | Location | Latitude | Population (#) |
|---|---|---|---|---|
| Dimitry (1935) | 5.1 | New Orleans | 30° | County Hospital (1000) |
| Norn (1982) | 12.0 | Aqaba, Jordan | 30° | Local civilian (127) |
| Reed (1959) | 1.6 | Canada | 60° | Eskimos (503) |
| Norn (1979) | 8.6 | Greenland | 65° | Eskimos (659) |
| Norn (1979) | 0.7 | Copenhagen | 55° | Local civilian (810) |
| Moran, Hollows (1984) | 3.4 | Australia | 23° | Rural Aborigine (64314) |
| Moran, Hollows (1984) | 1.1 | Australia | 23° | Rural non-Aborigine (40799) |

The "chronic keratitis" theory has many proponents.[6,37,38,50] Paton[37] postulates that actinic keratoconjunctivitis develops, calling forth "a poorly understood biochemical process" which causes the formation of a pterygium. Wong speculates a "pterygium angiogenesis factor." Paton feels a pterygium is further exacerbated by elevation of the pterygium head, dellen formation, dryness, and pterygium progression. This suggests tear function abnormalties as a cause for pterygium. However, Biedner et al.,[5] found no Schirmer test evidence for dryness in 60 patients with unilateral pterygium. Jensen failed to demonstrate the tear break-up time abnormalities, which might explain pterygium genesis. Pinkerton et al.,[38] found IgE (100 percent) and IgG (73 percent) deposited in pterygium connective tissue stroma. Also, plasma cell and lymphocyte infiltration were seen in the same areas as the IgE and IgG. Whether chronic inflamation is a cause of pterygium or a secondary finding is unclear. More investigations are required to characterize the role of inflammation in pterygium etiology.

Pingueculum transformation, popularized by Fuchs, has been widely accepted because of similar histopathology and the common observation that pingueculum and pterygium are present in the same patients. Why a pingueculum crosses the limbus and progresses on the cornea is not understood. Recently, the International Society for Geographical Ophthalmology (Oulu, May 1984) found no association between pingueculum and pterygium in Labrador.[23] It seems that this hypothesis is currently falling from favor.

## PTERYGIUM MANAGEMENT

When a therapeutic plan is considered, the current biologic activity of the pterygium should be assessed. A very red, inflamed, swollen progressive pterygium is more difficult to manage than a white, thin, avascular, nonprogressive lesion. Many authors[24,48] suggest medical therapy to quiet this lesion before operating. Occasionally medical therapy will obviate the need for surgery.

Regardless of the treatment modality, chances of failure or recurrence are increased by reexposing patients to the pterygium generating factors. Postoperatively, the patient's eyes need to be followed closely and protected from UV light (e.g., sunglasses) and inflammation (e.g., steroids) to avoid excessive inflammation and subsequent recurrence.

### Nonsurgical Management

According to most of the current theories of pterygium pathogenesis, a chronic keratoconjunctivitis is the underlying cause. Hence, treatment objectives should minimize the continuation of the chronic irritation.

Acute inflammation of a pingueculum or pterygium will manifest as burning, redness, tearing, and mild photophobia. Examination reveals conjunctival inflammation, swelling, and fluorescein staining over the lesion. There may also be punctate epithelial erosion on the adjacent cornea. Treatment should soothe these areas of inflammation initially while a long-term plan is formulated.

Preventive measures, which should always be used both preoperatively and postoperatively, include screening the eye from UV exposure by brimmed hats and sunglasses, and changing whenever possible occupational exposure or geographic location. Lubrication with artificial tear drops or decongestant drops provides short-term comfort and cosmetic improvement. Artificial tears may be used for longer terms without danger. Topical steroid drops and ointment add an additional level of comfort and control of symptoms but are not advisable long-term solutions due to potential steroid complications.

Vasoconstrictive agents decrease redness and improve pterygium appearance but they can become habit-forming based on the vasoconstrictive rebound phenomenon. Most contain an artificial tear vehicle which is also beneficial. Antihistamines added to the decongestant drops aid in the removal of histamine associated edema and itching. If type 1 (IgE) hypersensitivity models[38] are correct, antihistamines may also aid in pterygium prevention.

Sunglasses are an inexpensive method of reducing light energy absorption by the ocular surface. In addition, they provide a protective shield against dust and wind irritation. Cameron noted a decrease in pterygium prevalence in patients who wore glasses continually (for vision purposes) since age 15 years or younger, which gives support to this form of treatment and/or prevention.

### Surgical Management

Most surgeons consider surgical management for pterygium when there is (1) visual obscuration, (2) symptomatic, induced astigmatism, (3) motility restriction causing diplopia, or (4) extreme cosmetic disfigurement. As with any surgery, the risks (e.g., recurrence, infection, scarring, etc.) must be less than the benefits.

Although numerous surgical procedures have been proposed for treating pterygium, none is sure to provide a cure. Recurrence is the most problematic outcome and the motivation for the evolution of surgical approaches. Current procedures can be categorized by the following three surgical methodology decisions: (1) excision of the pterygium off the cornea by either avulsion or lamellar keratectomy, (2) disposition of the pterygium head by either transposition or excision, (3) leaving bare sclera or closing the remaining conjunctival defects to reestablish normal limbal histologic borders. These can augmented by adding postoperative radiation or chemical cauterization.

Avulsion is probably the oldest form (Aetius, sixth century A.D.)[6] of surgical removal because it does not require microsurgery, is least invasive, and is most consistent with earliest surgical instruments. Recent proponents of this technique point out its advantages: simplicity, safety, and rapidity. Zolli[53] prefers local anesthesia with epinephrine under the pterygium body (Fig. 10-3A). After dissecting the body off the sclera to the limbus with blunt Wescott scissors (Fig. 10-3B), the head is grabbed with stout Graefe forceps and avulsed off the cornea against counter pressure exerted at the opposite limbus (Fig. 10-3C). Often a small amount of tissue

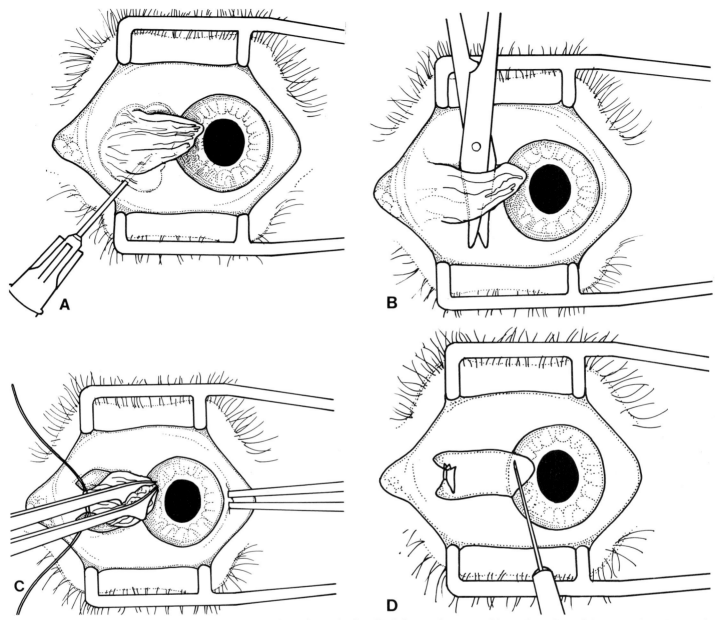

**Fig. 10-3.** Avulsion excision technique. (A) Injection of anesthetic. (B) Scissors sharp and blunt dissection of the pterygium body. (C) Suture strangulation and avulsion of pterygium head and neck. (D) Lamellar keratectomy excision of any residual pterygium tissue.

is left on the cornea and must be removed with a Beaver blade (Fig. 10-3D). Other avulsion techniques have used a squint hook, wire, suture, or horsehair.[6] Zolli[53] does not advise this technique for recurrent pterygium as the underlying corneal thickness cannot be evaluated. Larger, more broad-based pterygiums are more difficult to remove in one avulsive attempt because of its strong superficial corneal invasion and adherence. Long-term success rates have been poor (50 percent recurrence[6]) and may be the reason for the more intricate procedures which are practiced currently.

Lamellar keratectomy begins with conjunctival cautery to outline the proposed margins of pterygium body excision, as pterygium anatomy can be distorted once bleeding begins (Fig. 10-4A). Next, a corneal incision is made axial to the pterygium head and surrounding the neck (Fig. 10-4B). The incision depth should be just below Bowman's layer or as

shallow as possible to undermine the superficial invasion of the pterygium. A guarded corneal trephine (set at less than 0.2-mm depth) may be used to begin the lamellar keratectomy in attempt to obtain a more uniform initial keratectomy depth. Because of the superficial invasion of the pterygium, there is no need for deep incisions and the associated risk of perforation. Caution is always advised when reoperating previously keratectomized pterygiums.

Once this incision is accomplished, the lamellar keratectomy portion of the procedure is accomplished by either sharp or dull dissection. Scraping with the sharp side of the blade oriented perpendicular to the cornea (Figs. 10-4C and 10-4D), without slicing, will result in less knife serration and a very smooth corneal excision defect with all of the pterygium tissue removed. Sharp dissection (Fig. 10-4E) is more difficult but also produces excellent results. The sharper the

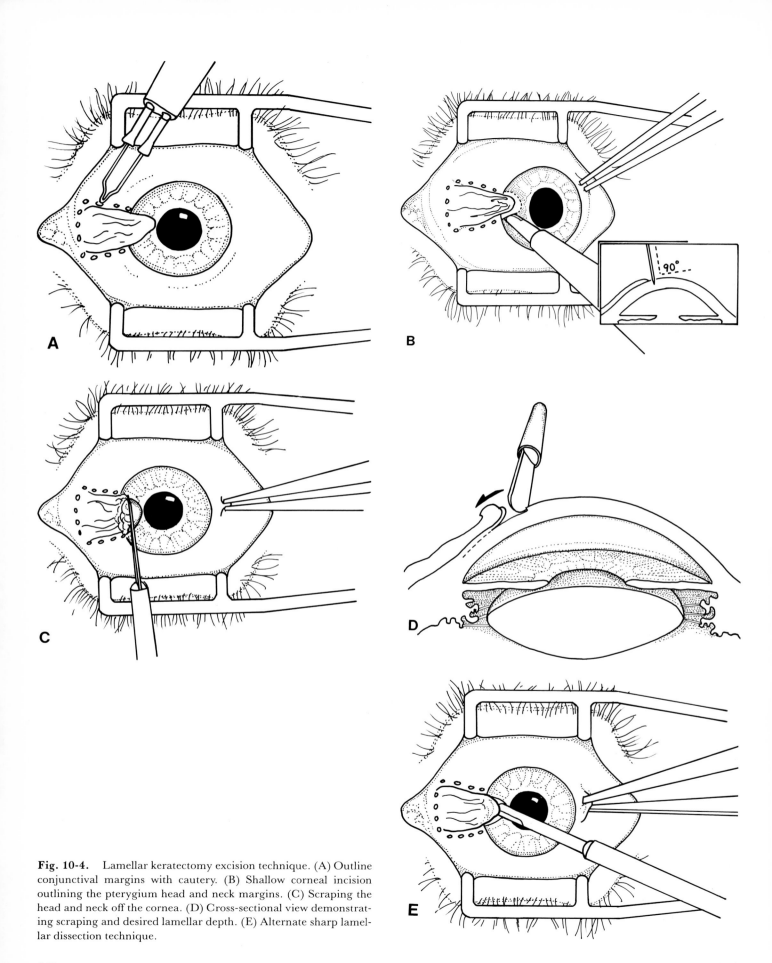

**Fig. 10-4.** Lamellar keratectomy excision technique. (A) Outline conjunctival margins with cautery. (B) Shallow corneal incision outlining the pterygium head and neck margins. (C) Scraping the head and neck off the cornea. (D) Cross-sectional view demonstrating scraping and desired lamellar depth. (E) Alternate sharp lamellar dissection technique.

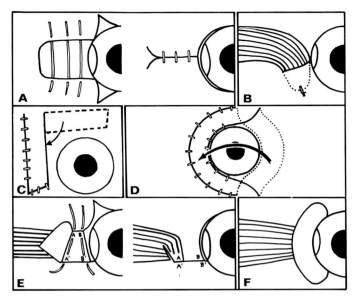

**Fig. 10-5.** Various conjunctival closure techniques. (A) Primary conjunctival anstomosis closed with 8-0 chromic collagen or 10-0 nylon, with radial conjunctival relaxing incisions. (B) Diversion of the pterygium head without excision, after McReynolds. (C) Transposed pedicle conjunctival flaps fashioned from a distal site after Aratoon. (D) Transposed conjunctival bridge flap from the opposite limbus after Forster. (E) Released contiguous conjunctival flap with radial conjunctival relaxing incision after Bangerter. (F) Bare sclera with conjunctival stabilization to episclera after McGavic.

dissection technique the more likely the chance for perforation. Kenyon et al. advise the use of a rotating diamond burr to smooth a rough keratectomy defect.

Following pterygium head and neck removal from the cornea, it is commonly either excised or "diverted," an attempt to change its direction of growth away from the cornea. Currently, most surgeons excise the head, neck, and much of the body.

In 1902, McReynolds published his popular diversion technique (Fig. 10-5B) which was used extensively for 50 years. In this technique the pterygium head is shaved off the cornea and tucked under the subconjunctival connective tissue and maintained in that position by a suture from the head out through the inferior conjunctival fornix. Care is taken to not leave bare sclera or limbus as this was thought to promote recurrence. Others[4,11] developed similar tuck procedures.

Conversely, bare sclera techniques[14,29] were originally developed in various forms to manage the problem of recurrence. There was considerable concern that the pterygium head was "transformed tissue" and would continue to grow if not excised. McGavic felt the abnormal conjunctiva and underlying Tenon's fascia should be excised. The normal conjunctiva is also recessed up to 5 mm from the limbus, is sutured to the sclera (Fig. 10-5F), and the sclera left bare to "allow the faster growing conjunctiva to fill in (the defect) before the abnormal connective tissue could form"[29] leading to recurrence. Others have had significant recurrences after

this technique.[6] Many of the bare sclera enthusiasts now use this technique in combination with beta radiation or topical thio-tepa (triethylenethiophosphoramide) to try to prevent recurrences. Bare sclera surgery is the least time consuming of all excision techniques.

When excising an inflamed pterygium and underlying fibrovascular tissue it is difficult to know how much tissue to remove or what is safe to leave behind (Fig. 10-6; see color insert following page 139). Many pterygiums involve the plica semilunaris, caruncle, inferior and superior conjunctival fornices and removal of all this tissue is probably an unnecessary waste of conjunctiva. Most authors[20,26,48] advise removing only the most inflamed conjunctiva, or that which is proximal to the pterygium body and adjoining limbus, conserving the remaining conjunctiva to reestablish the conjunctival fornices, replace the caruncle, and avoid any ocular motion restrictions. The underlying connective tissue can be widely excised to promote a very clean bare sclera excision and remove the unsightly thickened appearance of very aggressive lesions. Many authors[27,48] emphasize the need to remove all this reactive subconjunctival connective tissue as it's most histologically similar to the reactive fibrovascular tissue of recurrent pterygium. Care should always be used to avoid the underlying rectus muscle(s) and orbital fat.

The techniques of conjunctival closure (Fig. 10-5) of the post-excision defect are even more controversial and varied than the need for excision. Many surgeons favor some form of conjunctival closure to prevent recurrence by reestablishing the normal conjunctival–corneal limbal anatomy. Primary anastomosis,[27,52] pedicle grafts,[1,3,7,11] bridge grafts,[16] and various tissue transplant grafts have all been attempted. While no method is free of failure, we prefer conjunctival anastomosis for small, primary, or less-inflamed pterygiums and conjunctival transplantation for aggressive or recurrent lesions.

Primary conjunctival anastomosis (Fig. 10-5A) can be accomplished by blunt dissection to undermine the adjacent conjunctival tissue off the underlying Tenon's fascia, and suturing the free conjunctival edges together and to the underlying episclera to completely cover the scleral defect without corneal encroachment (Fig. 10-5A). Adding superior and inferior limbal conjunctival radial incisions (after Bangerter) allows limbal conjunctival relaxation and a smoother anastomosis.

Conjunctival pedicle grafts (Figs. 10-5C, 10-5D and 10-5E) can be helpful when a defect cannot be closed by primary anastomosis. A pedicle graft can be released from above or below similar to Bangerter (Fig. 10-5E) or transposed from above or below similar to Aratoon (Fig. 10-5C). A complete bridge flap (Forster) (Fig. 10-5D) from the opposite limbus, similar to a Gunderson conjunctival flap, has also been very successful. These pedicle and bridge flaps do require a large amount of normal conjunctiva from areas that already may be involved by the more advanced and aggressive pterygiums. Cosmetic appearance is often less if large amounts of tissue are diverted or dragged into the defect.

Autologous conjunctival transplant grafts have been proposed and used successfully by many authors.[15,20,26,48,49] The grafts are designed to fill the excisional defect with distant, uninflamed, normal conjunctiva to promote normal limbal anatomy with a superior cosmetic result. Free conjunctiva has been used for other reconstructive purposes besides pterygium[20,47,49] and graft failure or rejection has rarely been a problem. Recurrence of pterygium is also rare in most published conjunctival transplant series. Compared to bare sclera with beta-radiation, tissue transplantation is much more time consuming and tedious.

This surgical technique begins by a standard lamellar keratectomy excision (Figs. 10-4A–10-4E) of the pterygium as described above. Meticulous dissection of the underlying involved subconjunctival connective tissue should result in a clean, smooth, bare scleral tissue plane. This dissection is more difficult when a recurrent lesion is excised and the episcleral tissue planes are more difficult to establish and often the corneal stroma is very thin. Extraocular motions should be checked and reestablished if restricted by underlying connective tissue. The resulting conjunctival defect is measured (Fig. 10-7A) just prior to harvesting the graft.

The conjunctival graft is obtained from the superior bulbar conjunctiva, which is best exposed by a 7-0 silk suture placed at the superotemporal limbus and the eye drawn inferonasally (Fig. 10-7B). Measurements of the required conjunctival graft are marked with the cautery (Fig. 10-7B). A thin "conjunctiva-only" graft is then carefully dissected off the underlying Tenon's fascia (Fig. 10-7C). Subconjunctival injection of saline or anesthetic agent with epinephrine will aid this dissection. A small rim of intact conjunctiva is left at the superior limbus to avoid corneal epithelialization problems. The amputated free conjunctival graft is then carefully slid into position over the conjunctivoscleral defect, maintaining its shiny conjunctival side externally and the grayish, fibrous side toward the globe. The graft is then sutured into position using multiple interrupted 8-0 chromic collagen sutures, many with anchoring episcleral bites, especially at the limbus (Figs. 10-7D and 10-7E).

Postoperatively, the conjunctival graft progresses through a thrombotic, edematous stage, and revascularizes from its peripheral conjunctival anastomoses and deep episcleral vessels. The conjunctival graft finally thins and blanches to a natural conjunctival appearance (Figs. 10-8 and 10-9; see color insert following page 139). Most grafts require 2–3 months of topical steroid medication (e.g., sulfasteroid one drop three times each day) to reduce inflammation and to allow a quieter healing process. More inflamed tissues may require more steroids. All inflamed pterygiums should be treated preoperatively with topical steroid to reduce postoperative inflammation. The conjunctival donor sites are left open and gradually reepithelialize. Occasionally, a donor site pyogenic granuloma will occur and resolve without intervention. Some surgeons prefer the addition of a high-speed diamond burr to polish the lamellar corneal defect. With careful lamellar corneal dissection the corneal epithelium heals with remarkable corneal regularity (Figs. 10-8 and 10-9).

Lamellar keratoplasty has been used with excellent success by many ophthalmologists to prevent pterygium recurrence. Its success is thought to be explained by the reestablishment of a normal Bowman's layer.[44] Either complete circular[39] trephined lamellar tissue or semicircular,[44] freehand grafts have been used with equal success. This technique requires somewhat more risky, deeper dissection and suturing but is safe for most anterior segment surgeons. Recurrences have also been infrequently observed.[8] Final cosmetic appearance is not as favorable as with conjunctival transplant because the hypertrophic pterygium body recurs up to the transplanted cornea. But this procedure is reserved for recurrence control with cosmesis a secondary consideration.

The lamellar corneal graft technique begins with the standard lamellar keratectomy technique described above (Figs. 10-4A–10-4E), or with modified lamellar keratectomy using a trephine for the initial corneal incision. The limbal conjunctival defect is measured to determine the size of the donor lamellar graft needed (Fig. 10-10A). Generally, 8 mm is the largest round graft possible in order to avoid entering the pupillary axis and the rectus muscle at the same time. Caution should be used when dissecting near the rectus muscles where the sclera is only 0.3 mm thick. The trephine, set at less than 0.2 mm depth for safe lamellar dissection of the pterygium, is applied surrounding the head and limbal margins of the pterygium (Fig. 10-10B). The trephine should be tilted to make the incision predominantly corneal avoiding the conjunctiva and sclera or occasionally a complete 360° cut. The lamellar dissection is then completed (Figs. 10-10C). The cornea, conjunctiva, sclera and rectus muscles are all freed of involved pterygium and scar tissue and the bleeding is controlled.

The lamellar corneal graft can be taken from fresh or glycerin-stored tissue. The trephine is set at 0.2–0.3 mm and the tissue is dissected free with a lamellar dissector (Fig. 10-10D). Careful hemostasis is obtained with electrocautery. The graft is then sutured into position (Fig. 10-10E) with 10-0 nylon sutures on the cornea and degradable suture in the sclera. No sutures should approach or enter the visual axis. Poirier[39] recommends closure of the conjunctiva over the scleral portion of the lameller graft. Corneal sutures are removed at 2–3 months. Postoperative steroid–antibiotic drops are also recommended to control inflammation. Larger limbal conjunctival defects must be closed either with free-hand lamellar corneal grafts (Figs. 10-11A and 10-11B) or conjunctival grafts.

Buccal mucous membrane, skin, and amniotic membrane have also been used with success as transplant tissue.[6] Skin grafts are potentially removable but produce an unsightly discharge when in place. Oral mucous membrane results in an unsightly, red, beefy appearance. Keratopatch (Allergan Medical Optics, Irvine, CA), a lypophilzed corneal tissue substrate to be used instead of fresh eye bank lamellar corneal tissue, has recently entered the market.

We believe that any of these surgical procedures can be successful if the pterygium excised is not very active. We prefer to close conjunctival defects, to reestablish a normal

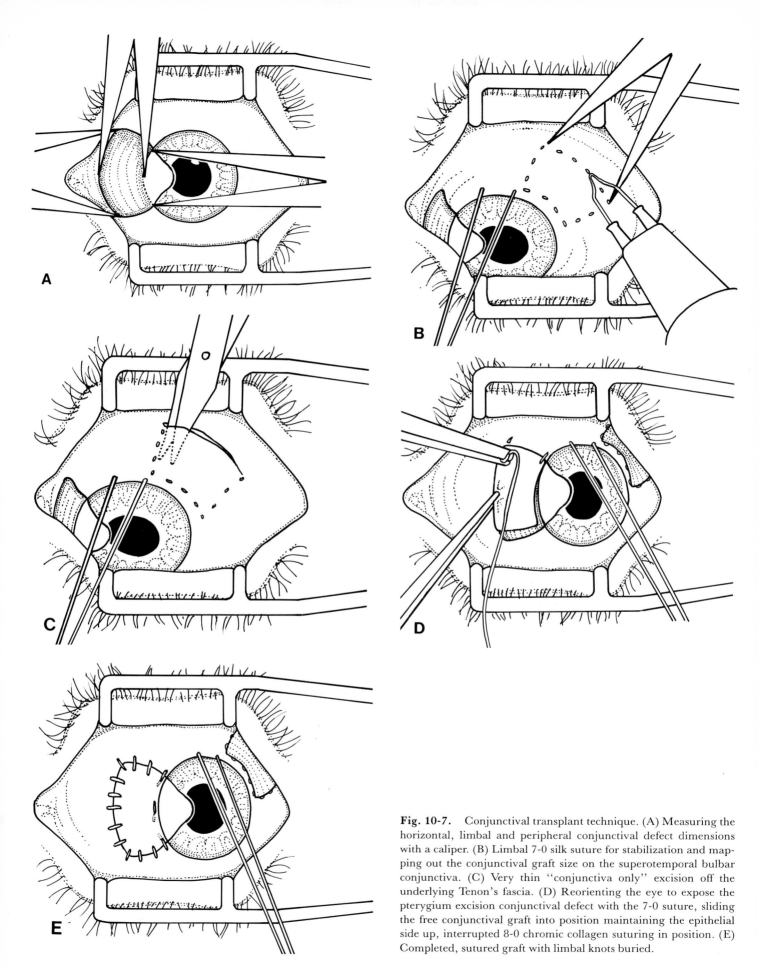

**Fig. 10-7.** Conjunctival transplant technique. (A) Measuring the horizontal, limbal and peripheral conjunctival defect dimensions with a caliper. (B) Limbal 7-0 silk suture for stabilization and mapping out the conjunctival graft size on the superotemporal bulbar conjunctiva. (C) Very thin "conjunctiva only" excision off the underlying Tenon's fascia. (D) Reorienting the eye to expose the pterygium excision conjunctival defect with the 7-0 suture, sliding the free conjunctival graft into position maintaining the epithelial side up, interrupted 8-0 chromic collagen suturing in position. (E) Completed, sutured graft with limbal knots buried.

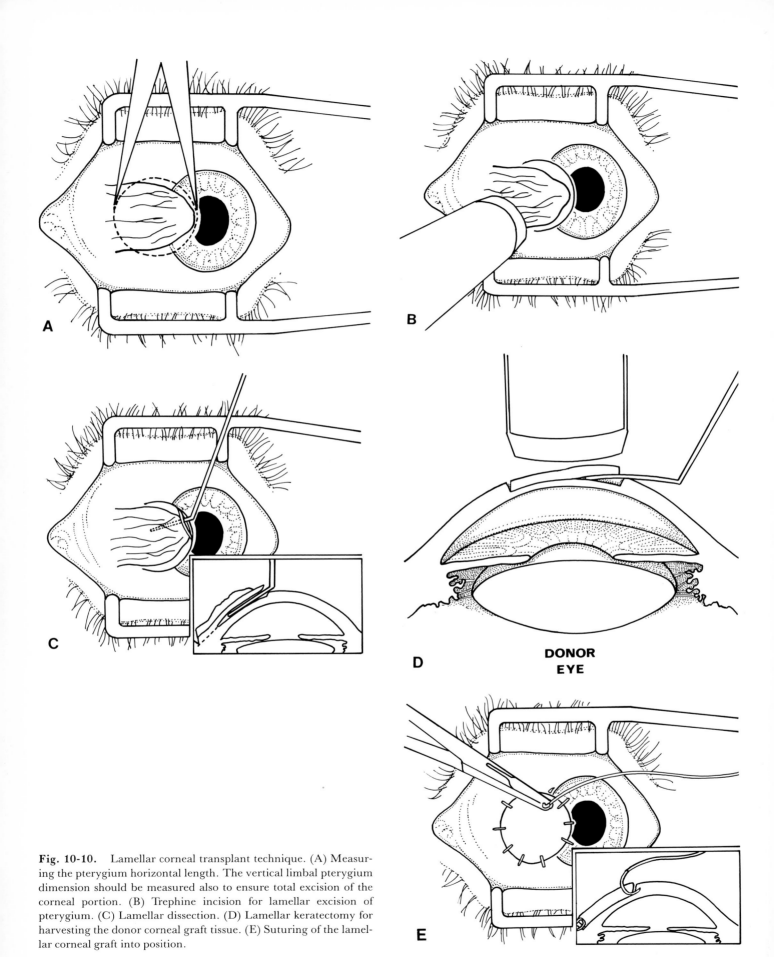

**Fig. 10-10.** Lamellar corneal transplant technique. (A) Measuring the pterygium horizontal length. The vertical limbal pterygium dimension should be measured also to ensure total excision of the corneal portion. (B) Trephine incision for lamellar excision of pterygium. (C) Lamellar dissection. (D) Lamellar keratectomy for harvesting the donor corneal graft tissue. (E) Suturing of the lamellar corneal graft into position.

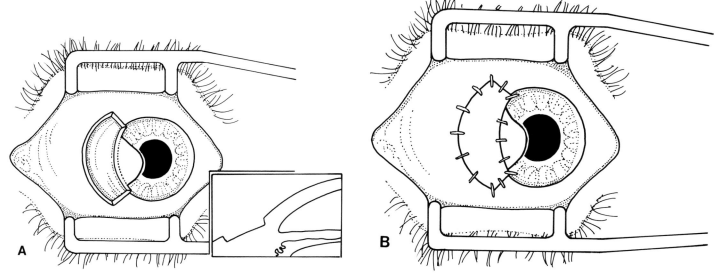

**Fig. 10-11.** Free-hand corneoscleral lamellar technique. (A) Limbal keratectomy. (B) Free-hand corneal graft sutured into position.

limbus, because recurrence seems to occur more frequently if sclera is left bare. Transplantation has been more useful, in our experience, when a large active primary or recurrent pterygium is encountered.

## POSTOPERATIVE MANAGEMENT

In an effort to reduce recurrences, additional treatments postoperatively have included: topical steroids, beta radiation, and thio-tepa. The many different additive treatments combined with varying surgical techniques again emphasize the inability of any one technique to be universally effective.

Topical steroids are well recognized anti-inflamatory medications which also inhibit collagen synthesis, stabilize vascular permeability, and inhibit vascularization. Their effect is not strong enough to prevent the recurrence of pterygium and they are used as an important adjunct to other forms of treatment.

Beta radiation has achieved strong popularity. It causes an obliterative endarteritis and inhibits fibroblast proliferation. Most surgeons, using beta radiation, prefer a bare sclera pterygium excision followed by strontium (Sr) 90 beta irradiation to be the exposed denuded limbal area. The total dose varies by report and clinical situation from 600 to 8800 rads/eye (median; 2000 rads/eye). The recommendations also vary with respect to application schedule (during surgery, within 4 days after surgery, within 3 weeks after surgery). Divided doses over 3 weeks to total 1500 rads/eye is probably safest to prevent cataracts or scleral necrosis. This dose usually allows the possibility of another treatment if there is a pterygium recurrence requiring reexcision. Proper application of beta radiation requires that the Sr 90 probes are tested frequently to ascertain their emission strength. Each individual dose is then calculated based on the probe's strength.

Sr 90 is the preferred energy source because it is a pure beta emitter, has a long half-life (28 years), and dissipates its energy over a short distance, preventing complications. The equator of the crystalline lens is exposed to only 20 percent of the total corneoscleral dose.

Infrequent complications have occurred from beta radiation including chronic pain and photophobia, scleral necrosis, secondary cataract, scleral infectious ulceration, and even endophthalmitis.[46] Most serious complications result after large or multiple doses of beta radiation are used for multiple recurrent lesions. Tarr and Constable[46] reported delayed (9 and 10 years later) scleral necrosis and ulceration, which led to pseudomonas endophthalmitis and evisceration. They recommend surgical repair of radiation scleral necrosis.

Thio-tepa is a nitrogen mustard alkylating agent with antimitotic and radiomimetic activity which suppresses endothelial and fibroblast proliferation. It has, therefore, been used to inhibit pterygium and corneal neovascularization both experimentally[42] and clinically.[2,19,32] It has worked well with recurrences ranging from zero to 7.7 percent. This is comparable to results obtained from other methods; however, thio-tepa has not received the same popularity as beta radiation. Harrison et al., in a double-blind study, compared thio-tepa to beta radiation and found only one ($n = 25$) recurrence in the beta radiation group versus none ($n = 24$) in the thio-tepa group.

The dosage of thio-tepa is very consistent in the literature at 1/2000 dilution (15 mg/30 cc Ringers lactate), one or two drops to the postoperative eye every 3 hours while awake for 6–8 weeks. This medicine must be stored in the refrigerator between uses.

Thio-tepa complications include red eye, conjunctival pigmentation, and skin and lash depigmentation.[2] Poor corneal transplant wound healing[42] has been seen but only one case of scleral ulceration[2] following thio-tepa has been recorded.

## COMPLICATIONS

Recurrence, defined as fibrovascular reinvasion of the cornea, represents the most dreaded complication of pterygium surgery. Its frequency is reported to be from between zero and 69 percent, depending on the definition of recurrence, adequacy of follow-up efforts, and the nature of the populations studied. Zauberman feels that the rate of recurrence may reflect the above parameters more than the nature of any surgical procedure.[51] He has classified recurrences based on the degree of hyperemia, volume of the head, and extension of the cap (ilots de Fuch's). The most aggressive and recurrent cases were seen in younger patients and had the worst prognosis. The older patients with more atrophic pterygiums had a lesser recurrence rate and better prognosis. There were no significant differences between the sexes.

The majority of recurrences may be seen in the first month whereas fewer will be seen after a long delay. Some very delayed recurrences may be true pterygiums which have recurred after successful treatment, but they are rare. Most recurrences seen in the first few months are preceded by blood vessels from the cut edge of the conjunctiva and are oriented in the same axis as the original pterygium. Seen initially on the conjunctiva, they progressively extend out onto the cornea. The postoperative treatments described above may limit the progression of any recurrence and should be tried. Others believe that immediate reoperation is necessary once a recurrence is identified.[6] Most prefer conservative management before reoperating.

Vision-compromising corneal scarring is a possible complication if the pterygium is not excised before it crosses the visual axis. A large lamellar keratoplasty may be performed to clear the superficial scarring and try to prevent recurrence.

Extraoccular motion restrictions are seen after multiple recurrences or surgeries. Conjunctival or mucous membrane grafts are probably required to prevent another recurrence. Large amounts of mobilized transplant tissue are needed to cover the large area of scarred conjunctiva excised.

Induced astigmatism is usually completely reversed by excision of the pterygium and prevention of its recurrence. Irregular corneal astigmatism may be corrected with a contact lens or rarely a full lamellar corneal transplant.

## CONCLUSIONS

The cause of pterygium is still poorly understood but probably is related to a chronic keratoconjunctivitis induced by UV exposure, at least initially. The mechanisms of its progression and recurrence are even less understood. Prevalence, treatment, successes and failures are poorly comparable between authors due to varying geographic locations, environmental exposure, population, and definition biases. We prefer excision with primary conjunctival closure for initial, small, uninflamed pterygiums and excision with conjunctival transplant for recurrent or aggressive lesions. Flexibility to try another management technique may be necessary on the occasional, aggressively recurrent lesion.

## REFERENCES

1. Aratoon V: Surgery of pterygium by conjunctival pedicle flap. Am J Ophthalmol 63:1778, 1967
2. Asregadoo ER: Surgery, thio-tepa, and corticosteroid in the treatment of pterygium. Am J Ophthalmol 74:960, 1972
3. Bangerter A: Pterygium operation and covering of conjunctival defects. Ophthalmologica 106:316, 1943
4. Berens C: New method for transplanting pterygium. Arch Ophthalmol 21:30, 1939
5. Biedner B, Biger Y, Roghkoff L, et al.: Pterygium and basic tear secretion. Ann Ophthalmol 11:1235, 1979
6. Cameron ME: Pterygium Throughout the World. Springfield, Thomas, 1965
7. Campodonico E: A new procedure in the excision method of pterygium operation. Int Cong Ophthalmol 1:201, 1922
8. Dake CL, Crone RA, De Keizer RJW: Treatment of recurrent pterygium oculi by lamellar keratoplasty, Doc Ophthalmologica, 48:223, 1979
9. Darrell RW, Bachrach CA: Pterygium among veterans. Arch Ophthalmol 70:158, 1963
10. DeKeizer RJW: Pterygium excision with or without postoperative radiation, a double blind study, Doc Ophthalmologica 52:309, 1982
11. Desmarres LA: Traite Theoretique et Pratique des Maladies des Yeux (ed. 2). Paris, Germer Bailliere, 1855, p. 168
12. Detels R, Dhir SP: Pterygium: A geographical study. Arch Ophthalmol 78:485, 1967
13. Dimitry TJ: Pterygium geography for the United States of America. Eye Ear Nose Throat 14:45, 1935
14. D'Oombrain A: The surgical treatment of pterygium. Br J Ophthalmol 32:65, 1948
15. Dowlut MS, Laflamme MY: Les pterygions recidivants: frequence et correction par autogreffe conjunctivale, Can J Ophthalmol 16:119, 1981
16. Forster RK: Personal communication.
17. Fuchs, E: Uber das pterygium. Graefes Arch Clin Exp Ophthalmol 38:1, 1892
18. Goldman KN, Kaufman HE: Atypical pterygium, Arch Ophthalmol 96:1027, 1978
19. Harrison M, Kelly A, Ohlrich J: Pterygium, Thio-tepa versus beta radiation, a double-blind trial. Tr Aust Coll Ophthalmol 1:64, 1969
20. Hartman DC: Use of free grafts in correction of recurrent pterygia, pseudopterygia and symblepharon. Calif Medicine 75:279, 1951
21. Hochbaum DR, Moskowitz SE, Wirtschafter D: A quantitative analysis of astigmatism induced by pterygium. Biomechanics 10:735–746, 1977
22. Jensen OL: Pterygium, the dominant eye and the habit of closing one eye in the sunlight. Acta Ophthalmologica 60:568, 1982
23. Johnson GJ: Etiology of spheroidal degeneration of the cornea in Labrador. Br J Ophthal 65:270, 1981
24. Kamel S: Pterygium, Its nature and a new line of treatment, Br J Ophthalmol 30:549, 1946
25. Karai I, Horiguchi S: Pterygium in welders, Br J Ophthalmol 68:347, 1984
26. Kenyon KR, Wagoner MD, Hettinger ME: Conjunctival autograft transplantation for advanced and recurrent pterygium, Ophthalmology 92:1461, 1985
27. King, JH Jr.: The pterygium. Arch Ophthalmol 44:854, 1950
28. Lerner S: Radiant Energy and the Eye. New York, Macmillan, 1980

29. McGavic, JS: Surgical treatment of recurrent pterygium. Arch Ophthalmol 42:726, 1949

30. McReynolds JO: The nature and treatment of pterygia. JAMA 39:269, 1902

31. McReynolds JO: Pterygium operation. South Med J 28:823, 1935

32. Meacham CT: Triethylene Thiophosphoramide; In prevention of pterygium recurrence, AM J Ophthalmol 54:751, 1962

33. Merigot de Treigny, Coirre: Le Pterygion. Bull Soc Ophthalmol Fr 1:152, 1933

34. Moran DJ, Hollows FC: Pterygium and ultraviolet radiation: A positive correlation, BR Ophthalmol 68:343, 1984

35. Norn MS: Spheroid degeneration, pinguecula and pterygium among arabs in the red sea territory, Jordan. Acta Ophthalmologica 60:949, 1982

36. Norn MS: Prevalence of pinguecula in Greenland and in Copenhagen and its relation to pterygium and spheroid degeneration. Acta Ophthalmologica 57:96, 1979

37. Paton D: Pterygium management based upon a theory of pathogenesis. Trans Am Acad Ophthalmol Otolaryngol 79:603, 1962

38. Pinkerton OD, Yoshitsugi H, Shigrmura BA: Immunologic basis for the pathegenesis of pterygium. Am J Ophthalmol 98:225, 1984

39. Poirier RH, Fish JR: Lamellar keratoplasty for recurrent pterygium. Ophthalmic Surg 7:38, 1976

40. Poulsen JT, Staberg B, Wulf HC, et al.: Dermal elastosis in hairless mice after UV-B and UV-A applied separately or simultaneously. Br J Dermatol 110:531, 1984

41. Ramsay AM: Atlas of External Diseases of the Eye. Glasgow, MacLehose, 1898

42. Rock RL: Inhibition of corneal vascularization by triethylene thiophosphoramide (thio-tepa), Arch Ophthalmol 69:330, 1963

43. Reed H, Hildes JA: Corneal scarring in canadian eskimos, Can Med Assoc J 81:364, 1959

44. Reeh MJ: Corneoscleral lamellar transplant for recurrent pterygium, Arch Ophthalmol 86:296, 1971

45. Spencer WH: Ophthalmic Pathology, An Atlas and Textbook. Philadelphia, Saunders, 1985

46. Tarr KH, Constable IJ: Late complications of pterygium treatment. Br J Ophthalmol 64:496, 1980

47. Thoft RA: Conjunctival transplantation, Arch Ophthalmol 95:1425, 1977

48. Vastine DW, Demartini DR, Free autologous conjunctival patch grafts for repair of active primary and recurrent pterygium. Poster Presentation at the Meeting of the American Academy of Ophthalmology Meeting, Chicago, IL, 1983

49. Vastine DW, Stewart WB, Schwab IR: Reconstruction of the periocular mucous membrane by autologous conjunctival transplantation. Ophthalmology 89:1072, 1982

50. Wong WW: A hypothesis on the pathogenesis of pterygiums, Ann Ophthalmol 10:303, 1978

51. Zauberman H: Pterygium and its recurrence. Am J Ophthalmol 62:1780, 1967

52. Ziegler SL: The subconjunctival excision of pterygium, in International Congress of Ophthalmology (ed. 12). Philadelphia, William F. Fell Co., 1922, p 205

53. Zolli CL: Experience with avulsion technique in pterygium surgery. Ann Ophthalmol 11:1569, 1979

# 11

# Superior Limbic Keratoconjunctivitis

## Ronald N. Gaster

Superior limbic keratoconjunctivitis was first described by Theodore in 1963.[14] It is a specific clinical entity which represents a chronic, recurrent keratoconjunctivitis and may be misdiagnosed or go unrecognized unless the clinician is familiar with the condition or has a high index of suspicion. Appropriate therapy can frequently alleviate the patients' discomfort and symptoms; however, remissions, recurrences, and spontaneous exacerbations can occur.

## CLINICAL FEATURES

Superior limbic keratoconjunctivitis is characterized by a number of distinctive clinical features: (1) marked inflammation and papillary hypertrophy of the tarsal conjunctiva of the upper lid, (2) inflammation and hyperemia of the superior bulbar conjunctiva, (3) fine punctate staining with fluorescein or rose bengal at the superior corneoscleral limbus, (4) proliferation with keratinization of the superior limbal and bulbar conjunctival epithelium, and (5) filaments at the superior limbus or cornea in approximately one-third to one-half of patients (Figs. 11-1 and 11-2; see color insert following page 139).[1,11,14,15,18]

The inflammation of the bulbar conjunctiva extends usually from 10:30 to 1:30 o'clock. It is most intense at the limbus and fades gradually over the superior 8–10 mm. The superficial punctate corneal staining associated with this condition extends superiorly for 4–5 mm onto the bulbar conjunctiva and involves the corneal area within 2 mm at the superior limbus.[17]

The superior corneal limbal epithelium can proliferate with hypertrophic thickened conjunctival epithelium. This proliferation can appear grey or raised and fleshy.[15] The inflamed limbus may appear congested or boggy and bulge down over the superior cornea.[1] The inferior cornea and conjunctiva are not affected.

Filaments are seen at the superior limbus and adjacent cornea in one-third to one-half of all cases. Their appearance is usually associated with noticeably increased discomfort

and irritation by the patient. Removal of the filaments is accompanied by corneal epithelial defects.

Typically, the symptoms associated with superior limbic keratoconjunctivitis are out of proportion to the clinical findings. Patients can have severe ocular irritation and complain of pain, burning, foreign body sensation, and photophobia. Blepharospasm has been noted, particularly in unilateral cases.[1]

Superior limbic keratoconjunctivitis typically follows a chronic course with remissions and recurrences and can last 1–10 years. It is seen most commonly in patients 20–70 years old. There is a somewhat greater incidence in women than in men.[15] The condition is usually bilateral, though it may occur unilaterally or be asymmetrically involved. Furthermore, one eye may be affected at one time and the other eye may develop a recurrence subsequently.

## ETIOLOGIC CONSIDERATIONS

The etiology of superior limbic keratoconjunctivitis is unknown. Theodore[14] and Thygeson[19] originally considered viral causation to be involved; however, viral cultures have been negative and ultrastructural studies have shown no histologic evidence of viral involvement.[3] Similarly, bacterial and fungal cultures have not been helpful. Scrapings from the involved superior bulbar conjunctiva that have been Giemsa-stained have shown marked keratinization of the epithelial cells, with degenerated nuclei and hyalinized cytoplasm, and polymorphonuclear leukocytes.[18] Epithelial scrapings from the superior palpebral conjunctiva demonstrate normal epithelial cells with a polymorphonuclear reaction. Biopsy specimens from the involved superior bulbar conjunctiva support the findings from scrapings and reveal epithelial keratinization with varying degrees of acanthosis, dyskeratosis, cellular infiltration, and nuclear balloon degeneration.[18] Palpebral conjunctiva biopsy specimens exhibit an infiltration of inflammatory cells including polymorphonuclear leukocytes, lymphocytes, and plasma cells. It is of note that there is an absence of eosinophils, basophils, and viral inclusion bodies in the scrapings and biopsy specimens.[18] Of interest, it was shown that the keratinization process of the conjunctiva in superior limbic keratoconjunctivitis has the same ultrastructural features as that occurring in normal skin.[2] It has been reported that in Papanicolaou-stained cells from scrapings of the superior bulbar conjunctiva of patients with superior limbic keratoconjunctivitis there is an unusual serpiginous appearance of the condensed chromatin within the nuclear membrane.[21] These findings were similarly seen in patients with keratitis sicca.[6]

There have been several reports noting an association between possible thyroid disease or elevated thyroid function tests and superior limbic keratoconjunctivitis.[1,11,12,16] These may suggest an immunologic basis to superior limbic keratoconjunctivitis. Treatment of the thyroid abnormality has not, however, been shown to improve the condition.

## MEDICAL TREATMENT

Since his original description of superior limbic keratoconjunctivitis, Theodore has recommended the use of locally applied 0.5% silver nitrate solution moistened on a cotton-tipped applicator as the mainstay of treatment.[14,15] Theodore advises touching the upper tarsal conjunctiva in three places only and then, while the patient looks down, touching the superior bulbar conjunctiva in all affected areas. Finally, the inferior conjunctiva should be treated.

The silver nitrate should be touched to these areas, not rubbed or scrubbed. The cornea itself should not be treated. Because there is little discomfort, no topical anesthetic is necessary (Theodore, personal communication). In a large number of patients, this treatment alone will allow relatively rapid relief of symptoms and, eventually, loss of all signs of the condition. Recurrences often develop and repeated treatments are usually necessary. The use of a silver nitrate applicator stick to cauterize the base of a surgical bed after chalazion removal has been associated with a severe corneal burn and opacification requiring penetrating keratoplasty.[5] These solid-tipped applicators should not be used near the cornea.

Any treatment for superior limbic keratoconjunctivitis may work for a while, but it may later be necessary to change to a different treatment. N-acetylcysteine allowed for subjective and objective improvement in 65 percent of patients in one study.[22]

The use of pressure patching alone or in combination with therapeutic soft contact lenses has been shown to eliminate both the signs and symptoms of superior limbic keratoconjunctivitis.[7] This treatment regimen may be initially successful by eliminating the mechanical rubbing of the lid on the globe by the pressure patching and subsequently by protecting the superior limbus and adjacent conjunctiva by the soft contact lenses. The use of a pressure patch for an initial 1 week prior to soft contact lens use was found to interrupt long-standing blepharospasm which was felt to aggravate the condition.[7] Other investigators, however, have implicated soft contact lens wearing as a causative factor in a syndrome similar to superior limbic keratoconjunctivitis.[4,9,10] It is

unclear at present what role thimerosal may have in the etiology of this particular syndrome.

The use of topical ocular decongestants, artificial tears, antibiotics, idoxuridine, and steroids have provided only brief symptomatic amelioration of symptoms in some patients and are usually not successful.[1,3,11,14,15]

## SURGICAL TREATMENT

Mechanical scraping of the upper palpebral and bulbar conjunctiva may be of benefit in some patients. It has been suggested that this debridement of surface cells may decrease the limbal engorgement and allow for adequate moistening of the conjunctiva and cornea.[3,22]

Recession of the bulbar conjunctiva was initially suggested for patients unresponsive to topical therapy.[13] The surgical technique involves first anesthetizing the conjunctiva with a topical anesthetic and then injecting a local anesthetic under the superior bulbar conjunctiva. A superior limbal peritomy from 10:30 to 1:30 o'clock is made with superior extensions radially long enough to recess the conjunctiva 4 mm superiorly (Figs. 11-3A and 11-3B). The conjunctiva is dissected from underlying Tenon's fascia. The former limbal edge of the conjunctiva is then sutured to the sclera with interrupted 7-0 chromic sutures (Fig. 11-3C). Topical antibiotic drops may be used postoperatively. This may eliminate symptoms in some difficult cases.

Resection of involved superior bulbar conjunctiva has similarly been found to be successful in difficult cases.[3,8] Removal of thickened excessive conjunctiva allows for the reestablishment of a normal limbal area and provides relief of symptoms in patients unresponsive to medical therapy. The surgical technique is similar to that of conjunctival recession, described above (Figs. 11-3A and 11-3B), except that the involved bulbar conjunctiva is excised and not sutured to the sclera. (Figs. 11-3D and 11-3E). Superior tarsal conjunctiva resection has been associated with only short-term relief of symptoms.[3] Preoperative tear production testing was helpful in predicting success with conjunctival resection in some patients. Those patients with normal tear production had a higher success rate with conjunctival resection.[8]

The focal application of thermal cauterization of the superior bulbar conjunctiva has recently been reported as an additional mode of therapy for superior limbic keratoconjunctivitis.[20] It is postulated that cautery produces transiently increased vascularity, plus epithelial migration and/or differentiation from surrounding "normal" conjunctiva, thereby disrupting the inflammatory cycle and restoring goblet cells. The technique requires both topical and subconjunctival anesthesia of the superior bulbar conjunctiva prior to applying the thermal cautery burns (Fig. 11-4A). A disposable microsurgical cautery is used to deliver from 30 to 50 focal applications that extend from the superior limbus horizontally over 3–4 clock hours and posteriorly for approximately 8 mm (Fig. 11-4B). Each burn involves full-thickness conjunctiva to produce focal shrinkage; it does not, however, extend down to the sclera. Postoperatively, topical antibiotic ointment such as erythromycin is applied.

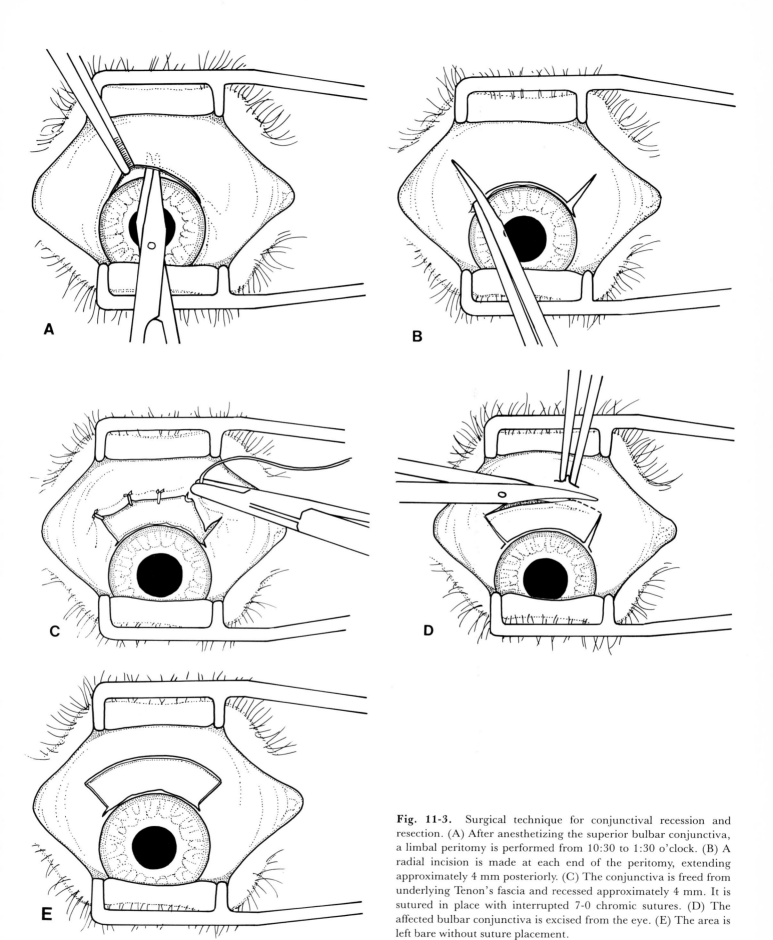

**Fig. 11-3.** Surgical technique for conjunctival recession and resection. (A) After anesthetizing the superior bulbar conjunctiva, a limbal peritomy is performed from 10:30 to 1:30 o'clock. (B) A radial incision is made at each end of the peritomy, extending approximately 4 mm posteriorly. (C) The conjunctiva is freed from underlying Tenon's fascia and recessed approximately 4 mm. It is sutured in place with interrupted 7-0 chromic sutures. (D) The affected bulbar conjunctiva is excised from the eye. (E) The area is left bare without suture placement.

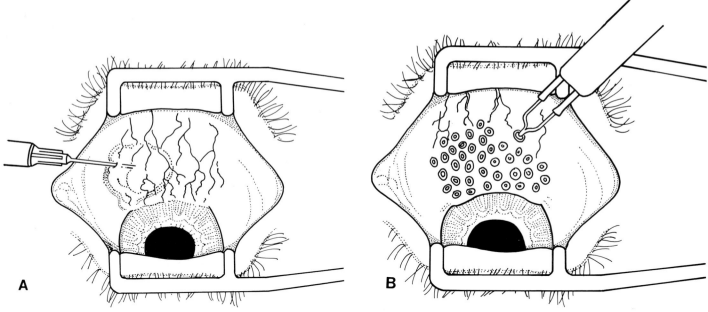

**Fig. 11-4.** Technique for thermocauterization of the bulbar conjunctiva. (A) After instillation of topical anesthetic drops, 2% xylocaine is injected beneath the superior bulbar conjunctiva with a 30-gauge needle. (B) A disposable microsurgical cautery is used to apply focal burns to the conjunctiva in the affected area.

## REFERENCES

1. Cher I: Clinical features of superior limbic keratoconjunctivitis in Australia. A probable association with thyrotoxicosis. Arch Ophthalmol 82:580–586, 1969
2. Collin HB, Donshik PC, Foster CS, et al.: Keratinization of the bulbar conjunctival epithelium in superior limbic keratoconjunctivitis in humans. An electron microscopic study. Acta Ophthalmol 56:531–543, 1978
3. Donshik PC, Collin HB, Foster CS, et al.: Conjunctival resection treatment and ultrastructural histopathology of superior limbic keratoconjunctivitis. Am J Ophthalmal 85:101–110, 1978
4. Fuerst DJ, Sugar J, Worobec S: Superior limbic keratoconjunctivitis associated with cosmetic soft contact lens wear. Arch Ophthalmol 101:1214–1216, 1983
5. Grayson M, Pieroni D: Severe silver nitrate injury to the eye. Am J Ophthalmol 70:227–229, 1970
6. Marner K: "Snake-like" appearance of nuclear chromatin in conjunctival epithelial cells from patients with keratoconjunctivitis sicca. Acta Ophthalmol 58:849–853, 1980
7. Mondino BJ, Zaidman GW, Salamon SW: Use of pressure patching and soft contact lenses in superior limbic keratoconjunctivitis. Arch Ophthalmol 100:1932–1934, 1982
8. Passons GA, Wood TO: Conjunctival resection for superior limbic keratoconjunctivitis. Ophthalmology 91:966–968, 1984
9. Sendele DD, Kenyon KR, Mobilia EF, et al.: Superior limbic keratoconjunctivitis in contact lens wearers. Ophthalmology 90:616–622, 1983
10. Stenson S: Superior limbic keratoconjunctivitis associated with soft contact lens wear. Arch Ophthalmol 101:402–404, 1983
11. Sutherland AL: Superior limbic keratoconjunctivitis. Trans Ophthalmol Soc NZ 21:89–95, 1969
12. Tenzel RR: Comments on superior limbic filamentous keratitis: Part 2. Arch Ophthalmol 79:508, 1968
13. Tenzel RR: Resistant superior limbic keratoconjunctivitis. Arch Ophthalmol 89:439, 1973
14. Theodore FH: Superior limbic keratoconjunctivitis. Eye Ear Nose Throat 42:25–28, 1963
15. Theodore FH: Further observations on superior limbic keratoconjunctivitis. Trans Am Acad Ophthalmol Otolaryngol 71:341–351, 1967
16. Theodore FH: Comments on findings of elevated protein-bound iodine in superior limbic keratoconjunctivitis: Part 1. Arch Ophthalmol 79:508, 1968
17. Theodore FH: Diagnostic dyes in superior limbic keratoconjunctivitis and other superficial entities, in Turtz AI (ed): Proceedings of the Centennial Symposium, Manhattan Eye, Ear and Throat Hospital, vol 1, Ophthalmology. Mosby, St. Louis, 1969, pp 260–266
18. Theodore FH, Ferry AP: Superior limbic keratoconjunctivitis. Clinical and pathological correlations. Arch Ophthalmol 84:481–484, 1970
19. Thygeson P: Observations on filamentary keratitis. Transactions of the American Medical Association, Section on Ophthalmology, 112th Annual Meeting. Chicago, AMA, 1963, pp 49–55
20. Udell IJ, Kenyon KR, Sawa M, et al. Treatment of superior limbic keratoconjunctivitis by thermocauterization of the superior bulbar conjunctiva. Ophthalmology 93:162–166, 1986
21. Wander AH, Masukawa T: Unusual appearance of condensed chromatin in conjunctival cells in superior limbic keratoconjunctivitis. Lancet 2:42–43, 1981
22. Wright P: Superior limbic keratoconjunctivitis. Trans Ophthalmol Soc UK 92:555–560, 1972

# 12

# Mucous Membrane Abnormalities

## Michael W. Belin    Sadeer B. Hannush

Visual function is dependent, in part, on clear optical media. Corneal transparency requires a healthy ocular surface. The ocular surface, a continuous sheet of epithelium and subjacent tissues, lines the inside of the eyelids, covers the globe, and extends over the cornea.[96] The ocular surface thus includes corneal, limbal, and conjunctival epithelial cell layers. The protective tear film requires an adequate acqueous component from the main and accessory lacrimal glands, as well as sufficient mucin production from the conjunctival goblet cells. Normal lid anatomy and function, including an intact palpebral conjunctiva, insure proper resurfacing of the cornea and maintenance of corneal clarity. Ocular surface integrity is, thus, affected adversely by mucous membrane abnormalities. These may have a variety of etiologies from autoimmune phenomena in ocular cicatricial pemphigoid, to toxic reactions in Stevens-Johnson syndrome, to infectious processes in trachoma, and physical trauma in chemical injuries. Regardless of the underlying etiology, mucous membrane abnormalities affecting the eye share many features, including scarring of the conjunctiva with decreased conjunctival goblet cell density, loss of normal lid architecture, tear film abnormalities, and scarring and vascularization of the cornea.

Many mucous membrane diseases may involve the eye, including pemphigus, bullous pemphigoid, cicatricial pemphigoid, erythema multiforme, toxic epidermal necrolysis, epidermolysis bullosa, and dermatitis herpetiformis. In this chapter, cicatricial pemphigoid, Stevens-Johnson syndrome, trachoma, and chemical injuries are discussed. These conditions can have significant destructive effects on the mucous membranes of the eye, to the extent that medical treatment may not suffice, and surgical correction may become necessary. Each clinical entity and its medical management is discussed separately, followed by a discussion of surgical techniques.

Cicatricial pemphigoid and Stevens-Johnson syndrome are both diseases of the skin and mucous membranes with a high predilection for severe ocular involvement. Despite their distinct pathologic and immunologic characteristics, they share several ocular features that include conjunctival shrinkage and scarring, entropion, trichiasis, and xerosis. Both may result in blindness due to opacification of the cornea.

## CICATRICIAL PEMPHIGOID

*Cicatricial pemphigoid* (also known as *ocular pemphigoid, essential shrinkage of the conjunctiva,* and *benign mucous membrane pemphigoid*) is an autoimmune cicatricial disease of the conjunctiva and, to a lesser extent, other mucous membranes and skin. It is a disease of late life with an average age of onset of 58 years,[37] and it affects women more than men.[87] It is generally believed to exhibit type II hypersensitivity reactions. IgG, IgA, and complement have been demonstrated along the epithelial basement membrane of the conjunctiva by direct immunofluorescence,[30] and circulating autoantibodies have been detected by indirect immunofluorescence.[108] An HLA–B12 association has been demonstrated in cicatricial pemphigoid.[62]

### Clinical Manifestations

Mucous membrane involvement includes the conjunctiva, nose, oral cavity, pharynx, larynx, esophagus, anus, and vagina. The conjunctiva is eventually involved in approximately 75 percent of patients with cicatricial pemphigoid.[37] Ocular pemphigoid is a bilateral disease. Although it frequently starts in one eye, the other eye is usually affected after an interval of less than 2 years.[24] The initial symptoms are those of chronic conjunctivitis with irritation, burning, and tearing. The chronic conjunctivitis may be aggravated by bacterial infections resulting in erroneous diagnoses. The basic destructive process is fibrosis beneath the conjunctival epithelium.[24,31,50] Symblepharon formation starts with the inferior fornix. The fornices gradually shrink, impairing the motility of the globe. With progressive shrinkage, ankyloblepharon develops. Ocular cicatricial pemphigoid is asso-

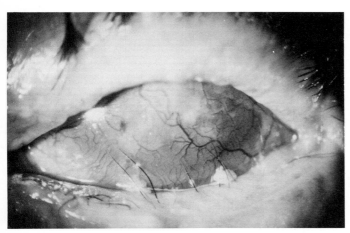

**Fig. 12-1.** End-stage ocular cicatricial pemphigoid exhibiting entropion with trichiasis, and corneal opacification and vascularization (Courtesy of Steven P. Dunn, M.D.).

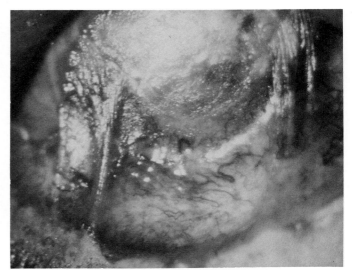

**Fig. 12-2.** End-stage ocular cicatricial pemphigoid with xerosis and symblepharon formation.

ciated with a diminished and unstable tear film.[6] There is a decrease in the aqueous components secondary to fibrous occlusion of the ducts of the lacrimal and accessory lacrimal glands, as well as a mucin deficiency because of destruction of goblet cells.[47,49,67,82] In the late stages corneal involvement leads to decreased vision.

Although primary corneal involvement with vesicular and bullous formation has been reported,[31,50] corneal erosions most commonly occur from entropion with trichiasis, lagophthalmos with abnormal blinking and exposure, and the abnormal tear film. This eventually leads to corneal neovascularization and opacification (Figs. 12-1 and 12-2).

## Histopathology and Immunology

In cicatricial pemphigoid the bullous formation occurs in a subepithelial location without acantholysis but with conjunctival metaplasia of the normal columnar epithelium into squamous epithelium with parakeratinization, keratinization,[1] and loss of mucous-producing goblet cells.[1,82] Recent studies indicate the sensitivity of conjunctival goblet cells as an indicator of primary ocular surface disease.[49,67] Eyes with cicatricial ocular pemphigoid and Stevens-Johnson syndrome demonstrate a profound loss of goblet cells in the conjunctiva. Thoft et al. hypothesize a hyperproliferation of conjunctival epithelium with concurrent failure of normal conjunctival differentiation.[101] Immunoglobulin deposition on the conjunctival basement membrane in a linear fashion is considered characteristic of ocular cicatricial pemphigoid.[59,60] It is not always present nor is it diagnostic.

## Differential Diagnosis

The diagnosis of ocular cicatricial pemphigoid is one of exclusion. Other causes of conjunctival scarring, shrinkage, and symblepharon include radiation and chemical burns, conjunctivitis secondary to adenovirus types 8 and 19, herpes simplex, diphtheria, and beta-hemolytic streptococci.[15,30]

All of these causes, however, have a rather acute self-limited course. Conjunctival shrinkage and symblepharon have been associated with the systemic use of practolol,[47] topical epinephrine,[53] echothiophate iodide, pilocarpine, and IDU.[73] Symblepharon has been also reported in Sjogren's syndrome,[46] sarcoidosis,[25] and trachoma, although trachomatis changes usually occur in the superior fornix. Other bullous diseases affecting the conjunctiva include epidermolysis bullosa, erythema multiforme, toxic epidermal necrolysis, and dermatitis herpetiformis.

## Treatment

Artificial tears, preferably preservative free, are helpful in the early stages. Topical antibiotics can be used to treat secondary bacterial infections. The role of topical and subconjunctival corticosteroids is limited. Systemic corticosteroids are of definite value in the treatment of acute manifestations of the disease, preventing rapid conjunctival shrinkage during periods of acute exacerbation.[61]

The chronic use of steroids is of limited value in halting the progression of the disease and is impractical in the older age groups. Rogers et al.[86] found that more than 80 percent of patients showed a beneficial response to the oral administration of dapsone in a dosage of 100 mg/day. A 4-week trial may be attempted. The major complications are hemolytic anemia, skin rashes, and arthralgias. Recently, Foster[26] has shown that cyclophosphamide and prednisone used in combination can halt the progression and bring improvement to patients with cicatricial pemphigoid. Mondino and Brown[64] further studied the efficacy of systemic immunosuppression using cyclophosphamide with prednisone, cyclophosphamide alone, azathioprine alone, and prednisone alone. Although immunosuppressive therapy did inhibit conjunctival shrinkage in all treatment groups, some eyes in each group progressed despite treatment, and there were many serious complications secondary to these agents. Their recommendation, therefore, is not to subject elderly patients with limited life spans to the risks of immunosuppressive therapy unless their eyes are at least at a moderate or advanced stage with ongoing progression.[64] Tseng et al.[104] recently demonstrated the beneficial effects of short-term topical vitamin A therapy in various dry eye disorders including cicatricial pemphigoid.

Entropion and trichiasis may be corrected earlier in the disease by oculoplastic surgical techniques with care not to shorten an already shrunken fornix. Trichiasis may also be treated with electrolysis, cryotherapy, and hyfercation. Therapeutic contact lenses may offer some help in protecting the cornea from drying and trichiasis, although the increased threat of infection in an already compromised host is evident. Any surgical procedure such as lysis of symblepharon, lid procedures, or intraocular procedures may increase the risk of acute exacerbation of the disease.[65] In the final stage with ankyloblepharon and keratinization of the ocular surface a keratoprosthesis may be useful in restoring some sight to these otherwise blind patients.

## STEVENS-JOHNSON SYNDROME

*Erythema multiforme* is an acute, usually self-limited, inflammatory disorder of the skin and mucous membranes. In its minor form, erythema multiforme primarily involves the skin. The major form is characterized by mucosal and cutaneous lesions, toxemia with fever and prostration, and severe ocular involvement. The major form is known as Stevens-Johnson syndrome (SJS). Some studies have described the following diagnostic criteria for SJS: (1) skin lesions; (2) erosive involvement of two or more mucous membranes; and (3) systemic toxicity, usually including malaise, fever, and prostration.[111] The minor variant of the disease may last 2 or 3 weeks, while the major form lasts an average of 6 weeks with individual skin lesions having life cycles of 2 weeks. The disease has no racial or geographical predilection, affects men more than women, and peaks in the second and third decades of life.[6,40,102] Mortality rates between 5 and 20 percent have been reported in SJS.[14,70]

### Etiology

SJS has been attributed to a wide variety of biological and pharmaceutical precipitating factors. It has been associated with various infections, particularly herpes simplex and Mycoplasma pneumonia; malignancies; and exposure to sunlight, cold, and x-rays. It has also been described as an allergic or toxic reaction to drugs, such as sulfonamides, phenytoin, penicillin, barbiturates, salycilates, mercury, arsenic and phenylbutazone.[2,6,11,70,102] The development of SJS after immunization with polio, smallpox, tetanus, diphtheria, and influenza vaccines has also been documented.[4,70]

## Clinical Manifestations

The prodromal symptoms of SJS include malaise, fever, prostration, symptoms of upper respiratory infection, and headaches, followed by mucous membrane and skin involvement. The characteristic lesion is the "iris" or "target" lesion, which consists of a red center surrounded by a pale zone with another red ring peripheral to the pale zone. Tense bullae develop from these lesions. Severe mucosal involvement is found, with the mouth and eye having the highest frequency of involvement.[6] The mucosal and cutaneous lesions disappear without scarring except for the conjunctiva.[102,111] Other complications include pneumonitis, septicemia, myocarditis, myositis, and glomerulonephritis.[14] Recurrences occur in approximately 20 percent of cases.[14]

Diffuse, bilateral conjunctivitis is a characteristic finding and lasts 2-4 weeks.[23] Conjunctival involvement may include formation of vesicles,[40,74] membranes, and pseudomembranes on both the palpebral and bulbar conjunctiva. Secondary bacterial infections may ensue. The conjunctival surfaces may heal with scarring and symblepharon or ankyloblepharon. This may result in entropion, trichiasis, lagophthalmos, and exposure. As in cicatricial pemphigoid, there is a profound destruction of conjunctival goblet cells.[67] This, together with fibrotic obstruction of the ducts from the lacrimal and accessory lacrimal glands, results in a dry eye condition. In some severe cases conjunctival and corneal keratinization may be found. Corneal complications include erosions, pannus, ulcers, opacification, and perforation. An anterior uveitis has also been described.[23,40,74]

Reports have shown that the severity of the systemic disease and ocular involvement, rather than treatment, determines the severity of late ophthalmic complications.[4] Of importance here is the self-limited nature of the acute process during which conjunctival shrinkage, symblepharon, and lid distortion occur. Unlike cicatricial pemphigoid, progressive scarring does not continue indefinitely. Further destruction of the eye is the result of complications resulting from the acute event including entropion with trichiasis, and a dry eye condition with its propensity for secondary infections, ulceration, scarring and perforation.

## Histopathology and Immunology

Not unlike cicatricial pemphigoid, formation of subepithelial bullae occur together with adjacent lymphocytes, histiocytes, and a few neutrophils and eosinophils.[52] The conjunctiva is involved in a nonspecific inflammatory reaction with a perivascular infiltration of lymphocytes.[40] Pseudomembranes may form from fibrous exudate, inflammatory cells, and necrotic epithelial cells.[24] True membranes may result from sloughing of the conjunctival epithelium and subepithelial layer. Immunologically, as in cicatricial pemphigoid, an immune complex mechanism is speculated to be important in the pathogenesis.[110]

## Treatment

No specific treatment is presently available for Stevens-Johnson syndrome. It is crucial that any suspected etiological agent be eliminated, as in the case of nonessential drugs, or treated, as in the case of underlying infections. The role of supportive care should be emphasized. Systemic cortico-steroids have been recommended for the general manifestations of SJS and may be life-saving in certain cases.[102] The starting regimen is 60–80 mg of prednisone daily until improvement is noted, with gradual tapering over 3–4 weeks. This has shown some improvement in systemic conditions, but little beneficial or harmful effects on the ocular problem.[35] The value of systemic steroids is by no means proven and has been challenged.[85] Local treatment does not seem to have significant influence on the severity of ophthalmic complications.[4] Periodic irrigation of the eye to wash out the exudate, along with gentle removal of loose membranes may be of benefit.[35] The effectiveness of early and frequent lysis of symblepharon (with a sterile glass rod) is questionable.[6,35] Early use of topical steroids has been advocated by some, but their benefit is questionable, too.[4] Stromal destruction with corneal perforation is not uncommon. The use of topical corticosteroids may be indicated in cases of moderate to severe anterior uveitis.[35]

Although the use of prophylactic antibiotics is controversial, secondary bacterial and fungal infections of the conjunctiva and cornea should be treated appropriately. Insertion of a scleral shell in hopes of maintaining the conjunctival fornices may be of value. Late management is that of the dry eye, including artificial tears, closure of lacrimal puncta, destruction of aberrant lashes by electrolysis or cryotherapy, and soft contact lenses to protect the cornea from drying and trichiasis.[65] Recent studies have advocated the use of topical vitamin A for various dry eyes disorders.[104] The surgical management in SJS, as in cicatricial pemphigoid, is directed toward correction of entropion, trichiasis, shrunken fornices, and, in late stages, opacified corneas.

## TRACHOMA

*Trachoma,* a chronic infectious keratoconjunctivitis, continues to be a major cause of preventable blindness in the world. It presents as a follicular conjunctivitis with superficial keratitis and corneal vascularization, later progressing to conjunctival scarring and lid distortion. The blinding sequelae are a result of damage to the cornea from early inflammation, and later from corneal exposure and trauma secondary to entropion and trichiasis. In its communicable, inflammatory phase the disease is characterized by the presence of lymphoid follicles surrounded by papillary hypertrophy in the conjunctiva, and by vascular pannus in the cornea. Trachomatis inflammation may undergo spontaneous resolution or may progress to conjunctival scarring and corneal opacification, the final visual acuity ranging from normal vision to total blindness.

## Etiology

Chlamydia trachomatis is the specific etiologic agent of trachoma, although other microorganisms contribute to the disease process. Chlamydia trachomatis eye infections occur in two distinct epidemiologic settings. The first pattern is the classic disease of developing countries, also known as "endemic trachoma," that is spread by eye to eye transmission, and is thought to be caused by serotypes A, B, or C of chlamydia trachomatis.[109]

The second pattern is an infection of the eye by sexually transmitted chlamydia trachomatis (usually serotypes D through K), which produces an eye disease often indistinguishable from the early inflammatory phases of endemic trachoma.[107,109] The sexually transmitted chlamydia trachomatis has sometimes been given the label paratrachoma to include inclusion conjunctivitis of the adult, neonatal inclusion conjunctivitis, pneumonitis, and gastrointestinitis.[107] All serotypes A through K are sometimes referred to collectively as TRIC (trachoma-inclusion conjunctivitis) agents. The lymphogranuloma venereum (strains L1, L2 and L3) variant does not replicate in the epithelium, but rather in deeper lymphoid tissues, where it is one of the causes of Parinaud's oculoglandular conjunctivitis.[19,107,109]

## Epidemiology

With a worldwide distribution, trachoma still represents a major public health problem in parts of Africa, the Middle East, and the dry regions of the Indian subcontinent and Southeast Asia. In the United States it is prevalent among the American Indians of the southwestern part of the country. Many cases are located in the "trachoma belt" of Arkansas, Missouri, Oklahoma, West Virginia, and Kentucky. Trachoma is associated with poverty. Its highest incidence is in unhealthy, dirty, and crowded conditions. It is transmitted from eye to eye by way of fingers, fomites, and water. In endemic areas most children are infected by the age of 1–2 years with a decrease in prevalence of active disease after 5 years of age. Blinding lesions are the late sequelae of severe inflammatory disease that occurs earlier in life.[19]

## Pathogenesis

Chlamydia trachomatis cannot be identified in all cases of clinically active trachoma. In Giemsa-stained conjunctival smears chlamydial inclusions are found most frequently in severe cases (50–60 percent), less often in moderate cases (10–20 percent), and least in mild cases (5 percent).[22] More sensitive tests such as fluorescent antibody staining or isolation techniques yield higher rates of ocular infection. Chlamydial infections activate a cell-mediated and a humoral response. Immunofluorescent techniques are the most sensitive today to detect the antibody response to most chlamydial serotypes.[109]

In most studies of chronic trachoma the IgG antibodies are present at highest titers. IgM antibodies occur rarely and indicate recent infection.[45,109] Secondary bacterial infections play a major role in the pathogenesis of trachomatis infections. The predominant pathogens include *Hemophilus aegyptius, Streptococcus pneumoniae, Moraxella species,* and *Staphylococcus aureus.*[19,105] The importance of reinfection in the development of the late stage cicatrizing picture in endemic trachoma has been well-established.[19,94]

## Clinical Features

Trachoma is a chronic follicular conjunctivitis that leads to conjunctival and corneal scarring. An acute onset is rarely observed. In isolated cases, however, it has been noted that incubation time is 1–3 weeks from inoculation until onset of the acute follicular conjunctivitis.[16] The most common initial symptom among children is photophobia. In the first year of life only a severe papillary conjunctivitis may be recognized, but later lymphoid follicles become a regular feature of trachoma. This follicle formation in the conjunctiva of the upper tarsus is one of the cardinal signs of trachoma.[19] MacCallan[58] divided the clinical course of trachoma into four stages based on the developmental changes in the follicles, papillary hypertrophy, and scar formation. Although corneal signs must be present to make a diagnosis of trachoma, the MacCallan classification is based on the findings in the conjunctiva only. It is useful for categorizing the stage of the disease, but it does not grade the intensity of the inflammatory process, and provides no prognostic value.

In MacCallan stage I, immature follicles are present on the upper tarsus with minimal papillary hypertrophy. Faint corneal subepithelial opacities occur with diffuse punctate keratitis and early pannus formation. Fibrovascular tissue may grow into the cornea underneath epithelium and destroy Bowman's layer.

In stage IIa, there is a predominance of mature, well-developed follicles on the upper tarsus, more advanced keratitis, and the presence of limbal follicles. The pannus advances and may be associated with subepithelial infiltrates and corneal haze.

In stage IIb, there is marked papillary hypertrophy of the upper tarsus obscuring the follicles. This stage is primarily an intense inflammation of the upper tarsal conjunctiva. The follicles give the appearance of "sago" grains. Large macrophages with phagocytized debris (Leber's cells) appear in the conjunctival substantia propria. There is further advancement of the pannus and infiltrates from the upper limbus, and necrosis of follicles on the tarsal conjunctiva and the limbus.

Stage III is the scarring and cicatrizing stage. The limbal corneal follicles necrose and cicatrize, and the area is covered with thickened transparent epithelium (Herbert's pits). These pits are diagnostic of trachoma. Scarring in the palpebral conjunctiva is manifest clinically by the appearance of stellate scars and horizontal linear scars, which in the upper tarsal conjunctiva are known as Arlt's line.

Stage IV marks the healing phase with resolution of the inflammatory activity and follicular reaction, diminishing of corneal infiltrates and staining, and the manifestations of

scarring: entropion, trichiasis, symbelpharon, and corneal opacification. The disease is no longer infectious.

To establish the diagnosis of trachoma in a given community where it is strongly suspected, Dawson[19] suggests that at least two of the following signs be present:

1. Follicles on the upper tarsal conjunctiva.
2. Limbal follicles or their sequelae, Herbert's pits.
3. Typical conjunctival scarring (e.g., Arlt's line).
4. Vascular pannus marked at the superior limbus.

More recently, Dawson and his associates[17,18] developed a classification system that describes the intensity of the disease. This classification has been shown to parallel the rate of recovery of the chlamydial agent from the infected tissue and is of prognostic value in individual cases.

Of diagnostic value in the laboratory are the following factors:

1. Giemsa-stained conjunctival smears, which generally have a low yield. They show the basophilic, intracytoplasmic, epithelial inclusion bodies (Halberstaedter-Prowazek bodies) similar to those seen in inclusion conjunctivitis.
2. Complement fixation, which measures antibodies to the chlamydial group antigen, but is not specific for *Chlamydia trachomatis.*
3. Indirect immunofluorescent technique (micro IF), which has been used to identify the various serotypes of chlamydial strains and is the most sensitive method available at this time.

## Treatment

The control of trachoma should include both chemotherapy and surgical intervention to correct lid deformities. The ideal treatment is with a full, oral dose of tetracycline, sulfonamide, or erythromycin for 3 weeks. Tetracycline can be used in total daily dose of 1.0–1.5 grams for 3 weeks, and is the drug of choice.[16,18,34] Triple sulfa (sulfadiazine, sulfamethazine, and sulfamerazine) can be used in cases resistant to tetracycline, but not as a primary drug due to the high incidence of ontoward reactions. In adults the dose is 2–4 grams loading, followed by a maintenance of 2–4 grams daily in three to four divided dosages for at least 3 weeks. In children a loading dose of 35 mg/Kg followed by a maintenance dose of 150 mg/kg/day not exceeding 6 gm/day in three to four divided dosages for 3 weeks. Neither tetracycline nor sulfa should be used in pregnant women, nursing mothers, or infants younger than 2 months of age in the case of sulfa or 7 years of age in the case of tetracycline.[34] Erythromycin is then the alternate drug of choice.[16,19,34]

Systemic therapy is very effective in individual cases or communities where seasonal epidemics of bacterial conjunctivitis are not a problem. However, in hyperendemic areas in which more than 50 percent of the children have active disease and especially those in which seasonal bacterial conjunctivitis is a major problem, the aim of therapy then becomes prevention of blindness.[18,19,34] Topical tetracycline given twice daily for 6–8 weeks or for 5-day courses monthly for 6 months seems to reduce or eliminate blinding complications.[34] At present the World Health Organization recommends the use of systemic antibiotics in addition to topical medication within endemic areas in selected cases with severe or moderate-intensity disease when these cases can be screened and monitored carefully.[18] It should be noted that no effective vaccine has been developed that provides long-lived protection. The surgical treatment is directed toward the correction of trichiasis and/or entropion. Once corneal opacity has occurred penetrating keratoplasty is indicated.

## CHEMICAL BURNS

Chemical burns are among the most urgent of ocular emergencies. They may occur as industrial accidents, in agriculture, or from household accidents. Although the great majority of chemical burns are fortunately minor, and usually not seen by ophthalmologists, the devastating effect of alkalies and acids on ocular tissue can be overwhelming.

Because of the more rapid penetration of alkalies into the cornea and anterior chamber, the results of alkali burns are usually more disastrous than those caused by acids. Alkalies react with fats to form soaps, damaging cell membranes and allowing rapid penetration through the corneal tissue.[3] Grant calculated the rates of penetration for the following alkalies: calcium hydroxide (slowest), potassium hydroxide (faster), sodium hydroxide (even faster), and ammonium hydroxide (fastest).[33] Calcium hydroxide does not penetrate well since the calcium soaps that are formed upon saponification are relatively insoluble and precipitate out, forming a barrier to further penetration.[83]

Acids have less ability to penetrate ocular tissues and cause less severe, more localized tissue damage. The corneal epithelium offers moderate protection against weak acids, and little damage is seen unless the pH is 2.5 or less.[33,83] Acids precipitate tissue proteins and thus set up physical barriers against further penetration. Buffering by surrounding tissue proteins also tends to localize the damage to the initial area of contact. The exceptions are burns from hydrofluoric acid and from acids containing heavy metals, which rapidly penetrate the cornea.[72]

### Clinical Manifestations

The benign chemical burns caused by weak acid or alkali have a similar appearance. Conjunctival hyperemia, diffuse chemosis, and mild corneal clouding or epithelial erosions are seen. The stroma may show mild edema and the anterior chamber may show minimal cell and flare. Because the clinical course of the milder alkali burns differs from the more severe burns it became important to have a classification to grade the severity of damage. Hughes proposed such a classification and based his grading on observable changes in the cornea, sclera, and conjunctiva.[42] Roper-Hall proposed the following scheme, which emphasizes limbal ischemia as a poor prognostic sign.[88]

Grade 1
  a.  Corneal epithelial damage
  b.  No conjunctival ischemia
  c.  Good prognosis
Grade 2
  a.  Hazy cornea, iris details seen
  b.  Less than one-third of limbus ischemic
  c.  Good prognosis
Grade 3
  a.  Total epithelial loss with stromal haze, iris details seen
  b.  One-third to one-half of limbus ischemic
  c.  Vision reduced, perforation rare

Grade 4
  a.  Cornea opaque, no details of iris seen
  b.  More than one-half of limbus ischemic
  c.  Poor prognosis, chronic course

The changes in the classification systems have followed the increased awareness that early changes in the cornea and conjunctival hyperemia are much less important in prognosis than changes in the limbal area. Injury to the limbal area is the single most critical factor in determining the severity of damage and prognosis for recovery. The two most important processes for repair of the chemically burned eye are vascularization and reepithelialization. Injury to the deep structures at the limbus may destroy the normal source for corneal reepithelialization and vascularization.

Hughes also distinguished three stages in the temporal sequence of events in alkali burns.[41,42] The immediate or acute phase lasts approximately 3 days and begins at the time of injury. There is necrosis of the corneal and conjunctival epithelium with rapid penetration of the alkali into the anterior chamber, ciliary body, and iris. There is an almost immediate rise in intraocular pressure, probably accounted for by immediate shrinkage of collagen fibers. There is conjunctival chemosis, injection, and possible limbal blanching. The cornea becomes opaque, the epithelium may slough, and there is widespread stromal edema.

The intermediate or subacute phase begins at about 3–7 days and is characterized by a prolonged period where the predominant factor is active inflammatory destruction of the eye. New blood vessels begin to invade the corneal stroma. Polymorphonuclear leukocytes (PMN) advance ahead of the vascularization, while fibroblasts parallel the vessel ingrowth. This leads to stromal ulceration and possible perforation in all but the mildest cases.[55] The conjunctival fornices are obliterated by symblepharon formation (Fig. 12-3).

The late or chronic phase is usually only seen in burns of a severe nature. Cicatrix formation limits both globe and lid movement and vision is reduced due to corneal vascularization and opacification. These eyes continue to have a propensity to ulcerate secondary to any insult (Fig. 12-4).

In severe acid burns the cornea and conjunctiva become rapidly white and opaque except for burns with nitric or chromic acids, which turn tissue yellow-brown. The epithelium may slough, leaving a relatively clear stroma. The clear cornea may mask the severity of the burn and eventual

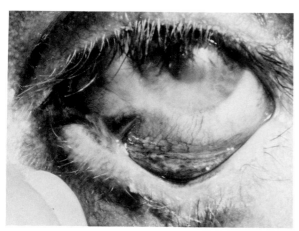

**Fig. 12-3.** Alkali burn exhibiting mild inferior corneal opacification, inferotemporal limbal blanching, and symblepharon.

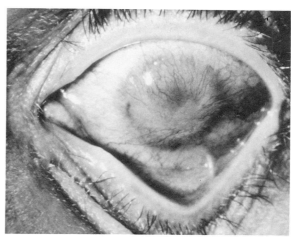

**Fig. 12-4.** Alkali burn with complete corneal opacification and vascularization (Courtesy of Jay H. Krachmer, M.D.).

opacification. The most severe acid burns exhibit complete corneal anesthesia, limbal pallor, and uveitis.[83]

## Control of Ulceration via Chemical Mediators

One of the most serious consequences in alkali-burned corneas is the appearance of corneal ulcerations within weeks of the initial injury. It is the progression of corneal ulceration to perforation that accounts for many of the lost eyes. Recent studies have focused on enzyme inhibition, collagen synthesis, and inhibition of polymorphonuclear leukocytes as a means of preventing future ulceration.

Corneal ulceration occurs when collagenolytic activity is greater than fibrillogenesis. The two events, degradation and removal of necrotic debris and replacement of the collagenous matrix, proceed simultaneously in the repair process.[79] The corneal periphery remains intact because of the balance between collagen production by the incoming fibroblasts and collagenase induced destruction. Centrally, however, there are no fibroblasts and without collagen synthesis the balance is in favor of destruction, ulceration, and eventual perforation.[10]

Much of the early speculation on collagenase activity in the human cornea was based on the inhibition of collagen lysis by known collagenase inhibitors. Derivatives of ethylenediamine-tetracetic acid (EDTA) were found to have anticollagenase activity in vitro.[44,90] Subsequently both L-cysteine and N-acetyl-L-cysteine (acetylcysteine; Mucomyst, Mead Johnson Pharmaceutical, Evansville, IN) were shown to have in vivo activity against collagenase.[11,91] Acetylcysteine has the advantage of being more stable and readily available (Mucomyst®, available in both 10% and 20% in 4-, 10-, and 30-ml dropper bottles).

Steroids have been reported to decrease the ability of tissue to produce collagenase.[51] It has been our clinical experience, however, that local corticosteroid application enhances corneal melting. Corticosteroids inhibit fibroblasts from repopulating the acellular stroma and potentiate colla-

genolytic activity by a general antianabolic effect, even in the face of decreased collagenase production.[29,83] Corticosteroids should be avoided during the second and third weeks after an alkali burn. It appears that during the first week collagenase activity has not peaked and after 4–5 weeks the inhibition of collagen synthesis is less deleterious.

Progesterone appeared to offer the advantage of suppressing synthesis without a general antianabolic effect. Medroxy-progesterone (topical, subconjunctival, or parenteral), was effective in preventing corneal ulceration in alkali-burned rabbit corneas.[68] Nortestosterone decanoate, an androgen as well as progestational hormone, reduced the incidence of ulceration in animals receiving weekly injections.[79]

Selective immunosuppression has recently been shown to be effective in preventing corneal ulcerations in alkaliburned guinea pigs. Neutrophils are capable of producing collagenase and selective neutrophil suppression was an effective means of preventing corneal ulceration. Neutrophil depletion after the onset of ulceration halted further progression.[27] The role of neutrophils in corneal ulceration is probably more complex than the simple reduction in the level of collagenase.

Ascorbic acid is involved in the biosynthesis and maintenance of collagen.[32] In order to form collagen, ascorbic acid is required for the hydroxylation of proline and lysine. Ascorbate is actively transported by the ciliary body into the aqueous. In severe alkali burns, damage to the ciliary body results in a decrease in the active transport of ascorbate and a relative scorbutic state of the anterior segment.[57] In the scorbutic state, impaired hydroxylation results in the formation of unstable collagen molecules which are very vulnerable to the action of proteolytic enzymes.[43] It follows that exogeneous supplementation by ascorbic acid may reverse the relative ascorbate deficiency and prevent corneal ulceration. Ascorbic acid given subcutaneously, parenterally, and topically raised aqueous ascorbate levels and decreased the incidence of corneal ulceration in alkali-burned rabbit corneas.[57,76,77]

Topical sodium citrate has also been shown effective in preventing ulceration in experimentally burned rabbit corneas.[78] All eyes were severely burned. Severely burned eyes in past studies have shown a poor response probably due to an absence of fibroblast activity. The capacity of citrate to act favorably suggested that its mechanism of action might be on the prominent cell type present, the PMN. Citrate chelates extracellular calcium causing a deficiency of this important intracellular second messenger.

Recently, systemic tetracycline has been shown to have anticollagenolytic activity. A small clinical trial in patients with persistent epithelial defects, and animal studies with alkali-induced burns had favorable responses. The ease of its use (250 mg po q.i.d.) may warrant its administration.[75]

There are few data supporting the usefulness of chemical mediators in controlled human studies. Their clinical use appears justified based on experimental animal studies and the uniformly poor prognosis of severe alkali burns once ulceration begins.

## Intraocular Pressure Response

Significant changes in intraocular pressure have been demonstrated following chemical burns. The ocular pressure response varies according to the severity of the injury and the time from the injury. In experimentally burned rabbit corneas there was an immediate elevation in intraocular pressure.[36] This acute rise was attributed to collagen shrinkage. This effect is not evident until the pH reaches 11 and is maximal when the pH is more than 12.[92] A second pressure rise is seen within the first few hours and is thought to be caused by the intraocular release of prostaglandins. A similar pressure response is seen after acid burns.[71]

Late pressure changes were divided into two groups: those exhibiting elevated pressure and those exhibiting low pressure. Both groups demonstrated damaged or blocked outflow channels, first as a result of mechanical obstruction in the trabecular meshwork and aqueous veins, and later by fibrous proliferation in the angle, which damaged the outflow channels irreversibly.[92] The hypotensive group, those with more severe burns, also exhibited vascular changes in the deep sclera, trabeculum, iris, and ciliary body. The more mildly burned eyes showed persistent pressure elevation, possibly the result of continued formation of aqueous by the ciliary body in the presence of an occluded angle.[55]

## Treatment of Chemical Burns

Chemical burns of the eye can be devastating. Therapy needs to be directed toward preventing further damage and preserving ocular structures. Realizing that there is much overlap, three phases can be defined: (1) the acute phase beginning at the time of injury and lasting approximately 1 week, (2) the intermediate stage beginning at 1 week and representing the period of inflammatory destruction of the eye, and (3) the chronic or cicatricial stage.[83]

### Acute Phase

Copious irrigation should be the initial treatment for every chemical eye burn regardless of the etiologic agent. Topical anesthetic (0.5% proparacaine) and lid retractors or a lid speculum will facilitate continuous irrigation. At times, severe orbicularis spasm may require a lid block in order to accomplish adequate irrigation. If needed, systemic analgesics are preferable to repeated use of topical anesthetics. If the nature of the chemical injury is unknown the use of pH paper is helpful in determining whether the agent was basic or acidic. Irrigation should continue for at least 30 minutes or 2 liters of irrigant in mild cases and 2–4 hours or 10 liters of irrigant in severe cases. The pH should again be checked to show that it is back within a normal range (7.3–7.7), and checked again in approximately 30 minutes to ensure that it has not changed. This is particularly important in alkali burns in which particulate matter can slowly dissolve and cause a persistent elevation in the pH. Prolonged irrigation can be accomplished with the use of a polymethylmethacrylate scleral lens with an attached perfusion tube (Medi-Flow or Morgan Therapeutic Lens),[66] by a perforated silicone tube designed to fit into the conjunctival fornices (Oklahoma Eye Irrigating Tube),[93] or by placement of an Angiocath inserted percutaneously into the conjunctival fornix. Due to the extremely rapid penetration of alkali through the cornea and into the anterior chamber, the irrigant of choice remains the one most-readily available (tap water or saline). Because most chemical burns occur outside the physician's office, initial therapy is usually carried out by nonmedical persons.

In calcium hydroxide burns (fresh lime, mortar, and plaster) there may be some benefit in irrigating with 0.024 M disodium EDTA (0.5 M Endrate with 20 parts normal saline), which chelates the calcium and helps loosen particles lodged in the fornices. Anterior chamber paracentesis remains controversial. Its use is suggested in moderate to severe burns if performed within one hour from time of accident.

Once irrigation is complete a careful search must be made for any retained particles. A topical anesthetic should be utilized. The lids should be doubly everted and the fornices swabbed with a cotton applicator moistened with ointment or EDTA. Larger particles can be removed with smooth forceps. Any redundant conjunctiva should be unfolded, as these areas are likely to hide particulate matter.

All but the mildest chemical burns are associated with a significant uveitis. For relief of pain and prevention of posterior synechiae adequate cycloplegia is essential. Atropine 1% or scopolamine 0.25% 2 or 3 times a day are probably the drugs of choice. The mydriatic phenylephrine is contraindicated since its vasoconstricting properties can worsen already preexisting perilimbal ischemia.[81] Intraocular pressure responses after chemical burns may vary. Elevated pressure in the initial postburn period can be managed with carbonic anhydrase inhibitors and/or timolol. Acetazolamide 250 mg every 6 hours or methazolamide 50 mg every 8 hours can be utilized, though smaller doses may be effective. Antibiotic ointment (chloramphenicol) and bilateral semipressure patches are applied. The goal is to promote epithelialization as rapidly as possible. The eyes are examined daily and the fluorescein staining pattern drawn. Only if inflammation is severe are corticosteroid drops applied. Moderate to severe burns may be started on ascorbic acid. Exact dosages are not known. Pharmacologic doses may be given orally, or a topical 10% solution can be given hourly.

## Intermediate Phase

The goal of therapy in the intermediate phase is the prevention of ulceration and/or perforation, and the limiting of symblepharon formation. The final goal in severe cases is not adequate vision but an intact globe that will maximize the chance of a successful corneal transplant in the future.

Collagenase inhibitors are initiated if epithelialization stops despite patching. Of the collagenase inhibitors discussed, Mucomyst® (N-acetyl-L-cysteine) has the advantage of being readily available from most pharmacies, easy to administer, and relatively nontoxic. Mucomyst® 20% can be given by dropper as often as every hour. The medication should be kept refrigerated and has an offensive odor, similar to rotten eggs. Ascorbic acid seems to reduce ulceration by promoting collagen synthesis. Dosages outlined in the acute phase should be continued. Guidelines for human dosages of medroxyprogesterone (Provera, Upjohn, Kalamazoo, MI) are not available. On the basis of experimental data, anticollagenase agents should be used until the epithelium has healed or for a minimum of 6 weeks. Close observation is needed on cessation of therapy because ulceration can supervene.

Therapy needs to be directed toward promoting corneal epithelial healing. In mild cases all that might be needed is an effective semipressure patch or bandage lens. Some clinicians advocate almost immediate mucosal grafting to replace necrotic conjunctiva. The most severe cases, those that would benefit most from mucosal grafting,[5,20,69] are associated with extensive scleral necrosis which limits the visibility of the graft.[55]

Soft bandage lenses also aid in epithelialization. There are numerous bandage lenses currently available. The lens should be large enough to cover limbus to limbus at all times. There should be adequate movement, approximately 1–2 mm, during a blink. Because severe alkali burns are also associated with destruction of the tear-producing elements of the eye, an ultra-thin, low-to-moderate water content lens may have some benefit over a high water content lens.

Within a few days following a severe chemical burn, fibrin formation begins to obliterate the conjunctival fornices. Areas of the bulbar and palpebral conjunctiva that are denuded of epithelium form adhesions. The fibrinous bands are then replaced by fibrovascular tissue. A glass rod lubricated with ointment can be used to sweep the fornices and lyse adhesions once or twice daily. The use of scleral shells to prevent apposition of tissue has met with only minimal success. Whether these procedures result in less symblepharon formation when active inflammation is finished is debatable.

Small perforations can be treated with a bandage lens or the application of tissue adhesive (cyanoacrylate). No tissue adhesive is FDA approved. Histo-acryl-Blau (butyl-2-cyanoacrylate, B. Brown Melsungen A.G.) is not available in the United States but can be obtained in Canada. The area to be sealed needs to be debrided of necrotic tissue and dried. A small amount of glue is applied via a polyethylene disc or thin tube and allowed to polymerize.[9] The cornea is then covered with a hydrophilic bandage lens.

Perforations too large to be sealed with tissue adhesive require either penetrating keratoplasty or a blowout patch. Techniques of corneal transplantation are discussed later. In performing a blowout patch some familiarity with handling corneal donor tissue and techniques of transplantation are required. Free-hand cutting of both donor and recipient tissues may be needed. If the anterior chamber can be reformed with a viscoelastic substance, this will often enable gentle trephining with a super sharp trephine (Superblade trephine, Pharmacia, Piscataway, NJ). Closure should be with interrupted 10-0 nylon with all knots buried. A soft bandage lens should be placed at the conclusion of the case. Steroids should be avoided but collagenase inhibitors continued.

### Late or Chronic phase

The treatment of the late stage begins when the inflammatory destruction of the intermediate stage ends. The major goals of therapy include supplementation of a deficient tear film, reestablishment of normal lid anatomy, and restoration of a clear visual axis.

Extensive involvement of the conjunctiva in advanced alkali burns results in the development of a severe dry eye. The aqueous component is decreased by obstruction of the main and accessory lacrimal glands, and the mucin component is decreased by widespread injury to the conjunctiva, resulting in almost complete destruction of the goblet cells. What follows is a severe dry eye, rendered unwettable by a lack of mucin. Frequent tear supplementation with some of the newer mucomimetic tear replacements is helpful. Lacriserts (Merck Sharp & Dohme, West Point, PA) may be of help in patients whose fornices are not obliterated. A thin, low-water content bandage lens may also be of help.

Another prerequisite for maintaining the precorneal tear film is periodic resurfacing by the lids. Symblepharon that restricts lid movements, cicatricial entropion and trichiasis, and obliteration of the fornices, all make proper corneal wetting impossible.[54] Before penetrating keratoplasty can be performed normal lid and conjunctival anatomy need to be restored if possible.

Corneal transplantation in the severely burned eye has been fraught with difficulties. Delayed healing, ulcer formation, vascularization, rejection, and lingering epithelial defects are more the rule than the exception. In addition, the inflammatory reaction that had been quiet for months or years may suddenly be reactivated.

Thoft recently developed the techniques of autotransplantation of healthy conjunctival tissue from the uninjured fellow eye,[95] and keratoepithelioplasty,[100] in which limbal tissue from a fresh donor eye is transplanted to serve as a source of new epithelium. In severe cases, those with markedly altered conjunctiva and lids, penetrating keratoplasty has an extremely poor prognosis. Keratoprosthesis surgery may offer the only chance for vision.

## SURGICAL TREATMENT

### Mucous Membrane Grafting

Ocular cicatricial pemphigoid, Stevens-Johnson syndrome, trachoma, and chemical burns are all associated with conjunctival shrinkage, symblepharon formation, entropion, trichiasis, exposure keratitis, and a severe dry eye. Various surgical procedures have been advocated in an attempt to restore a more normal lid and conjunctival anatomy. The results have been mixed, with the more severely affected eyes faring the poorest.

It is important to first correct any existing lid, lash, or conjunctival abnormality that may adversely affect the outcome of eventual corneal transplantation. Just as important, however, is to spare patients major oculoplastic reconstruction when there is little or no hope of eventual sight restoration. This is particularly true in patients with ocular cicatricial pemphigoid in which any surgical procedure may entail a risk of precipitating an increase in disease activity.[63] In addition, if a through-the-lid keratoprosthesis is to be considered as the initial sight-restoring procedure, then it is unnecessary to perform previous oculoplastic procedures. The goal of surgery is the prevention of the sequelae of long-standing lid, lash, and conjunctival abnormalities.

A dry eye may initially be treated with the frequent use of artificial tears. Artificial tears free of preservatives have theoretic benefits. Punctal occlusion will prolong the retention of tears. Many patients, however, have puncta already scarred closed by their underlying disease process. Mild trichiasis may be treated with a battery-powered electrolysis unit or hyfercation. More extensive trichiasis is best handled with cryoablation. Cicatricial entropion, in mild cases, may be repaired by one of many oculoplastic surgical techniques, but care must be taken not to shorten an already shrunken fornix. In more severe cases, mucous membrane grafting, free tarsal grafting, or preserved scleral grafting is necessary to reconstruct the shortened cul-de-sac.[63]

The best sources for mucous membrane grafting are the conjunctiva itself, the lower lip, the upper lip, and the cheek (in that order).[28,56] Often, patients with trachoma, mild to moderate chemical burns, or Stevens-Johnson syndrome have adequate available conjunctiva and/or tarsus to utilize for grafting.

Patients with moderate to severe chemical burns or Stevens-Johnson syndrome, and most patients with ocular cicatricial pemphigoid have inadequate conjunctiva and must rely on buccal mucosa as a source for mucous membrane grafting. In addition, patients with ocular cicatricial pemphigoid should have their disease stabilized prior to any

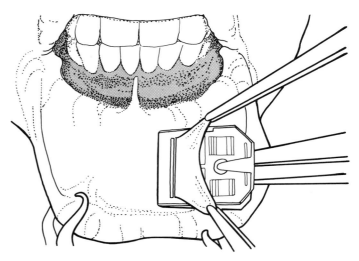

**Fig. 12-5.** Harvesting buccal mucosal graft with electrokeratome.

surgical manipulation. Immunosuppressive agents are often begun well in advance of anticipated surgery.

To obtain the buccal mucosal graft, the lower lip is first infiltrated with lidocaine and epinephrine (1:100,000), followed by saline to increase the firmness of the lip and facilitate removal of the graft. Towel clips can stabilize the lip during removal. The Castroviejo electrokeratome with the 0.3- or 0.4-mm shim is used for harvesting the split-thickness graft (Fig. 12-5). The thinner graft is utilized if the majority of the area to be covered is bulbar conjunctiva. The graft should be somewhat larger than the recipient bed to allow for shrinkage.[103] The denuded lower lip needs no suturing and will granulate in. The patient should be given a bland

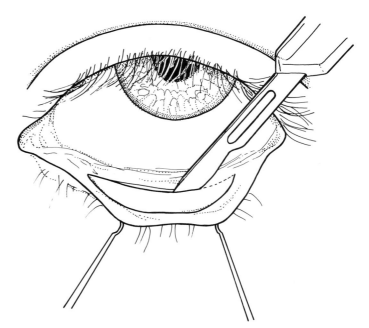

**Fig. 12-6.** Resection of lower tarsus to edge of meibomian glands.

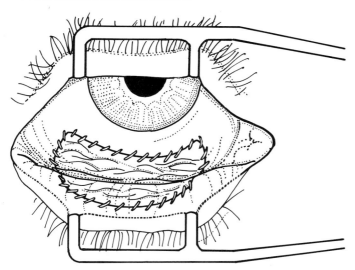

**Fig. 12-7.** Mucous membrane graft sutured in place.

mouthwash (hydrogen peroxide 1.5%–3.0%) t.i.d. and a soft diet. A regular diet can usually be resumed by the 10th day but the lip should be washed after each meal. Healing is usually complete by 2 weeks.[28]

The preparation of the recipient bed varies with the underlying lid abnormality. Symblepharon and conjunctival shortening may only require blunt dissection with removal of the abnormal conjunctiva. If the tarsus has undergone shortening with a loss of substance, it may be resected to the edge of the meibomian glands (Fig. 12-6). If a further degree of rotational correction is needed, preserved scleral grafts or free tarsal grafts are utilized to replace the excised, scarred, middle-third of the tarsus. The mucous membrane graft is

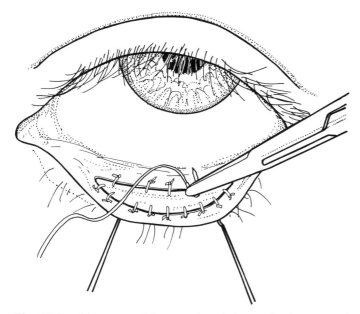

**Fig. 12-8.** Placement of free tarsal graft in previously prepared bed.

then placed in the cul-de-sac and sutured with 6-0 chromic (Fig. 12-7). A conformer is placed at the conclusion of the procedure and may be removed in 2–3 weeks.[8] In cases with minimal conjunctival shrinkage but severe tarsal scarring, a free tarsal graft with retained conjunctiva alone may give adequate anatomical correction (Fig. 12-8).

Vastine et al. recommended the use of large, free, autologous conjunctival grafts, when obtainable, for the reconstruction of the palpebral, bulbar, and forniceal conjunctiva. The stability of the epithelial surface and the lack of shrinkage and scarring were in contrast to their previous experience with buccal mucous membrane grafts.[106]

## Conjunctival Transplantation

A common endpoint to all the before-mentioned abnormalities is an eye scarred, vascularized, and prone to recurrent epithelial breakdown. Because the epithelium is diseased, its replacement is indicated. The previously mentioned mucous membrane grafting is at best able to restore the distorted anatomy but rarely yields acceptable visual results. Penetrating keratoplasty in an eye previously covered by mucous membrane grafting is no more successful than in the presence of the original injured ocular surface.[95] Two procedures, conjunctival transplantation and keratoepithelioplasty, have been developed in an attempt to restore to the corneal surface a more stable epithelial covering resembling corneal epithelium.

It is known that donor epithelial cells placed centrally by the usual keratoplasty techniques have a life expectancy of only 12–18 months.[48] The cells are eventually replaced by the host epithelium migrating centripetally. If the host epithelium is normal, this poses no difficulty, but when an abnormal ocular surface preexists, the normal donor epithelium is eventually replaced by the abnormal host surface. This corresponds to the recurrent epithelial defects and/or ulceration seen 1–2 years after a previously successful corneal transplant. Conjunctival transplantation attempts a more permanent resurfacing by peripheral placement of autologous donor conjunctival corneal cells.[100]

Conjunctival transplantation relies on the transformation of conjunctival epithelium into corneal epithelium. Conjunctival epithelium is an important source of mucin, with goblet cells making 5–10 percent of its cellular population. The corneal epithelium is devoid of goblet cells. Conjunctival epithelium varies in thickness from 3 to 15 cell layers and lacks the orderly progression from basal cells to squamous cells seen in the typical 5- to 6-cell layer corneal epithelium.[99] Conjunctival epithelium is nourished by an extensive subepithelial vascular network and lacks the rich stores of glycogen seen in corneal epithelium.[96] Conjunctival transplantation relies on the transformation of conjunctival epithelial cells into corneal epithelial cells to create an epithelial layer that tolerates the avascular corneal environment. As opposed to mucous membrane grafting in which healing is accomplished with a rich vascular network, conjunctival transplantation attempts to create an avascular epithelial ingrowth.

Conjunctival transformation has been studied in animals. Four to five weeks after conjunctival transplantation the epithelium has the histologic appearance of corneal epithelium.[89] Metabolic and functional transformation lags behind the morphologic transformation.[99] Months after transplantation the transformation is incomplete. When stressed, as by wounding, the transformed epithelium reacquires some of its original histologic characteristics.[97] Whether a true conjunctival to corneal transdifferentiation ever takes place remains unresolved.

The goals of conjunctival transplantation are (1) a rapid healing, secure epithelium with no tendency for recurrent epithelial defects, (2) a gradual clearing of the cornea with a regression of vascularization, and (3) a smoothing of the corneal surface.[98] Its use is limited to unilateral disease because a healthy supply of autologous conjunctival tissue is needed. Unilateral chemical or thermal injury is the most common indication.[99] It has been advocated before, after, or in conjunction with penetrating keratoplasty. The most favorable candidates are those whose unilateral scarring and vascularization are superficial enough to be removed by a lamellar keratectomy. The procedure cannot be recommended in bilateral disease such as bilateral chemical injury, cicatricial pemphigoid, or Stevens-Johnson syndrome in which a source of autologous conjunctiva is not available.

General anesthesia permits the comfortable operation on both eyes. The first step is a 360°, 5-mm wide, limbal conjunctival resection, followed by a total superficial keratectomy (Figs. 12-9 and 12-10). Careful preoperative evaluation with pachometry and slit-lamp examination should determine whether a keratectomy will be able to remove all the significant scarring vascularization. The thinnest portion of the keratectomized cornea should rarely be less than 0.3 mm. If it appears unlikely that a keratectomy will yield sig-

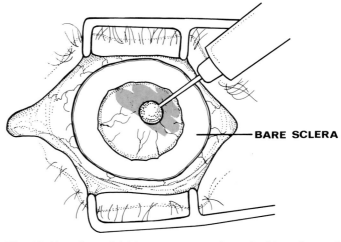

**Fig. 12-10.** Superficial keratectomy performed with a diamond burr on a gas-driven drill.

nificant optical improvement, then the keratectomy should be kept to a minimal depth, just exposing anterior stroma. This avoids graft–host edge thickness discrepancy if a penetrating keratoplasty is done at a later date. The keratectomy can be carried out with one of many available nitrogen gas-driven, foot-controlled drills (Stryker) utilizing a large (2.5–5 mm) diamond burr. The nitrogen gas pressure should be kept below the normal recommended level but should be enough to maintain a constant smooth rotation of the burr. The gas-driven drill enables the surgeon to perform quick, even keratectomy of increasing depth. The burr can also be used to smooth the sclera and limbal region.

Next, healthy conjunctival donor tissue is obtained from the intermuscular quadrants of the opposite eye in areas

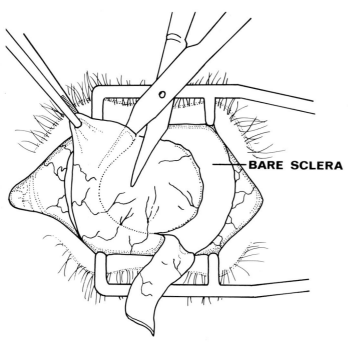

**Fig. 12-9.** A 360°, 5-mm wide, limbal conjunctival resection.

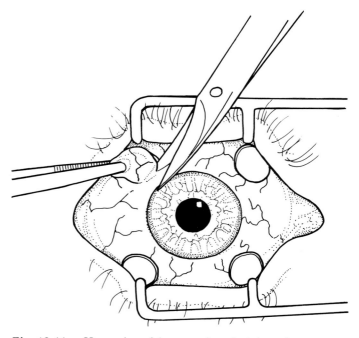

**Fig. 12-11.** Harvesting of donor conjunctival tissue from contralateral eye.

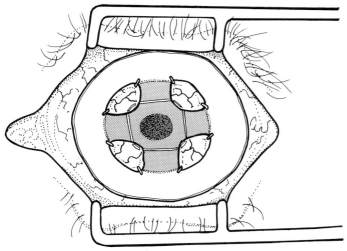

**Fig. 12-12.** Placement of donor grafts in recipient bed (see text).

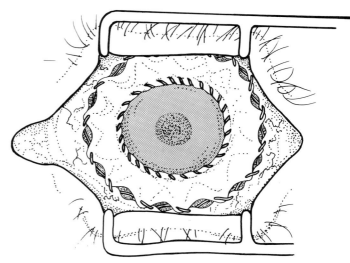

**Fig. 12-14.** Ring of donor conjunctiva sutured to limbus and resected conjunctival edge using running suture technique.

covered by the lids. The conjunctiva is elevated with smooth forceps and excised with scissors (Fig. 12-11). Four pieces 3–4 mm each are large enough to provide coverage. The donor sites may be left open or closed with absorbable suture. The grafts are then arranged around the periphery of the keratectomized cornea. Each graft is then secured with a two small bites of 10-0 nylon at the limbus. Finally a 10-0 nylon suture is passed through the apices of the grafts in purse-string fashion (Fig. 12-12). At the conclusion, a large-diameter, moderate-thickness bandage lens is placed. Postoperative care is limited to topical antibiotics and cyloplegics.

Herman et al. modified Thoft's original procedure by transplanting a 360° ring of autologous conjunctiva. He utilizes a Flieringa ring to act as a support for the donor graft (Fig. 12-13). The donor material is then secured to the prepared keratectomized host cornea as illustrated[39] (Fig. 12-14).

The clinical usefulness of the above procedures is severely limited by the requirement for healthy conjunctiva from the uninvolved eye. In an attempt to broaden the clinical applications Thoft devised keratoepithelioplasty in which lenticules of limbal tissue from fresh donor eyes are placed peripherally on a keratectomized cornea. Thoft envisions the limbal epithelium as a special transitional zone histologically different from both conjunctival and corneal epithelium. He believes the limbal epithelium has the ability to resurface the cornea without involvement of the conjunctival epithelium. Using a disposable Graefe knife, thin saucerlike lenticules of limbal tissue are carved from a freshly enucleated donor eye (Fig. 12-15). The lenticules are then sewn to the sclera around the limbus with two interrupted 10-0 nylon sutures per lenticule (Fig. 12-16). A bandage lens is placed at the conclusion of the case. Postoperative care is the same as outlined for autologous conjunctival transplantation except that low-dose, long-term topical steroids are necessary to prevent epithelial graft rejection.[100]

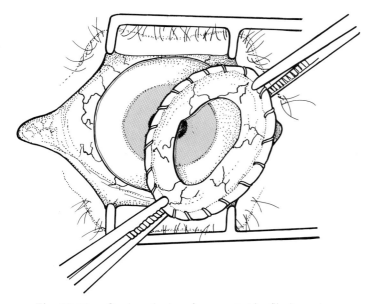

**Fig. 12-13.** Conjunctival graft supported by flieringa ring.

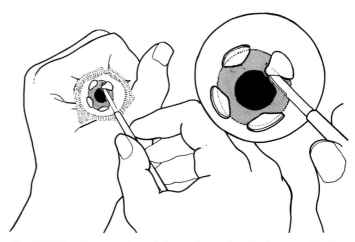

**Fig. 12-15.** Preparation of donor lenticules for keratoepithelioplasty.

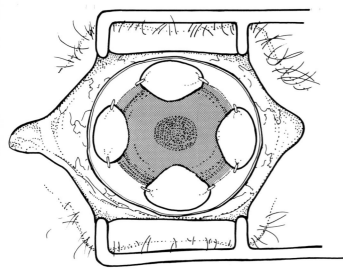

**Fig. 12-16.** Donor lenticules sutured in place (keratoepithelio-plasty).

## Corneal Transplantation

Corneal transplantation in patients with severe mucous membrane disorders has a uniformly poor prognosis. Delayed healing, ulcer formation, recurrent epithelial defects, and graft rejection are common. Initial concerns should be directed at correcting the lid, lash, and conjunctival abnormalities prior to corneal transplantation to insure proper resurfacing by the lids and adequate lubrication. Simple techniques such as punctal occlusion and cryoablation of lashes should not be ignored.

The timing of corneal transplantation in patients with Stevens-Johnson syndrome, trachoma, and chemical burns should be delayed until all acute activity has subsided, and after all lid, lash, and conjunctival procedures have been completed. Guidelines for patients with ocular cicatricial pemphigoid are less clear. Ocular cicatricial pemphigoid is a cyclic, chronically progressive disease. Intervention should occur when disease activity is at a minimum. Patients who are candidates for immunosuppression should have their disease activity minimized prior to surgery, because any surgery in patients with ocular cicatricial pemphigoid can cause a reactivation of the acute process. It is not known whether these patients are better managed with staged procedures (i.e., lids, conjunctiva, and penetrating keratoplasty) or one massive reconstruction involving lid reconstruction, mucous membrane grafting, and corneal transplantation. The role of conjunctival transplantation and epitheliokeratoplasty in patients needing eventual transplantation is also unclear. Whether these procedures should be done prior to transplantation, during transplantation, or only later, if epithelial breakdown occurs, is unknown. Patients with ocular cicatricial pemphigoid are not considered candidates for either conjunctival transplantation or epitheliokeratoplasty. Controlled long-term double-blind studies showing the efficacy of the above procedures are lacking. Finally, in some patients, particularly those with ocular cicatricial pemphigoid or severe chemical burns, a decision regarding when not to attempt

reconstructive surgery but to proceed instead to keratoprosthesis surgery needs to be made.

Major concerns regarding successful transplantation in patients with mucous membrane abnormalities include preservation of donor epithelium and maintaining the epithelium after surgery. Donor material should be carefully examined to rule out any epithelial irregularities. Time between enucleation of donor eyes and tissue utilization should be minimized. When possible, whole eye preservation and donor button removal from the epithelial surface prevent possible epithelial damage from the inverted punch technique. A coating of Healon on the donor epithelial surface appears to offer some protection during tissue handling. Because of the increased incidence of graft rejection and incidence of preexisting recipient corneal vascularization, donor buttons larger than 8.0 mm should be avoided.[7]

The recipient bed is first prepared by dissection of the inflammatory pannus and recession of the conjunctiva 4–6 mm behind the limbus. This reduces a source of vascularization. The bare sclera can be smoothed with a diamond burr as previously described. A Flieringa ring or other scleral supporter should be sutured to the globe. A partial-thickness trephinization is then performed. Because corneal opacification may preclude visualization of the anterior chamber, and previous inflammatory activity may have caused extensive anterior synechiae, it is hazardous to attempt full-thickness trephining. The anterior chamber can then be entered through a relatively clear zone, or dissection can be carried out to the level of the retrocorneal membrane if one exists. The retrocorneal membrane, which is more common in alkali burns, can then be removed with sharp dissection. Angled Kelman-McPherson and long-nosed Vannas scissors are well suited for this purpose. Extensive iridocorneal adhesions may require both blunt and sharp dissection, and an attempt should be made to reform the angle by synechialysis. Anterior synechiae that cannot be broken with blunt dissection can be cut with the long-nosed Vannas scissors.

Persistent bleeding from the iris and ciliary body are often encountered and may be controlled by careful use of a unipolar wetfield cautery or Mentor's wetfield pencil. Lens extraction should be considered even with moderate lens opacity to reduce the incidence of reoperations. When there is minimal distortion of the anterior chamber anatomy, extracapsular extraction is preferred. With extensive destruction of the normal anterior chamber architecture, lens extraction combined with an aggressive anterior vitrectomy is preferred. The use of intraocular lenses in patients with severe mucous membrane disease is unresolved. Their use is not recommended in patients who have had previous significant anterior chamber inflammation or in the presence of deep stromal vascularization. Healon placed between the iris and the recipient corneal rim will often physically keep the iris back. Though this has little, if any, effect on the functioning of the trabecular meshwork, grafts appear to do better with less iridocorneal adhesions.

The donor button is then secured using either a running or interrupted 10-0 nylon suture. A running suture has the advantage of stimulating less vascularization but is difficult to manage if one or more loops erode. In most cases, an interrupted closure is preferred. All knots should be buried on the donor side to keep the largest mass of suture away from the limbus. Prolene (polypropylene) suture and interrupted 11-0 nylon should be avoided because of the greater incidence of eroded sutures in vascularized corneas.

Postoperative care varies with the underlying pathology. Patients with trachoma and Stevens-Johnson syndrome are treated with long-acting cycloplegics and high-dose topical steroids. Frequent use of artificial tears or lubricants is necessary to protect the ocular surface. A partial tarsorrhaphy may be beneficial. In addition, patients with ocular cicatricial pemphigoid are continued on their systemic immunosuppression. Postoperative care of chemical burn patients varies in that only the minimal steroid necessary to control inflammation and prevent graft vascularization should be utilized. All patients need careful monitoring of intraocular pressure. Recommended hypotensive agents include Timoptic (Merck Sharp & Dohme, West Point, PA), Propine (Allergan, Irvine, CA), Diamox (Lederle, Wayne, NJ). Anticollagenolytic therapy should be instituted at the first sign of either corneal thinning or a persistent epithelial defect. Though the graft may initially stay clear, prognosis for long-term graft clarity is poor.

## Keratoprosthesis

In the presence of severe cicatricial changes with total loss of the fornices and deep corneal vascularization, penetrating keratoplasty has little if any chance of success. In those patients with bilateral disease keratoprosthesis surgery may afford the only hope for useful vision. Because the best results are obtained when keratoprosthesis is the initial procedure, patients should be spared massive anterior segment reconstruction when visual improvement is unlikely.[21]

The two major types of keratoprostheses are the "nut and bolt" and the "through and through" prostheses (Figs. 12-17A and 12-17B). The nut-and-bolt type is preferred in an eye with good anatomic integrity and a healthy conjunctiva. It may be useful in an eye that has had repeated graft failures.[12] Eyes with advanced xerophthalmia, obliterated fornices, and corneal vascularization as a result of ocular pemphigoid, Stevens-Johnson syndrome, trachoma or severe chemical burns are better served with a through-the-lid, through-and-through prosthesis.[2,21,84]

The through-and-through keratoprosthesis consists of two parts: (1) A methyl methacrylate optical cylinder with a dioptric power of +66, which is 3.5 mm wide and from 5.5 to 9.5 mm long, and is threaded along its entire length except for the last millimeter, and (2) the supporting plate, which is a perforated flexible Teflon skirt 8.5 mm in diameter, 0.2 mm thick, with a radius of curvature of 5.5 mm. The plate is perforated and threaded at the center to accept the optical cylinder.[12]

The operative procedure for a through-and-through, through-the-lid, modified Cardona keratoprosthesis is based on the original technique described by Castroviejo, Cardona, and DeVoe[13] and modified by Harris et al.[38] Under general anesthesia, the periorbital region and one lower leg

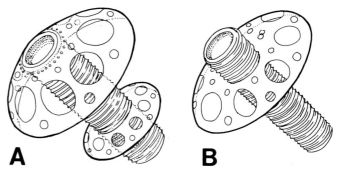

**Fig. 12-17.** Types of keratoprostheses: (A) nut-and-bolt and (B) through-and-through. (Redrawn with permission from Barraquer and Rutlar. *Microsurgery of the Cornea* Ediciones Scriba, Barcelona, Spain, 1984.)

are prepared and draped. A 4-cm vertical skin incision is made on the anteromedial surface over the tibia, approximately 4 cm below the patella, with a #15 Bard-Parker blade. The incision is carried down to the periosteum and the wound is opened with a self-retaining retractor. The #15 blade is used to incise a rectangle of periosteum 2.5 cm × 4 cm. A Freer elevator is then used to remove the rectangle of periosteum. After hemostasis, the subcutaneous tissue is closed with interrupted 3-0 chromic and the skin is closed with interrupted 6-0 silk. A modified pressure dressing and leg bandage are applied.[38]

Next, a total conjunctivectomy is performed removing all the bulbar and palpebral conjunctiva from limbus to lid margins. If the corneal integrity is such that the cornea will support a keratoprosthesis, a 3.5-mm partial-thickness trephinization is performed. A superior limbal incision is then made and an intracapsular cataract extraction (in phakic eyes), total iridectomy, and subtotal vitrectomy are performed. The wound is then closed with either running or interrupted 10-0 nylon. When the host tissue is inadequate to support the prosthesis, a 9.0-mm host/10.0-mm donor penetrating keratoplasty is performed. In these cases cataract extraction, total iridectomy, and vitrectomy are performed open sky. After the donor cornea has been secured, a 3.5-mm partial-thickness trephinization is performed.

The anterior chamber is then entered with a blade through the trephine incision, and the 3.5-mm button is removed with scissors. Any additional vitrectomy may be performed through the 3.5-mm wound. Two preplaced 9-0 nylon sutures are placed on opposite sides of the wound and the keratoprosthesis is then placed into the bed. A cyclodialysis spatula is used through either the cataract or keratoplasty incision to keep the cornea firmly against the flange. The preplaced sutures are tied, and additional 9-0 nylon sutures are placed to secure the flange against the cornea. The anterior chamber is then deepened with balanced salt solution. The 3.5-mm (or slightly smaller) trephine is used to punch a hole through the center of the periosteal graft. The periosteum is then fitted over the optical cylinder and secured to the episclera with 5-0 chromic sutures. The periosteum is closed around the keratoprosthesis with a single purse-string suture.

A 4-mm full-thickness horizontal incision is then made through the upper lid and tarsus. The keratoprosthesis is

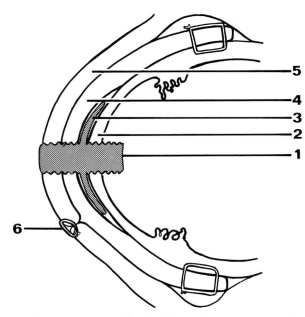

**Fig. 12-18.** Keratoprosthesis with interlamellar support. 1. Optical cylinder of the prosthesis threaded through the support. 2. Opaque host cornea. 3. Fenestrated support of plastic, platinum, etc. 4. Periosteum from the tibia of the same patient, sutured to the sclera near the insertion of the 4 rectus muscles. 5. Tarsal cartilage and skin of the upper lid. 6. Permanent tarsorrhaphy. (Redrawn with permission from Barraquer and Rutlar. *Microsurgery of the Cornea* Ediciones Scriba, Barcelona, Spain, 1984.)

then placed through the lid. A total tarsorrhaphy is performed using interrupted 6-0 silk (Fig. 12-18). A silastic washer is fashioned by punching a 3.5-mm hole in a 1 cm × 2 cm silastic sheet. A cut is then made into the trephined opening to allow the silastic washer to fit over the optical cylinder and under its lip. The silastic washer is then closed with two 6-0 silk sutures to form a gasket between the anterior lid surface and the exteriorized keratoprosthesis. The wound is dressed with antibiotic ointment and a doughnut-shaped gauze is fashioned to avoid pressure on the keratoprosthesis. A standard shield is placed. The silastic washer is removed in 2 weeks and the lid sutures in 3 weeks.[2,38]

Polack and Heimke reported on a small series of patients using a keratoprosthesis made of an aluminum oxide ceramic.[80] The material has excellent biocompatibility and allows for fibrous tissue ingrowth through the prosthesis perforations. Their surgical technique is similar to that previously outlined with the following modifications. (1) They recommend that the lacrimal gland be excised if any degree of tear production exists. (2) Cyanoacrylic glue is utilized to help form a watertight seal between the anterior corneal surface and the back of the prosthetic flange. And, (3) the horizontal rectimuscles are sectioned in an attempt to limit the movement of the prosthesis.[80]

Though short-term results have met with limited success, long-term results have been discouraging.[2] The through-and-through keratoprosthesis exteriorized through the upper lid has limited the most serious complication of extrusion to less than 20 percent but has made surgical reintervention difficult.[99] There is no adequate way of revising

the keratoprosthesis once it has been covered by periosteum and exteriorized through the upper lid. Other common and serious complications include sterile vitritis and the formation of a retroprosthetic membrane that effectively obscures vision. Because of the occurrence and severity of postoperative problems, a keratoprosthesis is indicated only when the prognosis for other reconstructive surgery is extremely poor. Yet for some patients, it represents the only hope for visual rehabilitation.

## REFERENCES

1. Anderson JR, Jensen OA, Kristensen EB, et al.: Benign mucous membrane pemphigoid: III. Biopsy. Acta Ophthalmologica 52:455, 1974
2. Aquavella JV, Rao GN, Brown AC, et al.: Keratoprosthesis. Ophthalmology 89:655, 1982
3. Arena JM: Treatment of caustic poisoning. Modern Treatment 8:613, 1971
4. Arstikaitis M: Ocular aftermath of Stevens-Johnson syndrome. Arch Ophthalmol 90:376, 1973
5. Ballen P: Mucous membrane grafts in chemical burns. Am Ophthalmol 55:302, 1963
6. Baum JL: Systemic disease associated with tear deficiencies. Int Ophthalmol Clin 13:157, 1973
7. Belin MW, Krachmer JW: Chemical burns of the cornea, in Easty DL, Smolin G: External Eye Disease. London, Butterworth 1985, pp 288–309
8. Beyer CK: The management of special problems associated with Stevens-Johnson syndrome and ocular pemphigoid. Transactions of the American Academy of Ophthalmology and Otolaryngology 83:1072, 1977
9. Boruchoff CH, Refojo M, Slansky HH, Webster RG, Freeman MI, Dohlman CH: Clinical applications of adhesives in corneal surgery. Transactions of the American Academy of Ophthalmology and Otolaryngology 73:499, 1965
10. Brown SI, Aliya S, Weller CA: Pathogenesis of ulcers of the alkali-burned cornea. Archives of Ophthalmology 83:205, 1970
11. Brown SI, Weller CA: Pathogenesis and treatment of collagenase-induced diseases of the cornea. Transactions of the American Academy of Ophthalmology and Otolaryngology 74:375, 1970
12. Cardona H, DeVoe AG: Symposium on keratoprosthesis-prosthokeratoplasty. Trans Am Acad Ophthalmol Otolaryngol 83:271, 1977
13. Castroviejo R, Cardona H, DeVoe A: Latest techniques of prosthokeratoplasty. Presented at the XXII International Congress of Ophthalmology, Paris, 1974
14. Chanda JJ: Erythema multiforme. Perspect Ophthalmol 3:183, 1979
15. Darougar S, Quinlan MP, Gibson JA, et al.: Epidemic keratoconjunctivitis and chronic papillary conjunctivitis in London due to adenovirus type 19. Br J Ophthalmol 61:76, 1977
16. Darougar S, Jones BR: Trachoma. Br Med J 39(2):117, 1983
17. Dawson CR, Whitcher JP, Lyon C, et al.: Response to treatment in ocular chlamydial infections (trachoma and inclusion conjunctivitis): Analogies with non-gonococcal urethritis, in Hobson D, Holmes KK (eds): Non-Gonococcal Urethritis and Other Infections. Washington, American Society for Microbiology, 1977, pp 135–139

18. Dawson CR, Jones BR, Tarizzo M: Guide to trachoma control.Geneva, World Health Organization, 1981

19. Dawson CR: Pathogenesis and control of blinding trachoma, in Duane TD (ed): Clinical Ophthalmology, (vol. 5). Philadelphia, Harper and Row 1984, Ch 60, pp 1–11

20. Denig R: Transplantation of mucous membrane of the mouth for various diseases and burns of the cornea. New York State J Med 107:1074, 1918

21. DeVoe AG: Symposium on keratoprosthesis-history, techniques and indications. Trans Am Acad Ophthalmol Otolaryngol 83:249, 1977

22. Dhermy P, Coscas G, Nataf R, et al.: Histopathologie des follicules au cours du trachome et des conjonctivite folliculaire. Rev Int Trach 4:295–398, 1967

23. Dohlman CH, Doughman DJ: The Stevens-Johnson syndrome, in Symposium on Cornea. Trans New Orleans Acad Ophthalmol. Mosby, St. Louis, 1972, pp 236–252

24. Duke-Elder S: System of Ophthalmology, vol 8. Diseases of the outer eye. Part I. Conjunctiva. Mosby, St. Louis, 1965, pp 498–527

25. Flach A: Symblepharon in sarcoidosis. Am J Ophthalmol 85:210, 1978

26. Foster CS: Immunosuppressive therapy for external ocular inflammatory disease. Ophthalmology 87:140, 1980

27. Foster CS, Zelt RP, Mai-phan T, et al.: Immunosuppression and selective inflammatory cell depletion. Arch Ophthalmol 100:1820, 1982

28. Fox SA: Mucous membrane grafts, in Ophthalmic Plastic Surgery. New York, Grune and Stratton, 1976, pp 77–107

29. Francois J, Feher J: Collagenolysis and regeneration in corneal burning. Ophthalmologica 165:137, 1972

30. Furney N, West C, Andrews T, et al.: Immunofluorescent studies of ocular cicatricial pemphigoid. Am J Ophthalmol 80:825, 1975

31. Gazala JR: Ocular pemphigus. Am J Ophthalmol 48:355, 1959

32. Gould BS: The role of certain vitamins in collagen formation, in Treatise on Collagen. London, Academic Press, 1968, p 323

33. Grant WM: Toxicology of the eye. Springfield, Thomas, 1974, pp 88–101

34. Grayson M: Oculogenital disease and related conditions, in Grayson M: Diseases of the Cornea. Mosby, St. Louis, 1983, pp 129–149

35. Grayson M: Stevens-Johnson syndrome (erythema multiforme), in Grayson M: Diseases of the Cornea. Mosby, St. Louis, 1983, pp 419–424

36. Gustavson KH: The chemistry and reactivity of collagen. New York, Academic Press, 1956, p 155

37. Hardy KM, Perry HO, Pingree GC, et al.: Benign mucous membrane pemphigoid. Arch Dermatol 104:467, 1971

38. Harris JK, Rao Gn, Aquavella JV, et al.: Keratoprosthesis: Technique and instrumentation. Ann Ophthalmol 16:481, 1984

39. Herman WK, Doughman DJ, Lindstrom RL: Conjunctival autograft transplantation for unilateral ocular surface diseases. Ophthalmology 90:1121, 1983

40. Howard GM: The Steven-Johnson syndrome: Ocular prognosis and treatment. Am J Ophthalmol 55:893, 1963

41. Hughes WF: Alkali burns of the eye. Arch Ophthalmol 36:189, 1946

42. Hughes WF: Alkali burns of the eye. Arch Ophthalmol 35:423, 1946

43. Hurych J, Chvapil M, Tichy M, et al.: Evidence for a faster degradation of an atypical hydroxyproline and hydroxylysine deficient collagen formed under the effect of 2.2-dipyridyl. Eur J Biochem 3:242, 1967

44. Itoi M, Gnadinger MC, Slansky HH, et al.: Collagenase in the cornea. Exp Eye Res 8:369, 1969

45. Jawetz E, Dawson CR, Schachter J, et al.: Immunoglobulin nature of antibodies in chlamydial infections, in Nichols R (ed): Trachoma and related disorders. Amsterdam, Excerpta Medica 1971, pp 233–242

46. Jones BR: The ocular diagnosis of benign mucous membrane pemphigoid. Proc R Soc Med 54:109, 1961

47. Jones DB: Prospects in the management of tear-deficiency states. Trans Am Acad Ophthalmol Otolaryngol 83:693, 1977

48. Kaye DB: Epithelial response in penetrating keratoplasty. Am J Ophthalmol 89:321, 1980

49. Kinoshita S, Kiorpes TC, Friend J, et al.: Goblet cell density in ocular surface disease. Arch Ophthalmol 101:1284, 1983

50. Klauder JV, Cowan A: Ocular pemphigus and its relation to pemphigus of the skin and mucous membranes. Am J Ophthalmol 25:643, 1942

51. Koob TJ, Jeffrey JJ, Elsen AZ: Regulation of human skin collagenase activity by hydrocortisone and dexamethasone in organ culture. Biochem Biophys Res Commun 61:1083, 1974

52. Korting GW, Denk R: Differential diagnosis in dermatology. Philadelphia, Saunders, 1976, pp 421–422

53. Kristensen EB, Norn MS: Benign mucous membrane pemphigoid: I. Secretion of mucous and tears. Acta Ophthalmologica 52:266, 1974

54. Lemp MA: Surfacing the precorneal tear film. Ann Ophthalmol 5:819, 1973

55. Lemp MA: Cornea and sclera. Arch Ophthalmol 92:158, 1974

56. Leone CR: Treatment of conjunctival diseases, in Silver B: Ophthalmic Plastic Surgery. San Francisco, American Academy of Ophthalmology and Otolaryngology, 1977, pp 105–115

57. Levinson RA, Paterson CA, Pfister RR: Ascorbic acid prevents corneal ulceration and perforation following experimental alkali burns. Invest Ophthalmol Vis Sci 15:986, 1976

58. MacCallan AF: Trachoma. London, Butterworths, 1936, pp 8–26

59. Mondino BJ, Ross AN, Rabin BS, et al.: Autoimmune phenomena in ocular cicatricial pemphigoid. Am J Ophthalmol 83:443, 1977

60. Mondino BJ, Brown SI, Rabin BS: Autoimmune phenomena of the external eye. Ophthalmology 85:801, 1978

61. Mondino BJ, Brown SI, Lempert S, et al.: The acute manifestations of ocular cicatricial pemphigoid: Diagnosis and treatment. Ophthalmology 86:543, 1979

62. Mondino BJ, Brown SI: Ocular cicatricial pemphigoid. Ophthalmology 88:95, 1981

63. Mondino BJ: Cicatricial pemphigoid and erythema multiforme. Int Ophthalmol Clin 23:63, 1983

64. Mondino BJ, Brown SI: Immunosuppressive therapy in ocular cica tricial pemphigoid. Am J Ophthalmol 96:453, 1983

65. Mondino BJ: Bullous diseases of the skin and mucous membranes, in Duane TD: Clinical Ophthalmology, vol 4. Philadelphia, Harper and Row, 1984, Ch 12, pp 1–16

66. Morgan LB: A new therapeutic scleral lens. Rocky Mountain Med J 68:26, 1971

67. Nelson D, Wright JC: Conjunctival goblet cell densities in ocular surface disease. Arch Ophthalmol 102:1049, 1984

68. Newsome DA, Gross J: Prevention by medroxyprogesterone of perforation in the alkali-burned rabbit cornea. Invest Ophthalmol Vis Sci 16:21, 1977

69. O'Connor GB: Early grafting in burns of the eye. Arch Ophthalmol 9:48, 1933

70. Ostler HB, Conant MA, Goundwater J: Lyell's disease, the Stevens-Johnson syndrome and exfoliative dermatitis. Trans Acad Ophthalmol Otolaryngol 74:1254, 1970

71. Paterson CA, Eakins KE, Jenkins RM, et al.: The ocular hypertensive response following experimental acid burns in the rabbit eye. Invest Ophthalmol Vis Sci 18:67, 1979

72. Paton D, Goldberg MF: Burns of the eye, in Management of Ocular Injuries. Philadelphia, Saunders, 1976, pp 163–180

73. Patten JT, Cavanagh HD, Allansmith MR: Induced ocular pseudopemphigoid. Am J Ophthalmol 82:272, 1976

74. Patz A: Ocular involvement in erythema multiforme. Arch Ophthalmol 43:244, 1950

75. Perry HD, Kenyon KR, Lamberts DW, et al.: Systemic tetracycline in the treatment of persistent epithelial defects. Presented at the American Academy of Ophthalmology. San Francisco, 1985

76. Pfister RR, Paterson CA: Additional clinical and morphological observations on the favorable effect of ascorbate in experimental ocular alkali burns. Invest Ophthalmol Vis Sci 16:478, 1977

77. Pfister RR, Paterson CA, Hayes SA: Topical ascorbate decreases the incidence of corneal ulceration after experimental alkali burns. Invest Ophthalmol Vis Sci 17:1019, 1978

78. Pfister RR, Nicolaro ML, Paterson CA: Sodium citrate reduces the incidence of corneal ulcerations and perforations in extreme alkali burned eyes. Invest Ophthalmol Vis Sci 21:486, 1981

79. Pfister RR: Chemical injuries of the eye. Ophthalmology 90:1246, 1983

80. Polack FM, Heimke G: Ceramic keratoprosthesis. Ophthalmology 87:693, 1980

81. Ralph RA, Slansky HH: Therapy of chemical burns. Int Ophthalmol Clin 4:171, 1974

82. Ralph RA: Conjunctival goblet cell density in normal subjects and in dry eye syndromes. Invest Ophthalmol 14:299, 1975

83. Ralph RA: Chemical burns of the eye, in Duane TD (ed): Clinical Ophthalmology. Philadelphia, Harper and Row, 1980, Vol 4, chapter 28, pp 1–25

84. Rao GN, Blatt HL, Aquavella JV: Symposium on keratoprosthesis results of keratoprosthesis. Trans Am Acad Ophthalmol Otolaryngol 83:284, 1977

85. Rasmussen JE: Erythema multiforme in children. Response to treatment with systemic corticosteroids. Br J Dermatol 95:181, 1986

86. Roger RS, Seehafer JR, Perry HO: Treatment of cicatricial (benign mucous membrane) pemphigoid with dapsone. J Am Acad Dermatol 6:215, 1982

87. Rook A, Wilkinson DS, Ebling FJG: Textbook of Dermatology, vol 2. Oxford: Blackwell Scientific, 1968, pp 1163–1192

88. Roper-Hall MJ: Thermal and chemical burns. Trans Ophthalmol Soc UK 85:631, 1965

89. Shapiro MS, Friend J, Thoft RA: Corneal re-epithelialization from the conjunctiva. Invest Ophthalmol Vis Sci 21:135, 1981

90. Slansky HH, Gnadinger MC, Itoi M, et al.: Collagenase in corneal ulcerations. Arch Ophthalmol 82:108, 1969

91. Slansky HH, Berman MB, Dohlman CH, et al.: Cysteine and acetylcysteine in the prevention of corneal ulcerations. Ann Ophthalmol 2:488, 1970

92. Stein MR, Naldoff MA, Dawson CR: Intraocular pressure response to experimental alkali burns. Am J Ophthalmol 75:99, 1973

93. Tan BG: Oklahoma eye irrigating tube. Trans Am Acad Ophthalmol Otolaryngol 74:435, 1970

94. Taylor HR, Pendergast RA, Dawson CR, et al.: An animal model for cicatrizing trachoma. Assoc Res Vis Ophthalmol 21(3):422, 1981

95. Thoft RA: Conjunctival transplantation. Arch Ophthalmol 95:1425, 1977

96. Thoft RA, Friend J: Biochemical transformation of regenerating ocular surface. Invest Ophthalmol Vis Sci 16:14, 1977

97. Thoft RA, Friend J, Murphy HS: Ocular surface epithelium and cornea vascularization in rabbits. Invest Ophthalmol Vis Sci 18:85, 1979

98. Thoft RA: Indications for conjunctival transplantation. Ophthalmology 89:335, 1982

99. Thoft RA: Conjunctival surgery for corneal disease, in Smolin G, Thoft RA: The Cornea. Boston, Little Brown, 1983, pp 465–476

100. Thoft RA: Keratoepithelioplasty. Am J Ophthalmol 97:1, 1984

101. Thoft RA, Friend J, Kinoshita S, et al.: Ocular cicatricial pemphigoid associated with hyperproliferation of the conjunctival epithelium. Am J Ophthalmol 98:37, 1984

102. Tonnesen MG, Soter NA: Erythema multiforme. J Am Acad Dermatol 1:357, 1979

103. Tse DT, Mandelbaum S, Epstein E, et al.: Mucous membrane grafting for severe palpebral vernal conjunctivitis. Arch Ophthalmol 101:1897, 1983

104. Tseng SC, Maumenee AE, Stark WJ, et al.: Topical retinoid treatment for various dry-eye disorders. Ophthalmology 92:717, 1985

105. Vastine DW, Dawson CR, Daghfous T, et al.: Severe endemic trachoma in Tunisia: I. The effect of topical chemotherapy on conjunctivitis and ocular bacteria. Br J Ophthalmol 58:833, 1974

106. Vastine DW, Stewart WB, Schwab IR: Reconstruction of the periocular mucous membrane by autologous conjunctival transplantation. Ophthalmology 89:1072, 1982

107. Viswalingam ND, Wishart MS, Woodland RM: Adult Chlamydial ophthalmia (paratrachoma). Br Med Bull 39(2):123, 1983

108. Waltman SR, Yarran D: Circulating autoantibodies in ocular pemphigoid. Am J Ophthalmol 77:891, 1974

109. Wang SP, Grayston JP, Kuo CC, et al.: Serodiagnosis of chlamydia trachomatis infection with the microimmunofluorescence test, in Hobson D, Holmes KK (ed): Nongonococcal urethritis and other infections. Washington, Am Soc Microbiol 1977, pp 237–248

110. Wuepper KD, Watson PA, Kazmierowski JA: Immune complexes in erythema multiforme and the Stevens-Johnson syndrome. J Invest Dermatol 74:368, 1980

111. Yetiv JZ, Bianchine JR, Owen JA: Etiologic factors of the Stevens-Johnson syndrome. South Med J 73:599, 1980

# 13

# Scleritis

## Edward J. Rockwood          David M. Meisler

*Scleritis* is a severe, painful, and potentially destructive inflammatory disorder of the sclera. Scleritis and its complications can result in visual loss and perforation of the eye. It is bilateral in as much as 45 percent of patients,[83] and is often recurrent.[85]

## PRESENTATION OF THE SCLERITIS PATIENT

The predominant symptom of scleritis is pain, unlike episcleritis, in which there may be an otherwise asymptomatic, diffusely or focally red eye. The pain associated with scleritis is often described as a deep, boring ache that can be referred to the ipsilateral brow, jaw, or temple. In one form of scleritis, scleromalacia perforans, however, there is bluing and thinning of the sclera with little evidence of active ocular inflammation and pain. Photophobia and lacrimation are common in scleritis; however, a discharge is not usually seen. The patient might not complain of loss of vision unless there is a serous retinal detachment secondary to posterior scleritis or unless there is a sclerokeratitis or corneal edema resulting from associated elevated intraocular pressure.

Scleritis can present with inflammation in the region of the visible anterior sclera, the posterior sclera, or both. Anterior scleritis can be focal (nodular) or diffuse. The necrotizing forms of scleritis are usually subdivided into necrotizing-with-inflammation or necrotizing-without-inflammation (scleromalacia perforans). The latter condition has most often been reported in association with rheumatoid arthritis,[83,87] and less commonly with Crohn's colitis[29] and other systemic conditions.

In anterior scleritis, there is a dilation of the deep episcleral vascular plexus in a radial pattern in conjunction with a dilation of the more superficial conjunctival and anterior episcleral vascular networks. Phenylephrine 10% applied topically to the eye will constrict the more superficial dilated vessels which are also seen in conjunctivitis and episcleritis, but usually will have less effect on the deep episcleral vessels

seen in scleritis and may help differentiate between the superficial and deep inflammatory processes.[85] An important finding in anterior scleritis is a thickening of the sclera from edema that can be appreciated on a well-focused, thin slit-lamp beam and can be palpated as a tender, firm, nonmobile mass. In more-advanced stages of scleral inflammation, there may be scleral thinning, necrosis, or both, which give the characteristic bluish coloration seen in scleritis (Fig. 13-1; see color insert following page 139). Even in the absence of scleral thinning, a violaceous hue which is seen most easily in bright daylight, can appear in areas of anterior scleritis.

The development of areas of avascularity in the conjunctiva or episclera overlying an area of scleritis is significant because it heralds the onset of a necrotizing phase of the disease (Fig. 13-2; see color insert following page 139). The ocular morbidity of necrotizing scleritis is markedly greater than in nonnecrotizing forms of the disease.

Posterior scleritis was formerly believed to be uncommon, comprising 2 percent of one large series of scleritis patients.[84] However, the relative incidence of posterior scleritis is probably greater.[87] Posterior scleritis has been misdiagnosed as other ocular conditions including choroiditis, central serous choroidopathy, retrobulbar tumors, and intraocular malignancy.[5,30,89] Posterior scleritis can present with proptosis,[42] motility disturbance, ptosis,[4] lid retraction, choroidal hemorrhage,[1] serous retinal detachments, choroidal folds,[5] and choroidal elevation or detachment[47,53,58,62] (Figs. 13-3 and 13-4), the last two of which often are seen in the fundus in an annular, peripheral configuration.[23] Secondary angle closure glaucoma has also been reported.[62] In the diagnosis of posterior scleritis an indication, in the absence of anterior disease, is a fundus elevation with the same color and pigmentary pattern as the normal adjacent fundus.[5] By contrast, choroidal lesions such as melanoma, metastatic tumors, or macular degeneration can be expected to produce choroidal and retinal pigment epithelial derangement that will contrast with the normal pigmentary pattern of the surrounding unaffected fundus.

SURGICAL INTERVENTION IN CORNEAL AND EXTERNAL DISEASES
ISBN 0-8089-1850-8

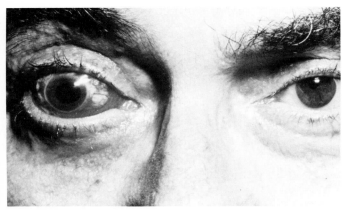

**Fig. 13-3.** Right proptosis in a 71-year-old male with anterior and posterior scleritis.

Echographic A-scan examination of posterior scleritis often reveals a thickening of the choroidal–scleral complex with high internal reflectivity, secondary to scleral edema and cellular infiltration. Additionally, an echo-free area is often seen posterior to the sclera, representing edema in the posterior, subtenons area adjacent to areas of scleral involvement in posterior scleritis.[5]

CT scanning of the orbit can show a thickened sclera that demonstrates contrast enhancement.[6] CT scanning and ultrasound can be particularly helpful when the differential diagnosis includes inflammatory orbital pseudotumor, thyroid orbitopathy, and orbital tumors.

## EVALUATION OF SCLERITIS

The investigation of scleritis demands a careful search for underlying systemic disease. A detailed medical history should be taken and a complete physical examination should

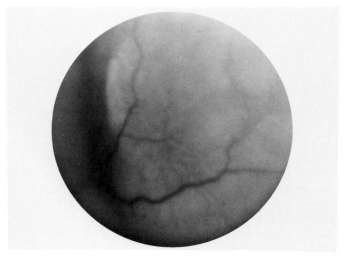

**Fig. 13-4.** Peripheral choroidal elevation temporally in the left eye of a 43-year-old female with posterior and anterior scleritis. Ultrasound revealed a greatly thickened sclera without evidence of choroidal fluid.

be performed. The presentation of a rash in a particular region or distribution can suggest a specific underlying disease such as syphilis. Arthralgias and arthritis might be a manifestation of rheumatoid arthritis, gout, or ankylosing spondylitis. Hemoptysis or pulmonary distress could be the result of tuberculosis or Wegener's granulomatosis. Other disorders associated with scleritis include ulcerative colitis,[9,49] Crohn's colitis,[29,44,49,61] herpes zoster,[49,59,66,88] relapsing polychondritis,[51] porphyria,[22] and giant cell arteritis.[43,48]

With these possible diagnoses in mind, the investigating ophthalmologist can plan an appropriate diagnostic battery. This may include a complete blood cell count with a differential, which may reveal a mild to moderate anemia or leukocytosis associated with chronic systemic disease. A Westergren sedimentation rate is a nonspecific test but indicates the level of systemic inflammation and may reflect the activity of scleritis.[46] Other tests should include a VDRL or RPR and an FTA-abs test (syphilis), urine analysis (renal disease in Wegener's granulomatosis), rheumatoid factor (rheumatoid arthritis), serum uric acid (gout), and a chest roentgenogram (tuberculosis, Wegener's granulomatosis). In the presence of lower back pain or arthritis, a sacroiliac roentgenogram series combined with an HLA B-27 (human lymphocyte antigen) would help confirm the diagnosis of ankylosing spondylitis. Extensive HLA testing, however, has not proved helpful in establishing the etiology of scleritis.[40,69,77] Whenever a clinical picture suggestive of scleritis is seen with a significant discharge or in association with a corneal ulceration, there must be an appropriate evaluation for microbial infection. Scleritis has been reported as an extension of *Pseudomonas aeruginosa* corneal infections.[63]

Tissue biopsy may confirm the diagnosis of a systemic illness associated with scleritis. Lung biopsy can confirm Wegener's granulomatosis. A nasal mucosal biopsy is, however, technically much easier and safer when there is evidence of nasal mucosal involvement. Temporal artery biopsy is indicated when giant cell arteritis is suspected.

Biopsy of scleral tissue may be associated with an increased risk of perforation. Histopathologic examination of excised scleral tissue usually does not establish a definitive diagnosis in scleritis. Often it only confirms the presence of scleral inflammation and necrosis.[72] Young and Watson[90] reported on the histopathology of eight eyes with three different types of scleritis. Two had scleromalacia perforans, three had an anterior necrotizing scleritis, and three had scleritis following ocular surgery. It was not possible for the authors to distinguish between these three categories histopathologically. Eyes in all three categories showed granulomatous inflammation of the conjunctiva, episclera, and sclera with a cellular infiltrate of lymphocytes, plasma cells and mast cells. However, a recent, comprehensive histopathologic study on 41 cases of scleritis by Rao, Marak, and Hidayat (1985)[66] suggested that different, distinct forms of necrotizing scleritis do exist. This question is not yet settled, but it is probable that different stages of inflammation and different systemic therapies could partially explain the variable results obtained by these investigators. Occasionally, a scleral biopsy may be indicated. In one case reported by Bloomfield et al.,[10] a scleral biopsy revealed a caseating granuloma of the sclera with acid-fast bacilli. A culture was positive for *Mycobacterium tuberculosis*. In this case, scleral biopsy led to the use of appropriate and specific therapy.

## THE MECHANISM OF SCLERAL MELTING

The pathophysiologic mechanism of scleral melting has not been determined with certainty. Many factors may play a role. The deposition of circulating immune complexes and vasculitis have been implicated. Sevel and McGavin et al[52,71] have noted that rheumatoid scleritis often began late in the course of arthritis, usually 10 to 13 years after its onset, and when the scleritis did occur, it often coincided with the development of extraarticular manifestations of rheumatoid arthritis.[38] The presence of circulating immune complexes with complement activation is associated with the presence of extraarticular manifestations of rheumatoid arthritis,[13] and may be a factor in the etiology of some cases of rheumatoid scleritis.

Scleritis was found in 6 of 113 patients with IgA nephropathy. Although scleral biopsy was not performed, renal biopsies demonstrated IgA deposits in the muscular arterioles and the mesangial areas of the kidneys.[28,56] It was not known whether the IgA was directed against scleral antigens or if an unknown antigen resulted in circulating immune complexes that may have led to renal and scleral disease.

Vasculitis can result from the effects of the deposition of circulating immune complexes in the microvasculature and activation of the complement cascade. The inflammation that occurs in the vessel walls can lead to blockage and ischemia. Normally, brief periods of ischemia induced by cryopexy, diathermy, and scleral buckling are tolerated well, without subsequent scleral damage, thinning, or necrosis. Sevel,[73] in 1968, demonstrated the relative resiliency of scleral tissue to an ischemic insult. Exclusion of vascular supply to the sclera for 8 weeks in an animal model failed to result in scleral necrosis. In each of these situations, there was no immunologic inflammatory component superimposed on the ischemic insult. Both the ischemia from vasculitis combined with an immunologically mediated inflammation may be necessary to produce scleral necrosis.

Immune responses directed against scleral tissue or scleral antigens might play a role in the etiology of scleritis in some patients. Rao et al.[65] have demonstrated that a group of 10 non-rheumatoid necrotizing scleritis patients showed evidence for both circulating immune complexes and lymphocyte transformation in the presence of solubilized human scleral antigen. A second group of 10 patients with rheumatoid scleritis failed to show evidence of in vitro cell-mediated or humoral immune responses to scleral antigen; only circulating immune complexes were identified.

The pathogenesis of postoperative scleritis also is not well understood. It is possible that the trauma and inflammation induced at the time of surgery might lead to immune sensitization to normal or altered scleral tissues and a subsequent antibody or cell-mediated response to the sclera. A second explanation might be that a patient with a preexisting circulating immune complex disorder might be more susceptible to the usually mild and well-tolerated ischemic insults that occur at the time of surgery from tissue cutting and cautery. This latter sequence of events could explain the development of postoperative scleritis in a patient discussed by Bloomfield et al.[11] The patient had a vasculitic syndrome, and developed bilateral scleritis after bilateral cataract surgery. Histopathologic examination of excised conjunctival and episcleral tissue revealed focal deposits of IgG, IgM, and $C_3$. Lyne and Lloyd-Jones[50] reported six cases of postoperative scleritis, all but one having occurred in patients 75 or older. One had a positive rheumatoid factor and an elevated antinuclear antibody titer; the other had only a positive antinuclear antibody titer, despite no evidence of systemic disease. Three different suture materials (nylon, silk, dacron) were used among their six cases that developed postoperative scleritis. It appeared unlikely that any single suture material could be incriminated as the inciting factor in these patients. Salamon et al.[70] failed to demonstrate a sensitivity to the suture material, by specific testing, in one patient who developed a postoperative scleritis.

*Pseudomonas aeruginosa*[24,27,36,41,63,80] and *Pseudomonas fluorescens*[63] scleritis have recently been reported. Corneal ulceration, often leading to perforation is the most common corneo-scleral manifestation of ocular pseudomonal infection. Pseudomonal scleritis usually occurs as a direct, localized extension of corneal disease.[24,27] The morbidity from ocular pseudomonal infections is high.[63] Keratolysis often continues unabated even after treatment with appropriate and intensive antibiotic therapy.

Scleral necrosis has been observed in a few instances in locations remote from the initial area of corneal ulceration.[7,24] In some cases, a scleral nodule or ulcer persisted or developed subsequent to initiation of antibiotic therapy. Cultures of necrotic areas usually revealed a persistence of pseudomonal organisms. In a few cases, the pseudomonal scleritis began in a recent postoperative setting,[7,63] but in others, no inciting or associated factors were identified. The keratolytic and sclerolytic damage of pseudomonal infections is believed to be a result of proteolytic enzyme release from the microorganism.[31] Corticosteroid therapy may play a role in the development of pseudomonal infections and pseudomonal keratolysis by suppressing inflammatory responses[19,78] and by potentiating the activity of corneal collagenases.[15]

Noninfectious and nonsystemic causes of scleral melting have included a tight-fitting soft contact lens[16] and postirradiation of a pterygium.[20] A severe alkali burn had preceded use of the contact lens in the former case. These cases may be analogous to the vasculitis-associated subgroup of scleritis in that the alkali burn and the β-irradiation might have caused compromised vascularity before the development of the scleral melt.

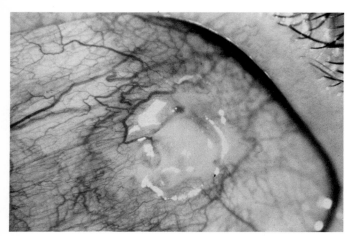

**Fig. 13-5.** Area of conjunctival necrosis and a bed of inflammatory exudate superotemporally in the left eye of the same patient in Figure 13-4.

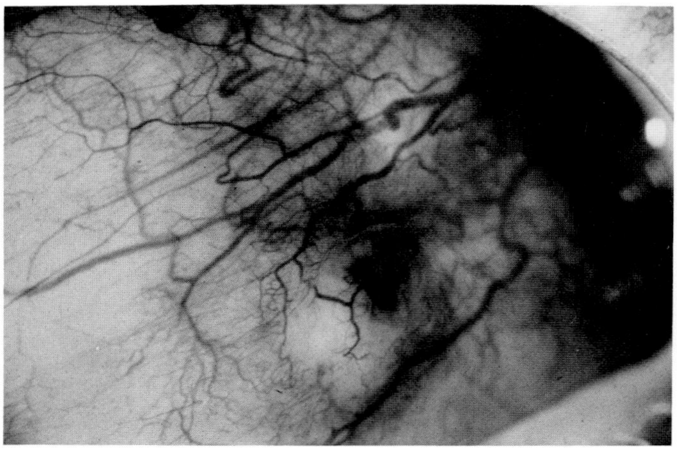

**Fig. 13-6.** Same area as in Fig. 13-5, 4 months after oral prednisone and topical fluoromethalone therapy. Note resolution of conjunctival defect.

## THE MEDICAL THERAPY OF SCLERITIS

The medical therapy of scleritis is determined by the presence or absence of necrotizing disease and the nature of any identifiable associated systemic ailment or etiologic agent.

A nonsteroidal anti-inflammatory agent is the preferred treatment for most cases of rheumatoid and nonrheumatoid inflammatory scleritis in the absence of conjunctival and episcleral avascularity or scleral necrosis. Watson,[86] in a consise article on the medical management of scleritis, preferred indomethacin in a suggested dosage of 100 mg daily and subsequent tapering to 75 mg daily. An alternative agent mentioned in the same article, oxyphenbutazone, is no longer available in the United States. By using nonsteroidal anti-inflammatory agents, the adverse effects of systemic corticosteroids (hyperglycemia, osteoporosis, and weight gain) can be avoided. The gastrointestinal disturbances caused by systemic corticosteroids and indomethacin can be reduced by taking the medication with meals or an antacid.

Therapy for necrotizing scleritis usually requires high-dose systemic corticosteroid therapy. Prednisone, 60–100 mg daily with a subsequent tapering dependent on the response to therapy, is appropriate. Dramatic relief of severe pain is often the first sign of response to therapy, followed by diminished inflammation and scleral edema. Systemic corticosteroid therapy should not only stop progression of the necrotizing process, but will often allow healing in areas of avascularity and necrosis (Figs. 13-5 and 13-6). Areas of previous scleral bluing will often show no change after treatment and resolution of scleral inflammation.

Topical corticosteroids alone are not sufficient to arrest the inflammatory process of scleritis. They may play a role in reducing a secondary intraocular inflammatory component. Subconjunctival corticosteroids are contraindicated in scleritis, according to some authors,[33,84] because of the risk of

precipitating a scleral perforation or melt at or near the site of injection.

Antimetabolite therapy is the treatment of choice in Wegener's granulomatosis.[35] The use of cyclophosphamide has reduced the mortality of Wegener's granulomatosis from about 50 percent to much lower levels.[25] Additional beneficial effects can be obtained in some patients with concomitant use of systemic corticosteroids.[27,18] However, steroid therapy alone might allow progression of the disease.[18] Foster et al.[32] have reported that the use of cytotoxic drugs, including cyclophosphamide, methotrexate, and azathioprine, reduces the mortality rate as well as improves the ocular prognosis in patients with seropositive rheumatoid arthritis. Appropriate management of the patient with Wegener's granulomatosis and any of the systemic vasculitidies is best achieved with the aid of a rheumatologist or other physician experienced in the administration or cytotoxic agents.

Topical, periocular, and, occasionally, systemic antibiotics are indicated in culture-proved or suspected pseudomonal scleritis. Topical aminoglycosides (gentamicin, tobramycin) usually provide good coverage for *Pseudomonas aeruginosa*. Syphilitic scleritis requires systemic penicillin therapy. Bloomfield et al.[10] reported successful treatment of their patient who had systemic and scleral tuberculosis with systemic isoniazid and rifampin in addition to subconjunctival streptomycin. Stenson et al.[75] successfully treated a patient who had scleritis associated with an *Aspergillus oryzae* meningitis with topical natamycin (5%), topical and subconjunctival amphotericin B, and systemic flucytosine and amphotericin B.

Gout responds well to colchicine and uricosuric agents (probenecid). Long-term probenecid and dietary restrictors are usually required to maintain an appropriately reduced serum uric acid level in patients with gout and the rare syndrome of gouty scleritis.

Other medical treatments have been tried in the therapy

of scleritis with varying or no success. The chelating agent EDTA[29,63] has been employed in an attempt to block the activity of lytic enzymes at the site of scleral necrosis. Subconjunctival heparin has been used to prevent some of the ischemic complications of scleritis secondary to a vasculitis.[17,29,37] The vaso-occlusion seen in these syndromes is, however, probably secondary to direct lumenal occlusion by inflammatory cells and fibrinoid necrosis[34] rather than thrombosis. Acetylcysteine,[47,61,63] 1-cysteine,[39] and d-penicillamine,[47,91] have also not given consistent results.

## SURGICAL MANAGEMENT

The majority of scleritis patients have a remission on an adequate medical regimen.[83] With appropriate and early therapy, perforation of the sclera is uncommon. The increased scleral lucency and bluing often seen in scleromalacia perforans is not an indication for surgery. Many patients develop a progressive worsening of appearance, which can be dramatic (Fig. 13-7; see color insert following page 139), yet the scleral coat remains intact. McGavin et al.[52] presented the results of ultra-sound measurements of the sclera in areas of increased translucency from scleritis in which they demonstrated that such areas were not always thinned. Small areas of scleral necrosis without perforation often heal inward after medical therapy. Healing of the area often results in new collagen deposition after conjunctival and episcleral revascularization has occurred.

Problematic scleral disease may, however, require surgical intervention. Historically, the surgical approach to scleral disease began with Van der Hoeve.[82] In his classic study of scleromalacia perforans, he described the use of a buccal mucosal graft and a conjunctival flap to cover bare uvea. Eber subsequently reported successful treatment with the latter method.[26] However, Renard et al.[67] reported the

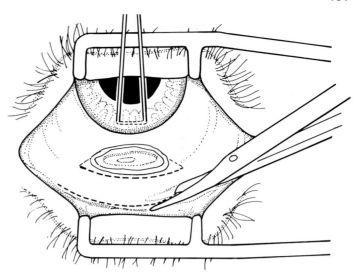

**Fig. 13-9.** The margins of the conjunctival flap are cut with scissors from the conjunctiva immediately adjacent to the defect. Tenon's fascia is not dissected from the conjunctiva.

unsuccessful application of buccal mucosa in treating perforations.

Free autologous conjunctival grafts have been used to close very small conjunctival and episcleral defects that have not responded well to medical therapy and may be developing an area of scleral sequestration. Conjunctival donor sites should not be areas of scleral thinning or inflammation. Conjunctival rotation flaps or "bucket-handle" grafts[20] can be fashioned if adjacent, unscarred conjunctiva is available (Figs. 13-8–13-10). The posterior incision for the "bucket-handle" flap should be made as far from the limbus as possible. Areas of frank necrosis and tissue softening should be debrided. A second conjunctival incision can be made near the diseased area and the flap is then slid into position. An

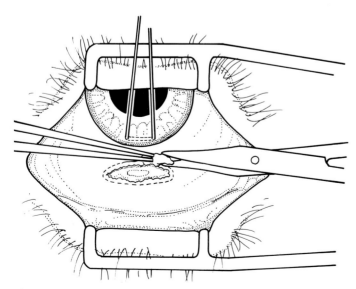

**Fig. 13-8.** Diagram of large conjunctival and episcleral defect in the inferior bulbar region. Necrotic tissue is debrided.

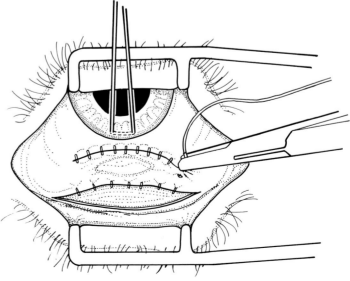

**Fig. 13-10.** The bucket-handle or bridge flap graft is sutured into position with an absorbable suture material (7-0 vicryl).

absorbable suture (e.g., 7–0 vicryl) can be used to suture the graft in place with as little tension as possible to avoid retraction.

Indications for tectonic surgery in scleritis include spontaneous or traumatic scleral rupture, progressive circumferential necrotizing scleritis unresponsive to medical therapy, and intractable pain resulting from an area of necrotizing scleritis.[84] Various materials have been used to reinforce the sclera.

Paufique[60] described the successful use of a scleral graft to repair a small scleral perforation. Subsequently, others have implemented repair with scleral tissue.[57,68,74] Today it remains a popular tissue for tectonic procedures, supplying a collagen framework that gives support to the globe. It can readily be fashioned from donor eyes and because it has no active cellular components, it does not necessarily have to be fresh for the graft to be accepted.[1] Preserved human donor (banked) sclera has been successfully used for the repair of moderate to sizable scleral defects or areas of severe thinning. It is readily obtainable, can be stored for long periods of time in alcohol, is flexible, and can easily be cut into the appropriate size and shape. Fresh cadaveric tissue probably has no advantages over the more convenient banked sclera. Before use, banked sclera should be soaked in sterile water, preferably overnight, to remove residual alcohol. (Lamellar autogenous scleral rotation flaps have been successfully used in treating marginal corneal disease such as Mooren's ulcer,[76] "paralimbic" scleromalacia,[21] and for closing aqueous fistulae in the sclera. However, the dissection and iatrogenic thinning of the sclera make this procedure inadvisable in patients with substantial areas of scleral thinning and necrosis).

There are many variations of the technique for scleral grafting. In one, conjunctival resection is performed prior to grafting to remove adjacent, inflamed, and necrotic conjunctiva from the site of scleral necrosis. The conjunctival incision can be either limbus or fornix based. Often this decision is affected by the location and amount of conjunctival–scleral necrosis. Alternatively, a combined limbus- and fornix-based flap can be dissected anteriorly and posteriorly away from the area of scleral and conjunctival necrosis. Necrotic or ischemic conjunctiva and episclera are often adherent to the sclera[79] and button-holing of the conjunctiva is a common event. Furthermore, in areas of scleral thinning and staphyloma formation, dissection of the conjunctiva should be done with a blunt intrument (blunt-tipped scissors or spatula) to avoid inadvertent scleral penetration.

Debridement of the conjunctiva, Tenon's fascia and episclera should be minimal and include only completely avascular and necrotic areas. Preservation of viable conjunctiva is necessary for covering the graft at the end of the procedure. Cauterization of actively bleeding vessels should be done sparingly because the episcleral vascular plexus is important in the subsequent vascularization of the graft. Attention is then directed to the scleral bed. In many instances, the scleral graft can be directly sutured into position as an onlay scleral graft,[57–74] leaving the recipient bed unaltered, especially when repairing areas of severe ectasia

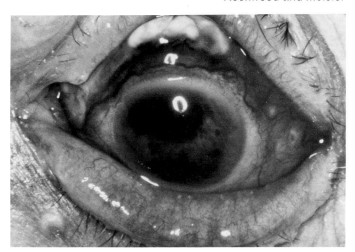

**Fig. 13-11.** Superior scleral perforation with prolapsed vitreous in the left eye of an 80-year-old female with rheumatoid scleritis.

or perforation without devitalized tissue (Figs. 13-11) and 13-12). Cautious use of electrocautery at a low setting has been used to remove adherent necrotic tissue to the sclera and to reduce the extent of scleral bulging before placement of the graft.[8,12,79,81] Scleral dissection may be occasionally necessary when the scleral inflammatory involvement is deep.

In cases of pseudomonal scleritis and sclerokeratitis, it is essential to undertake a thorough removal of any softened or necrotic tissue that could later serve as a nidus for recurrent infection. These areas can be larger than anticipated on clinical examination, so it is possible that a more extensive graft may be required. Cryotherapy of adjacent scleral tissue has been advocated to kill remaining pseudomonal organisms.[27] This should be performed prior to graft placement and a low temperature should be achieved ($-79°C$). Alpren et al.[2] found that a single freeze–thaw cycle to $-79°C$ resulted in a 99.9 percent reduction of pseudomonas organisms in infected rabbit and guinea pig corneas.

Scleral cryotherapy should also be implemented in areas surrounding vitreous prolapse from a scleral perforation pos-

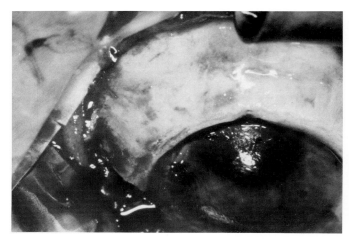

**Fig. 13-12.** Scleral graft in position prior to suturing in place.

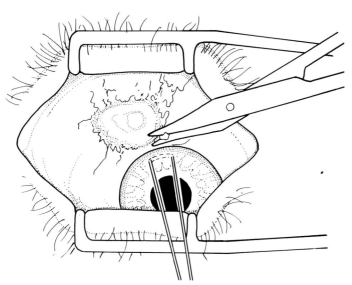

**Fig. 13-13.** Preoperative appearance of an eye with scleral necrosis and thinning.

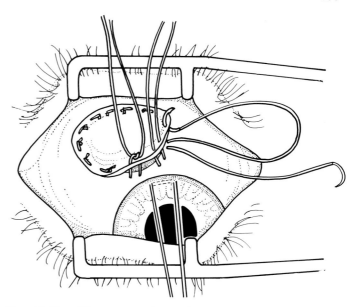

**Fig. 13-15.** The suture ends are then passed through the scleral graft and tied.

terior to the ora serrata to reduce the risk of rhegmatogenous detachment. Small vitreal herniations can be managed with a gentle "Weck-cel" vitrectomy. Larger defects with larger vitreal herniations may require a limited vitrectomy with the use of a suction-cutting device to remove vitreous from the perforation site. These measures minimize the risk of vitreal incarceration between the graft and the edge of the scleral bed.

The scleral graft is sized and fashioned. It should be of an adequate size to extend beyond the area of scleral necrosis or attenuation. This will allow suturing of the graft to stronger, thicker recipient tissue and reduce the possibility of penetration of the globe when passing the anchoring sutures. Interrupted, nonabsorbable material (silk, nylon) should be

used to suture the graft in place. Double-armed sutures may be used. After an initial pass through the recipient bed, these can be passed through the graft margin and tied in an interrupted fashion (Figs. 13-13–13-18).[57]

Proper covering of the graft with viable, vascularized conjunctiva is essential for graft retention. If conjunctival loss is significant, a rotation or bucket handle conjunctival flap can be used.

Scleral grafts occasionally fail, even after an uncomplicated procedure and successful covering by conjunctiva.[14,68,81] Breslin et al.[14] in 1977, suggested that a tissue-

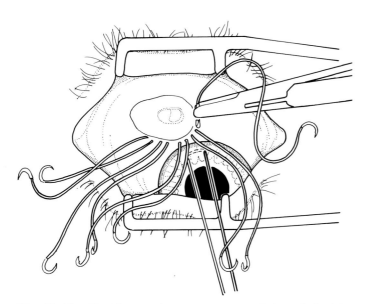

**Fig. 13-14.** Double-armed sutures are passed through healthy areas of recipient bed sclera surrounding the debrided scleral bed.

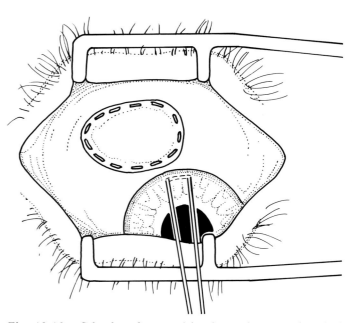

**Fig. 13-16.** Scleral graft sutured in place prior to conjunctival closure.

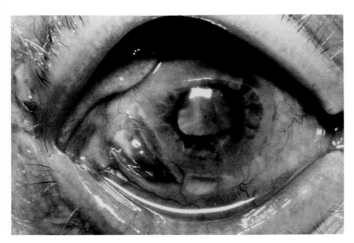

**Fig. 13-17.**   Corneoscleral melt with a small degree of uveal prolapse (Courtesy of Vincent deLuise, M.D.).

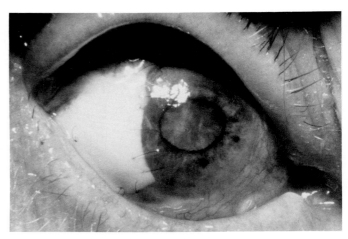

**Fig. 13-18.**   A scleral graft has been used to repair the corneoscleral defect of the patient in Figure 13-17 (Courtesy of Vincent deLuise, M.D.).

specific autoimmunity to sclera could be the pathogenetic mechanism of scleral graft failure. However, one case of Torchia et al.[81] had possible necrotic bacteria on a Gram-stained section of the failed scleral graft. Occurrence or reoccurrence of infection should be considered a possibility in any graft failure, and appropriate cultures should be taken and antibioic therapy implemented.

Autogenous fascia lata[3,8,12,79,81,91] or periosteum[14,45,64] have also been used as alternatives to sclera for primary repair of a scleral defect or subsequent to a failed scleral grafting procedure (Fig. 13-19; see color insert following page 139). Both tissues have the advantages of being living, autogenous tissues and, as such, are probably incorporated into the recipient bed faster than banked sclera. the use of autogenous tissue has a theoretical advantage of not inciting an immune response to foreign antigen, but this has not been a frequent problem with homologous scleral tissue. Periosteum and fascia lata are readily obtainable, durable, and very flexible. A disadvantage is that both require a second operative site with the attendant risks and morbidity.

Both fascia lata and periosteum grafts can be cut to fit any size or shape defect. A notch in the graft will allow it to be positioned around the rectus muscle insertion to cover ectatic sclera anterior and posterior to the muscle insertion. For an inaccessible, posterior lesion, it might be necessary to temporarily tag and sever the extraocular muscle to be resutured later.[57] Anteriorly the graft can be trimmed to fit flush with the limbus or beneath a limbus-based conjunctival flap. Suturing techniques can be similar to those used with banked scleral grafts, however, the more rapid incorporation of the graft allows the use of absorbable suture material. The flexibility of periosteum and fascia lata allows the surgeon to suture the graft in place under mild tension to reduce choroidal bulging in areas of ectatic sclera. When placing a graft along the edge of a rectus muscle tendon, the graft can be anchored to the tendon margin by two double-armed absorbable sutures (Fig. 13-20). Adequate suture placement in the graft is necessary to prevent migration.

A general surgeon's assistance is helpful for harvesting fascia lata and periosteum grafts. Autogenous fascia lata is obtained from the lateral thigh. After preparing and draping one side from the hip to the knee, a longitudinal skin incision is made at the beginning of the distal third of the lateral thigh. This is made 4–5 inches in length and dissected through subcutaneous tissues and fat down to the glistening, smooth, tendinous fascia lata. A section about 4 × 2 inches in size can be removed and the wound closed in two layers.[8,81]

For autogenous periosteum, one of the patient's legs is prepared in the sterile fashion from the knee to the foot. A large-cuff sphygmomanometer can be placed around the thigh and inflated to just over the systolic pressure to reduce the bleeding immediately prior to making an incision. An 8- to 10-cm vertical skin incision is made commencing at 8 cm distal to the anterior tibial tubercle and carried down to the level of the bone. A number 15-blade is used to outline a 7 cm × 2 cm strip of periosteum. A periosteal elevator is used to gradually free the periosteal strip from the tibial surface and scissors are used to complete the excision. The graft is kept moist in sterile saline-soaked gauze until used. The skin wound is closed in two layers and a penrose drain can be inserted.[14,45]

Other graft materials used, although not widely, include auricular cartilage[55,67] and aortic homografts.[54]

## GENERAL SURGICAL CONSIDERATIONS

In anticipation of surgery, systemic immunosuppression should be continued or implemented. Other preoperative measures should include systemic antibiotics to prevent infection and shielding of the eye to avoid direct pressure that could result in prolapse of intraocular contents. Analgesia and sedation, and perhaps a seventh nerve block, if necessary, can be used to reduce movement and blepharospasm,

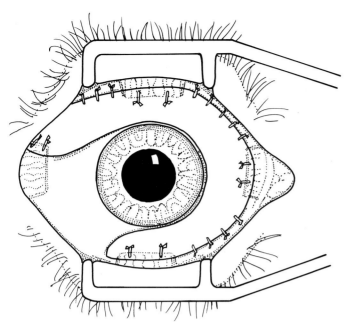

**Fig. 13-20.** Fascia lata has been anchored to the insertions of the four recti muscles and to the sclera with interrupted absorbable sutures. Note that the graft is larger than the underlying scleral defect. (Reprinted with permission from Bick MW: Surgical treatment of scleromalacia perforans, Arch Ophthalmol 61:907–917, 1959.)

thereby relieving unnecessary pressure on the globe. Preoperative administration of intravenous mannitol can be used to lower the intraocular pressure to reduce the risk of perforation when operating on an eye with ectatic sclera. General anesthesia is indicated to avoid possible scleral rupture from the pressure on the globe, which may be incurred from a retrobulbar injection. Blind passage of a superior rectus fixation suture should also be avoided. Proper positioning of the globe for surgical exposure can be achieved by placing one or two silk, peripheral corneal traction sutures.

At the end of the surgical procedure, a topical antibiotic, cycloplegic, and corticosteroid are instilled on the eye. Systemic immunosuppressant therapy should be continued. A pressure patch used initially will help keep the graft flat and reduce the possibility of hematoma formation at the operative site. Adequate control of postoperative intraocular pressure is important to prevent loosening and rupture of scleral sutures. Timolol or betaxolol and a carbonic anhydrase inhibitor, if necessary, should be used to treat pressure elevations.

## REFERENCES

1. Ahrendt N: Scleritis associated with central choroidal hemorrhage. Acta Ophthalmol 59:80–84. 1981
2. Alpren TVP, Hyndiuk RA, Davis SD, et al.: Cryotherapy for experimental *Pseudomonas* keratitis. Arch Ophthalmol 97:711–714, 1979
3. Armstrong K, McGovern VJ: Scleromalacia perforans with repair grafting. Trans Ophthalmol Soc Aust 15:110–121, 1955
4. Barr CC, Davis H, Culbertson WW: Rheumatoid scleritis. Ophthalmology 88:1269–1273, 1981
5. Benson WE, Shields JA, Tasman W, et al.: Posterior scleritis. A cause of diagnostic confusion. Arch Ophthalmol 97:1482–1486, 1979
6. Berger B, Reeser F: Retinal pigment epithelial detachments in posterior scleritis. Am J Ophthalmol 90:604–606, 1980
7. Berler DK, Apler MG: Scleral abcesses and ectasia caused by *Pseudomonas aeruginosa*. Ann Ophthalmol 14:665–667, 1982
8. Bick MW: Surgical treatment of scleromalacia perforans. Arch Ophthalmol 61:907–917, 1959
9. Billson FA, DeDombal FT, Watkinson G, et al.: Ocular complications of ulcerative colitis. Gut 8:102–106, 1967
10. Bloomfield SE, Mondino B, Gray GF: Scleral tuberculosis. Arch Ophthalmol 94:954–956, 1976.
11. Bloomfield SE, Becker CG, Christian CL, et al.: Bilateral necrotising scleritis with marginal corneal ulceration after cataract surgery in a patient with vasculitis. Br J Ophthalmol 64:170:170–174, 1980
12. Blum FG, Salamoun SG: Scleromalacia perforans: A useful surgical modification in fascia lata or scleral grafting. Arch Ophthalmol 69:287–289, 1963
13. Bourke BE, Moss IK, Mumford P, et al.: The complement fixing ability of putative circulating immune complexes in rheumatoid arthritis and its relationship to extra-articular disease. Clin Exp Immunol 48:726–732, 1982
14. Breslin CW, Katz JI, Kaufman HE: Surgical management of necrotizing scleritis. Arch Ophthalmol 95:2038–2040, 1977
15. Brown SI, Weller CA, Vidrich AM: Effect of corticosteroids on corneal collagenase of rabbits. Am J Ophthalmol 70:744–747, 1970
16. Brown SI, Rosen J: Scleral perforation; A complication of the soft contact lens. Arch Ophthalmol 93:1047–1048, 1975
17. Brubaker R, Font RL, Shepard EM: Granulomatous sclerouveitis; regression of ocular lesions with cyclophosphamide and prednisone. Arch Ophthalmol 86:517–524, 1971
18. Bullen CL, Leisegang TJ, McDonald TJ, et al.: Ocular complications of Wegener's granulomatosis. Ophthalmology 90:279–290, 1983
19. Burns RP: Pseudomonas aeruginosa keratitis: Mixed infections of the eye. Am J Ophthalmol 67:257–262, 1969
20. Cameron ME: The treatment of beta irradiation necrosis of the sclera. Aust J Ophthalmol 6:86–90, 1978
21. Cappin JM, Allen DW: Paralimbic scleromalacia; spontaneous scleral intercalary perforation. Br J Ophthalmol 57:871–872, 1973
22. Chumbley LC: Scleral involvement in symptomatic porphyria. Am J Ophthalmol 84:729–733, 1977
23. Cleary PE, Watson PG, McGill JI, et al.: Visual loss due to posterior segment disease in scleritis. Trans Ophthalmol Soc UK 95:297–300, 1975
24. Codere F, Brownstein S, Jackson WB: *Pseudomonas aeruginosa* scleritis. Am J Ophthalmol 91:706–710, 1981
25. Coutu RE, Klein M, Lessell S, et al.: Limited forms of Wegener's granulomatosis; eye involvement as a major sign. J Am Med Assoc 233:868–871, 1975
26. Eber CT: Fistula at limbus (Scleromalacia perforans). Am J Ophthalmol 17:921–923, 1934
27. Eiferman RA: Cryotherapy of *Pseudomonas* keratitis and scleritis. Arch Ophthalmol 97:1637–1639, 1979

28. Endoh M, Kaneshige H, Tomino Y, et al.: IgA nephropathy associated with myasthenia gravis and scleritis. Tokai J Exp Clin Med 6:421–425, 1981

29. Evans PJ, Eustace P: Scleromalacia perforans associated with Crohn's disease; treated with sodium versenate (EDTA). Br J Ophthalmol 57:330–335, 1973

30. Feldon SE, Sigelman J, Albert DM, et al.: Clinical manifestations of brawny scleritis. Am J Ophthalmol 85:781–787, 1978

31. Fisher E, Allen JH: Corneal ulcers produced by cell-free extracts of *Pseudomonas aeruginosa.* Am J Ophthalmol 46:21–27, 1958

32. Foster CS, Forstot SL, Wilson LA: Mortality rate in rheumatoid arthritis patients developing necrotizing scleritis or peripheral ulcerative keratitis; effects of systemic immunosuppression. Ophthalmology 91:1253–1263, 1984

33. Fraunfelder FT, Watson PG: Evaluation of eyes unucleated for scleritis. Br J Ophtlmol 60:227–230, 1976

34. Frayer WC: The histopatology of perilimbal ulceration in Wegener's granulomatous. Arch Ophthalmol 64:58–64, 1960

35. Haynes BF, Fishman ML, Fauci AS, et al.: The ocular manifestations of Wegener's granulomatosis; fifteen years experience and review of the literature. Am J Med 63:131–141, 1977

36. Jain IS, Gupta SD: Multiple scleral abcesses due to pseudomonas pyocyaneous. Orient Arch Opthalmol 7:326, 1969

37. Jampol LM, West C, Goldberg MF: Therapy of scleritis with cytotoxic agents. Am J Ophthalmol 86:266–271, 1978

38. Jayson MIV, Jones DEP: Scleritis and rhrumatoid arthritis. Ann Rheum Dis 30:343–348, 1971

39. Jayson MIV, Easty DL: Ulceration of the cornea in rheumatoid arthritis. Ann Rheum Dis 36:428–432, 1977

40. Joysey VC, Roger JH, Ashworth RF, et al.: Parallel studies of HLA antigens in patients with rheumatic heart disease and scleritis: Comparisons with three control populations. J Rheumatol [Suppl] 3:84–88, 1977

41. Kapoor S, Gupta AK, Sood M: An unusual case of scleral involvement by pseudomonas pyocyaneous. Indian J Ophthalmol 23:29–30, 1975

42. Kennedy AC, McGavin DDM: Rheumatoid scleritis producing exophthalmos. Br J Clin Pract 29:73–76, 1975

43. Kierlar RA: Exudative retinal detachment and scleritis in polyarteritis. Am J Ophthalmol 82:694–698, 1976

44. Knox DL, Schachat AP, Mustonen E: Primary, secondary and coincidental ocular complications of Crohn's disease. Ophthalmology 91:163–173, 1984

45. Koenig SB, Kaufman HE: The treatment of necrotizing scleritis with an autogenous periosteal graft. Ophthalmic Surg 14:1029–1032, 1983

46. Lachman SM, Hazelman BL, Watson PG: Scleritis and associated disease. Br Med J 1:88–90, 1978

47. Leveille AS, Morse PH: Combined detachments in Wegener's granulomatosis. Br J Ophthalmol 65:564–567, 1981

48. Long RG, Friedmann AI, James DG: Scleritis and temporal arteritis. Postgrad Med J 52:689–692, 1976

49. Lyne AJ, Pitkeathley DA: Episcleritis and scleritis; association with connective tissue disease. Arch Ophthalmol 80:171–176, 1968

50. Lyne AJ, Lloyd-Jones D: Necrotizing scleritis after ocular surgery. Trans Ophthalmol Soc UK 146:99–102, 1979

51. McAdam LP, O'Hanlan MA, Bluestone R, et al.: Relapsing polychondritis: Prospective study of 23 patients and a review of the literature. Medicine (Baltimore) 55:193–212, 1976

52. McGavin DDM, Williamson J, Forrester JV, et al.: Episcleritis and scleritis; a study of their clinical manifestations and association with rheumatoid arthritis. Br J Ophthalmol 60:192–226, 1976

53. Marushak D: Uveal effusion attending scleritis posterior; A case report with A-scan and B-scan echograms. Acta Ophthalmol 60:773–778, 1982

54. Merz EH: Scleral reinforcement with aortic tissue. Am J Ophthalmol 57:766–770, 1964

55. Nicholas MJG: Cure of a necrotic nodular scleritis by auricular cartilaginous graft. Bull Soc Ophthalmol Fr 72:981–982, 1972

56. Nomoto Y, Sakai H, Endoh M, et al.: Scleritis and IgA nephropathy. Arch Intern Med 140:783–785, 1980

57. Obear MF, Winter FC: Technique of overlay scleral homograft. Arch Ophthalmol 71:837–838, 1964

58. Oksala A, Koponen J: Choroidal detachment associated with scleritis—a case report with echograms. Ultrasound Med Biol 1:283–285, 1974

59. Ostler HB, Thygeson P: The ocular manifestations of Herpes zoster, varicella, infectious mononucleosis, and cytomegalovirus disease. Surv Ophthalmol 21:148–159, 1976

60. Paufique L, Moreau PG: La scleromalacie perforante aspect histologique traitement par greffe sclerale. Ann D'oculistique 186:1065–1076, 1953

61. Petrelli EA, McKinley M, Troncale FJ: Ocular manifestations of inflammatory bowel disease. Ann Ophthalmol 14:356–360, 1982

62. Quinlan MP, Hitchings RA: Angle-closure glaucoma secondary to posterior scleritis. Br J Ophthalmol 62:330–335, 1978

63. Raber IM, Laibson PR, Kurz GH, et al.: *Pseudomonas* corneoscleral ulcers. Am J Ophthalmol 92:353–362, 1981

64. Rao GN, Aquavella JV, Palumbo AJ: Periosteal graft in scleromalacia. Ophthalmic Surg 8:86–92, 1977

65. Rao NA, Hidayat AA: Pathogenesis of scleritis. ARVO Abstracts Invest Ophthalmol Vis Sci 22(Suppl):170, 1982

66. Rao NA, Marak GE, Hidayat AA: Necrotizing scleritis; a clinicopathologic study of 41 cases. Opthalmology 92:1542–1549, 1985

67. Renard G, Lelievre P, Mazel J: Scleromalacie perforante. Bull Mem Soc Fr Ophthalmol 66:243–251, 1953

68. Rosenthal JW, Willims GT: Scleromalacia perforans; as a complication of rheumatoid arthritis. Am J Ophthalmol 54:862–864, 1962

69. Saari M, Vuorre I, Kaila J, et al.: Family studies of ocular manifestations in arthritis. Can J Ophthalmol 13:144–151, 1978

70. Salamon SM, Mondino BJ, Zaidman GW: Peripheral corneal ulcers, conjunctival ulcers, and scleritis after cataract surgery. Am J Ophthalmol 93:334–337, 1982

71. Sevel D: Rheumatoid nodule of the sclera; (a type of necrogranulomatous scleritis). Trans Ophthalmol Soc UK 85:357–367, 1965

72. Sevel D: Necrogranulomatous scleritis; clinical and histologic features. Am J Ophthalmol 64:1125–1134, 1967

73. Sevel D: Necrogranulomatous scleritis; effects on the sclera of vascular deprivation. Br J Ophthalmol 52:453–460, 1968

74. Sevel D, Abramson A: Necrogranulomatous scleritis treated by an onlay scleral graft. Br J Ophthalmol 56:791–799, 1972

75. Stenson S, Brookner A, Rosenthal S: Bilateral endogenous

scleritis due to *Aspergillus oryzae*. Ann Ophthalmol 14:67–72, 1982

76. Stilma JS: Conjunctival excision or lamellar scleral autograft in 38 Mooren's ulcers from Sierra Leone. Br J Ophthalmol 67:475–478, 1983

77. Strimlan CV, Taswell HF, Kueppens F, et al.: HL-A antigens of patients with Wegener's granulomatosis. Tissue Antigens 11:129–131, 1978

78. Suie T, Taylor FW: The effect of cortisone on experimental pseudomonas corneal ulcers. Arch Ophthalmol 56:53–56, 1956

79. Taffet S, Carter GZ: The use of a fascia lata graft in the treatment of scleromalacia perforans. Am J Ophthalmol 52:693–696, 1961

80. Tarr KH, Constable IJ: Pseudomonas endophthalmitis associated with scleral necrosis. Br J Ophthalmol 64:676–679, 1980

81. Torchia RT, Dunn RE, Pease PJ: Fascia lata grafting in scleromalacia perforans; with lamellar corneal-scleral dissection. Am J Ophthalmol 66:705–709, 1968

82. Van der Hoeve J: Scleromalacia perforans. Arch Ophthalmol 11:111–118, 1934

83. Watson PG, Hayreh SS: Scleritis and episcleritis. Br J Ophthalmol 60:163–191, 1976

84. Watson PG, Hazelman BL: The sclera and systemic disorders. London: WB Saunders, 1976, pp 122–123, 409–410

85. Watson PG: Diseases of the sclera and episclera, in Duane TE (ed): Clinical Ophthalmology, vol 4. pp 1–39 Philadelphia, Harper and Row, 1979, pp 1–39

86. Watson PG: the diagnosis and management of scleritis. Ophthalmology 87:716–720, 1980

87. Watson PG: The nature and the treatment of scleral inflammation. Trans Ophthalmol Soc UK 102:257–281, 1982

88. Womak LW, Leisegang TJ: Complications of Herpes zoster ophthalmicus. Arch Ophthalmol 101:42–45, 1983

89. Yeo JH, Jakobiec FA, Iwamoto T, et al.: metastatic carcinoma masquerading as scleritis. Ophthalmology 90:184–194, 1983

90. Young RD, Watson PG: Microscopical studies of necrotising scleritis I. cellular aspects. Br J Ophthalmol 68:770–780, 1984

91. Zer I. Machtey I, Kurz O: Combined treatment of scleromalacia perforans in rheumatoid arthritis with penicillamine and plastic surgery. Ophthalmologica 166:293–300, 1973

# 14

# Management of Endophthalmitis

## William W. Culbertson          Harry W. Flynn, Jr.

Microbial endophthalmitis is a bacterial or fungal infection of the intraocular tissues that often results in severe visual loss. Although the exact nationwide incidence of endophthalmitis is unknown, we have estimated that endophthalmitis develops once following every 1000 routine cataract extractions performed in South Florida. Modern surgical techniques have probably decreased the likelihood of endophthalmitis following intraocular surgery. Increasing numbers of cases are, however, being referred to eye centers each year, probably because of an absolute increase in the amount of cataract surgery being performed nationwide.

Although much has been learned in recent years regarding the frequency of isolation of specific organisms causing endophthalmitis in various settings, there have been no properly randomized clinical trials comparing various treatment modalities (i.e., intraocular versus subconjunctival antibiotics, intraocular antibiotics and vitrectomy versus intraocular antibiotics alone, etc.). As a result, generally accepted treatment regimens are empirically derived formulas based on animal laboratory experiments and retrospective clinical reviews of human cases.

## PATHOGENESIS OF ENDOPHTHALMITIS

The infectious organism in endophthalmitis may originate from outside the eye (exogenous endophthalmitis) or from the blood stream (endogenous endophthalmitis). Exogenous endophthalmitis most commonly follows recent intraocular surgery such as cataract extraction, secondary intraocular lens implants, penetrating keratoplasty or pars plana vitrectomy. Virtually any procedure in which a potential pathway, however trivial, exists from outside to inside the eye may result in endophthalmitis including radial keratotomy, suture removal, surgical capsulotomy, or peripheral iridectomy. Endogenous endophthalmitis develops when organisms gain access to the blood stream, usually from intravenous lines.

The frequency of organisms isolated in cases of suspected postoperative endophthalmitis at the Bascom Palmer Eye Institute are listed in Table 14-1 along with their visual outcomes following treatment.[4,7] In general, the severity and rapidity of onset of postoperative endophthalmitis correlates with the type of organism causing the endophthalmitis. Typically, Gram-negative bacteria, *Streptoccus, Pneumococcus,* and *Staphylococcus aureus* cause a rapidly progressive virulent presentation within 2–4 days after surgery. Endophthalmitis caused by *Staphylococcus epidermidis* and some *Staphylococcus aureus* variants have a less toxic, less virulent, delayed onset 7–21 days after surgery. Fungal endophthalmitis has a slowly progressive course with a clinical onset 1–3 months postoperatively. Persistent intraocular anaerobic bacteria (*Propioniobacterium acni*) may cause a smoldering endophthalmitis persisting 6–12 months after surgery.

Another type of exogenous endophthalmitis occurs when bacteria enter the eye through an intact or leaking, thin-walled, conjunctival filtering bleb (Fig. 14-1).[5] The majority of cases of "through-the-bleb" endophthalmitis are caused by *streptococcus* and *hemophilus* species. The presence of an intact lens-zonular diaphragm does not appear to protect the vitreous cavity from infection in these cases. The ophthalmologist must suspect that endophthalmitis exists if otherwise unexplained intraocular inflammation develops in the presence of a filtering bleb.

Endophthalmitis may also complicate penetrating trauma such as a laceration or puncture of the globe by any object at any velocity.[1,2,6] The risk of infection is apparently greatest when the object is organic (such as a thorn) or has been in contact with organic material, soil, or water from a lake or stream. The visual prognosis in traumatic endophthalmitis is poor, probably as a result of a combination of several factors including delayed recognition, the intrinsic effects of the injury, the virulence of the organisms involved, and the potential for mixed infections. The most common organisms in traumatic endophthalmitis are *Staphylococcus, Streptococcus,* and *Bacillus* species.

SURGICAL INTERVENTION IN CORNEAL AND EXTERNAL DISEASES
ISBN 0-8089-1850-8

**Table 14-1**
Final Visual Results versus Culture Results:
Bascom Palmer Eye Institute Experience

| Organism | Percentage of Patients with 20/200 or Better |
|---|---|
| S. epidermidis | 75 |
| S. aureus | 45 |
| Streptococcus species | 25 |
| Gram negative | 10 |
| Culture negative ("Sterile") | 90 |

Microbial keratitis is a rare cause of endogenous endophthalmitis. Endophthalmitis only occurs in bacterial keratitis when the cornea perforates without effective topical antibiotic therapy. Corneal perforations occurring in bacterial keratitis after intensive topical antibiotic therapy do not result in endophthalmitis. Bacterial endophthalmitis does not occur in bacterial keratitis when there has not been a perforation. In contrast, fungal endophthalmitis may develop in fungal keratitis with or without perforation. This is because of the poor penetration of topical antifungal agents in deep fungal keratitis and because of the apparent ability of fungi to penetrate Descemet's membrane. In fungal keratitis, inflammation in the anterior chamber can be quite severe and should not be interpreted as a definite indication of progression of keratitis to endophthalmitis.

Endogenous endophthalmitis is most often the result of hematogenous fungal dissemination following in-dwelling intravenous lines for hyperalimentation or drug administration, the use of contaminated needles by drug addicts or following prolonged treatment of complications of major surgery in a debilitated patient.[3,8] The most common organism is candida species. Bacteria, usually streptococcus, staphylococcus or bacillus cereus are rare causes of endogenous endophthalmitis, typically occurring in the septicemic patient, in microbial endocarditis, following dental work, or in intravenous drug abusers. The organism circulates to the uveal tract or retina creating a focal area of inflammation, which may be observed ophthalmoscopically as a localized area of choroiditis or retinitis. The infection may extend into the vitreous gel causing true endophthalmitis or may be contained in the retina or uveal tract with sterile vitreous inflammation only.

Endophthalmitis occurs when organisms gain access to and proliferate within the vitreous gel. The interior of the eye, especially the vitreous cavity, has very limited defenses against microbial invaders. In fact, the vitreous gel itself may actively support the growth of microorganisms much as a bacterial culture media would. Leukocytes enter the vitreous in response to the infection and a purulent vitreous abscess may quickly form. Although the lens-zonular or posterior capsule-zonular membrane may provide some relative theoretical protection against microbial invasion of the vitreous from the anterior chamber, it is not enough to noticeably alter the incidence of endophthalmitis following extracapsular cataract extraction.

Visual loss and ocular injury in endophthalmitis are the combined results of the organisms's natural toxicity, the inflammation produced by the eye in response to the presence of the organism, and the side effects of the treatment of the infection by the ophthalmologist. The damage produced by the organism itself is the result of its own enzymes, proteases, collagenases and toxins as typified in *pseudomonas, serratia, proteus, staphylococcus aureus,* and *bacillus cereus endophthalmitis.* Polymorphonuclear leukocytes that are attracted by bacteria or fungi also produce collagenase. Tissue necrosis and vascular thrombosis are the result. Even when an eye with bacterial endophthalmitis has been sterilized by antibiotics, the toxic and enzymatic destructive factors produced by the bacteria and polymorphonuclear leukocytes continue to damage the eye. Once the eye has been successfully sterilized and the acute inflammation resolves, visual function may be compromised or lost by a combination of corneal opacification, glaucoma, retinal detachment, toxic retinal damage, or phthisis bulbi.

An important factor contributing to the ocular damage in endophthalmitis is the result of the adverse consequences of the treatment required to sterilize the eye. Intraocular antibiotics are relatively safe when given once in the proper dosages, but the cumulative retinotoxic effect of antibiotic injections into the inflamed eye is uncertain. Removing the vitreous may expose the retina to higher, more toxic, concentrations of antibiotic. In addition, vitrectomy performed in an inflamed endophthalmitis eye is usually more difficult because of compromised visibility and because of the presence of partially necrotic retina. These factors increase the risk for intraoperative hemorrhage or retinal detachment and consequent visual loss as compared to vitrectomy performed in a noninflamed eye with clear media.

## PREVENTION OF ENDOPHTHALMITIS

Awareness of the sources of microbial contamination in intraocular surgery may help to prevent some cases of endophthalmitis. In postoperative endophthalmitis, the

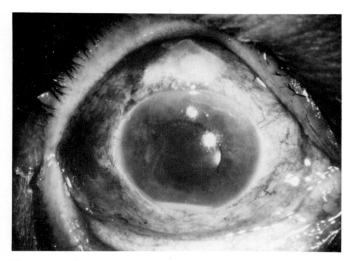

**Fig. 14-1.** Strep viridans endophthalmitis associated with a thin-walled glaucoma filtering bleb in a pseudophakic eye. Note the hypopyon in the bleb and in the anterior chamber.

organism may be present on the conjunctiva or lid and is washed into the eye at the time of surgery. Certain conditions contribute to the likelihood of pathogenic flora being present on the eye, including cicatricial conjunctival or lid disease, lacrimal drainage obstruction, conjunctival surface disease, chronic staphylococcal blepharitis, or the presence of a prosthesis in the other eye. Advanced age, debilitation, or poor personal hygiene are also contributory factors. Nonocular infection sources such as pharyngitis, otitis media, skin abscesses, or genitourinary infections can be foci for dis semination of bacteria to the region of the eye. Intraocular surgery should not be undertaken in a patient with possible bacterial conjunctivitis, keratitis, dacryocystitis, or rhinopharyngitis.

Patients with any of the underlying predisposing ocular abnormalities listed above should have preoperative cultures taken of the lids and conjunctiva of both eyes. The appropriate antibiotics are given topically and/or systemically to eradicate the infection. Posttreatment cultures of the lids and conjunctiva should be obtained prior to surgery to confirm sterility.

The routine use of preoperative topical antibiotics to reduce indigenous bacterial flora is controversial. Gentamicin or tobramycin drops may be given prophylactically four times a day beginning 3 days prior to surgery, but their efficacy is uncertain. More prolonged use of topical antibiotics could result in the emergence of resistant strains. Many ophthalmologists give subconjunctival prophylactic antibiotics either before or after intraocular surgery. A good choice is 20 mg of gentamicin for Gram-negative and sensitive Gram-positive coverage and 100 mg of cefazolin for *staphylococcus* or *streptococcus* coverage. If subconjunctival corticosteroids are also given, local allergic phenomena are unlikely. Either of these antibiotics should not be given if allergy to the drug or to a cross-reacting drug is known. Subconjunctival injections always carry the remote risk of scleral perforation so the ophthalmologist should weigh the risk versus the benefit.

Preoperative and intraoperative attention to technique designed to restrict access of bacteria to the conjunctival fornix and to the anterior chamber makes sense. The lid margin can be isolated from the conjunctival fornix by curving the edge of the plastic drape around the upper and lower lid margin with the lid speculum. The conjunctival fornix should be kept dry enough during surgery so that fluid does not wash in and out of the anterior chamber. Micropore filters can be used for any fluids injected inside the eye. Intraocular manipulation and fluid injections should be minimized. Another potential source of microbial organisms is contaminated instruments or fluids. Use of disposable fluids or medications in multiple patients should not be allowed because of possible cross-contamination between patients.

An uncommon, possibly preventable cause of endophthalmitis is suture removal. Sutures should not be removed if keratitis surrounds the suture, or if conjunctivitis is suspected. Instruments used to remove sutures in the office should be sterile.

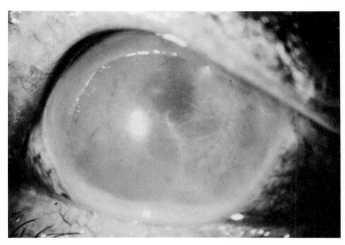

**Fig. 14-2.** Staph aureus endophthalmitis 4 days following ECCE with posterior chamber implant. Note the hazy cornea, hypopyon, fibrinoid exudate and vitreitis.

## DIAGNOSIS

Endophthalmitis is suspected in susceptible patients based on typical symptoms and ocular findings. The most common symptom is decreasing vision. Pain is an inconsistent symptom and the diagnosis of endophthalmitis should not depend on its presence or absence.

Patients with endophthalmitis usually demonstrate reduced visual acuity, a hypopyon, and vitreitis (Fig. 14-2). Visual acuity may deteriorate rapidly from better than 20/100 in the morning to light perception or worse by afternoon due to increasing vitreitis. The red reflex may be lost and the cornea may become opaque. When the retina can be visualized, multiple intraretinal petechial hemorrhages are an early finding.

Early diagnosis and prompt treatment are the most important factors in the management of endophthalmitis. Visual outcome following treatment of postoperative endophthalmitis is dependent on the virulence of the infecting organism, the rapidity of treatment, and the type of treatment in order of decreasing importance. Ophthalmologists have no control over the identity and virulence of the organism. They can only control the rapidity and type of treatment administered. By educating the postoperative patient to return for immediate examination in the event of decreasing vision or increasing pain, possible cases of endophthalmitis may be diagnosed earlier and treatment initiated. Timing a routine postoperative examination on the third or fourth postoperative day is also a useful screening exam for early signs of the more virulent types of endophthalmitis. In general, the more toxic and virulent organisms produce earlier and more rapidly progressive endophthalmitis presenting typically on the second to third postoperative day.

## TREATMENT

Any patient who develops decreased vision, a hypopyon, and vitreitis following any intraocular procedure must be suspected as having bacterial or fungal endophthalmitis until proven otherwise. The adverse visual consequences that result from delay in treatment with intraocular antibiotics are far greater than the potential hazards of therapy including intraocular antibiotic injection. Intraocular antibiotic injections and sterilization of the interior of the eye are essential features of therapy. In contrast to the treatment of bacterial keratitis, initial identification of the infecting organism is of less importance in managing endophthalmitis. If the eye is not sterilized with the first antibiotic injection, by the time the organism is identified on culture and antibiotic sensitivity is obtained (24–36 hours), serious further visual loss and ocular damage has occurred. Broad-spectrum intraocular bacteriocidal antibiotics should be given intravitreally initially after aqueous and vitreous have been obtained for culture. Intraocular antibiotic treatment of the patient should not be delayed in order to transfer the patient to a referral center for vitrectomy, for instance. An ophthalmologist who is capable of performing intraocular surgery is usually capable of safely performing an anterior chamber and vitreous paracentesis for culture purposes and injecting intraocular antibiotics.

## OBTAINING THE CULTURES

At the Bascom Palmer Eye Institute, all patients suspected of having bacterial or fungal endophthalmitis have lid and conjunctival cultures performed. Patients with relatively good vision (20/200 or better), a good red reflex, minimal to moderate vitreitis, and a slowly progressive course usually undergo a diagnostic aqueous or vitreous paracentesis with injection of intravitreal and subconjunctival antibiotics alone without vitrectomy. This may be performed either in the office or the operating room. A 25-gauge 5/8-inch needle on a 1.0-cc syringe is passed through the limbus into the anterior chamber and 0.2 cc of aqueous is aspirated for culture purposes. The anterior chamber is reformed with balanced salt solution. Similarly, a 23-gauge needle is introduced into the vitreous cavity through the pars plana 3.5 mm posterior to the limbus and 0.2 cc of liquid vitreous is aspirated and cultured. If vitreous cannot be aspirated with a 23-gauge needle, then a 21-gauge or larger needle is passed through the scleral puncture site. If vitreous cannot be aspirated through the needle, a small-diameter vitrectomy instrument is introduced through the same sclerotomy. Using minimal infusion, 0.2–0.3 cc of solid vitreous is aspirated. If a therapeutic pars plana vitrectomy is considered, an infusion cannula is sutured in place. The entire vitrectomy aspirate is collected for later culture.

Two to three drops of undiluted aqueous and vitreous samples obtained by simple paracentesis are dropped directly onto the solid culture media, and onto two clean microscopic slides for Gram and Giemsa stains. Drops are placed on blood agar, chocolate agar in a $CO_2$ jar, and thioglycolate broth and are incubated at 37° for bacterial isolation. Drops are also placed on blood agar and Saboraud's agar (without cyclohexamide inhibitor) at 25°C (room temperature) for fungal isolation. These slides and culture plates can be then taken to the hospital microbiology laboratory for incubation, identification, and antibiotic sensitivity assay. If a pars plana vitrectomy has been performed, the syringes of vitreous aspirate may then be concentrated by suctioning the aspirate through 0.45 micron pore-size filter paper. The microorganisms are collected on the top of this filter paper, which can be cut into sections and placed face up, directly on the culture material. Bacterial colonies grow at the edge and on the top of the filter paper. Alternately, drops of the vitreous aspirate can be placed directly on the culture plates without concentration but the yield of organisms will not be as high. Antibiotics are injected intraocularly immediately after the vitreous and aqueous samples are obtained. The Gram and Giemsa stains are reviewed but the initial antibiotic injection is not delayed for the stain results. In suspected endogenous endophthalmitis, blood cultures and medical consultations should be obtained.

## VITRECTOMY IN ENDOPHTHALMITIS

The efficacy of vitrectomy in suspected bacterial or fungal endophthalmitis has not been established in a control trial. Cases that initially undergo vitrectomy in published studies are typically more severe than the nonvitrectomized cases, so the effect of the vitrectomy alone cannot be established.[1-2] We have reserved vitrectomy for rapidly progressive cases with severe inflammation, dense vitreous infiltration, and vision of hand movements or worse. Less severe cases have anterior chamber and vitreous paracenteses and intraocular antibiotics are injected but do not undergo vitrectomy as a part of their initial therapy. If the eye shows distinctly more inflammation 24–36 hours after antibiotic injection, however, then therapeutic vitrectomy, reculturing and reinjection of antibiotics are considered.

Vitrectomy has the advantages of mechanically removing toxic debris, providing a larger quantity of vitreous for culture, permitting better antibiotic distribution, facilitating repeat vitreous paracentesis, and accelerating clearance of the vitreous cavity. Vitrectomy in severely inflamed endophthalmitis eyes with semiopaque media is, however, technically difficult and the risk of intraoperative complications is high. In addition to possibly delaying treatment, other technical difficulties of vitrectomy include limited visualization, intraoperative retinal detachment due to necrotic retina, and intraocular bleeding from sclerotomy sites in congested eyes. Vitreous surgeons with previous experience in vitrectomy in endophthalmitis are desirable but may not be readily available. The delay in referral to an experienced vitrectomy surgeon and in arranging for an operating room may negate any theoretical advantage of vitrectomy. Because pars plana vitrectomy in eyes with endophthalmitis is a hazardous procedure, this surgery should be performed only by an experienced posterior segment surgeon. This should not be the first vitrectomy performed by an anterior segment surgeon.

The ophthalmologist performing the vitrectomy must decide if the view through the anterior segment of the eye is adequate for visualization of the vitreous cavity during the procedure. Occasionally, fibrin debris accumulates in the pupil on the implant surface and must be periodically removed using irrigation in a sweeping motion with a cannula inserted through the limbus. The pars plana vitrectomy should begin in the anterior central vitreous cavity. Often, after the central vitreous has been removed, the retina can be visualized and the vitrectomy safely completed. If the retina cannot be visualized after the central vitreous cavity has been cleared, however, complete removal of the posterior cortical vitreous should not be attempted. If retinal detachment occurs during the course of vitrectomy for endophthalmitis, the prognosis for retinal reattachment is very poor. The vitrectomy in endophthalmitis cases should be performed quickly and the eye closed as rapidly as possible because of the bleeding hazards induced by low or negative intraocular pressure in a severely inflamed eye. When the eye is closed, 0.2 cc of vitreous fluid is aspirated and intraocular antibiotics are injected.

If corneal opacification impairs adequate visualization for a pars plana vitrectomy, an open sky vitrectomy can be considered. These eyes are usually severely inflamed with an extremely poor prognosis whatever the treatment. A 270° limbal incision is made and the cornea is retracted. The implant is removed and a central vitrectomy is quickly performed without infusion. The side wall of the eye tends to collapse especially in younger patients and careful avoidance of the retina is required during the procedure. After the central vitreous is removed, the limbal incision is closed, and the globe is reformed with infusion solution. The 0.2 cc of fluid is aspirated and antibiotics are injected into the central vitreous cavity through the limbal incision.

The presence of an intraocular lens does not appear to adversely affect the outcome of endophthalmitis treatment. But intraocular lenses should be removed if they interfere with the performance of the vitrectomy.

## ANTIBIOTICS

The selection of antibiotics to be used in treating suspected cases of endophthalmitis is based primarily on the specific clinical setting in which endophthalmitis has occurred. The goal is to sterilize the intraocular space as soon as possible with adequate doses of antibiotics to which most of the common endophthalmitis organisms are sensitive. A minimum of 30–36 hours usually elapses between the time the vitreous is initially cultured and antibiotic sensitivities are eventually obtained. During this time, progressive intraocular damage occurs if the offending organism was not sensitive to the originally injected antibiotics. In postoperative endophthalmitis, the most common organisms isolated are *Staphylococcus epidermidis, Staphylococcus aureus, proteus,* and *Pseudomonas.*

**Table 14-2**
Preparation of Intraocular Antibiotics

Gentamicin Sulfate: 0.1 mg in 0.1 ml
1. Withdraw 0.1 ml (4 mg) from a fresh vial of gentamicin sulfate for injection (40 mg/ml).
2. Add to this 3.9 ml sterile saline.
3. 4.0 ml of this solution contains 4 mg gentamicin sulfate and 0.1 ml contains 0.1 mg.
4. Slowly inject 0.1 ml of this solution into the vitreous cavity.

Cefazolin Sodium: 2.25 mg in 0.1 ml
1. Reconstitute the powder in a 500-mg vial using 2.0 ml of sterile saline.
2. Withdraw 1.0 ml of this solution (containing 225 mg cefazolin) and dilute up to 10 ml with sterile saline.
3. 10 ml of this solution thus contains 225 mg cefazolin and 0.1 ml contains 2.25 mg.
4. Slowly inject 0.1 ml of this solution into the vitreous cavity.

Vancomycin Hydrochloride: 1.0 mg in 0.1 ml
1. Reconstitute the powder in a 500-mg vial using 10 ml of sterile saline.
2. Withdraw 2.0 ml of this solution (containing 100 mg vancomycin) and dilute up to 10 ml with sterile saline.
3. 10 ml of this solution thus contains 100 mg of vancomycin and 0.1 ml contains 1.0 mg.
4. Slowly inject 0.1 ml of this solution into the vitreous cavity.

Clindamycin Phosphate: 1.0 mg in 0.1 ml
1. Withdraw 0.2 (30 mg) from a fresh vial of clindamycin phosphate for injection (150 mg/ml).
2. Add to this 2.8 ml sterile saline.
3. 3.0 ml of this solution contains 30 mg clindamycin phosphate and 0.1 ml contains 1.0 mg.
4. Slowly inject 0.1 ml of this solution into the vitreous cavity.

Amphotericin B:
1. Reconstitute the powder in a 50-mg vial using 10 ml of sterile nonbacteriostatic water.
2. Withdraw 0.1 ml of this solution and dilute up to 10 ml.
3. 10 ml of this solution thus contains 5 mg of Amphotericin-B and 0.1 ml contains .005 mg.
4. Slowly inject 0.1 ml of this solution into the vitreous cavity.

Gentamicin and cefazolin are chosen for initial antibiotic treatment because 95 percent of bacteria isolated in postoperative cases at the Bascom Palmer Eye institute have been sensitive to one or both of these antibiotics. Gentamicin 0.1–0.4 mg is given intravitreally and 20 mg of gentamicin is given subconjunctivally for Gram-negative coverage. Cefazolin 2.25 mg is given intravitreally and 100 mg is given subconjunctivally for Gram-positive coverage. Vancomycin, 1.0 mg intravitreally and 25 mg subconjunctivally may be substituted for cefazolin in patients with histories of allergy to either penicillins or cephalosporins. Preparation of antibiotics for intraocular use is listed in Table 14-2.

In cases of endophthalmitis associated with filtering blebs, the most common organisms are streptococcus species and hemophilus influenzae. Vancomycin, 1.0 mg intravitreally and 25 mg subconjunctivally may be substituted for cefazolin for optimal coverage of streptococcal species. Hemophilus influenzae are usually sensitive to gentamicin.

In posttraumatic endophthalmitis, *bacillus* species, *staphylococcus epidermidis,* Gram-negative organisms, streptococci, and fungi are seen. Clindamycin, 0.5–1.0 mg intravitreally and 50 mg subconjunctivally can be substituted for cefazolin for optimal *bacillus* species coverage and for gram-positive coverage. Gentamicin, 0.1–0.4 mg intravitreally and 20 mg subconjunctivally is given for Gram-negative coverage.

Amphotericin, 0.005 mcg is given intravitreally in cases in which a fungal organism has been isolated in culture, seen on smear, or when fungal endophthalmitis is *highly* suspected on clinical grounds.

Usually the vitreous cavity is sterilized after the first antibiotic injection and repeated taps and antibiotic injections are unnecessary. Intravitreal antibiotics are reinjected after 24–36 hours if an organism is cultured which is resistant to the antibiotic already injected or if the eye looks decidedly more inflamed after 24 hours. Repeat vitreous aspiration is performed at the time of repeat intraocular antibiotic injection.

Topical and intravenous antibiotics are of limited benefit in the management of exogenous endophthalmitis. The quantity of antibiotic that penetrates the eye by these routes is low when compared to intraocular and subconjunctival administration. Endophthalmitis cannot be treated with topical or intravenous antibiotics alone although intravenous antibiotics may help to maintain vitreous antibiotic levels after intraocular antibiotic administration. If an ongoing bacteremia or fungemia is suspected in endogenous endophthalmitis, the appropriate intravenous antibiotic should be given based on blood and vitreous culture results.

## CORTICOSTEROIDS

Topical, periocular, and intraocular corticosteroids may be used to suppress intraocular inflammation in bacterial endophthalmitis. Topical corticosteroids such as 1% prednisolone acetate may be given hourly after intraocular antibiotic injection. Triamcinolone, 20 mg may be injected subconjunctivally or as a posterior sub-Tenon's injection. In very severe cases of endophthalmitis, consideration should be given to the use of intraocular dexamethasone, 0.4 mg in 0.1 cc, at the termination of the vitrectomy.

## DIFFERENTIAL DIAGNOSIS

Several clinical disorders simulate endophthalmitis because they produce eye pain, decreased vision, and hypopyon. The most common example is bacterial keratitis in which a corneal ulcer with a corneal stromal infiltrate is associated with an hypopyon and inflammatory cells in the vitreous. Although bacterial corneal ulcers are usually associated with hypopya, they only *rarely* develop endophthalmitis even following corneal perforations. Eyes with pre-

sumed bacterial corneal ulcers should never be tapped because of the potential for the introduction of bacteria inside the eye. Occasional cases of deep fungal keratitis penetrate into the anterior chamber through the cornea after an extended period. Anterior chamber paracentesis may be required to establish the diagnosis in these cases.

A postoperative hyphema in the anterior chamber mixed with fibrin occasionally simulates a hypopyon. The bright red tinge of the hyphema and the absence of vitreitis differentiates this from endophthalmitis.

Infectious pseudomonas scleritis, especially when it occurs postoperatively, may present similarly to endophthalmitis with pain and a hypopyon. Careful examination of the sclera in the incision area shows necrotic, very tender sclera and abnormal thickening of the conjunctiva. Patients with this condition have severe pain radiating to the parietal area and minimal vitreitis.

Patients with a previous history of uveitis often have excessive intraocular inflammation immediately postoperatively with fibrin and cells in the anterior chamber and cells in the vitreous. The inflammation is expected, nonprogressive, and suppressible with topical corticosteroids in contrast to true infectious endophthalmitis.

## CONCLUSION

Microbial endophthalmitis is a vision-threatening disease, which is ideally managed through early recognition and prompt treatment with intraocular antibiotic injections. Vitrectomy is probably helpful in severe progressive cases. Some cases are possibly preventable by identification of high-risk eyes and prophylactic preoperative sterilization of these eyes.

## REFERENCES

1. Affeldt JC, Forster RK, Mandelbaum S, et al.: Traumatic endophthalmitis. Ophthalmology (in press) 1986
2. Brinton GS, Topping TM, Hyndiuk RA, et al.: Post-traumatic endophthalmitis. Arch Ophthalmol 102:547–550, 1984
3. Edmunds JE, Foos RY, Mongtomerie JZ, et al.: Ocular manifestations of Candida septicemia: Review of seventy-six cases of hematogenous Candida endophthalmitis. Medicine 53:47–75, 1974
4. Forster RK, Abbott RL, Gelender H: Management of infectious endophthalmitis. Ophthalmology 87:313–318, 1980
5. Mandelbaum S, Forster RK, Gelender H, et al.: Late onset endophthalmitis associated with filtering blebs. Ophthalmology 92:945–972, 1985
6. O'Day DM, Smith RS, Gregg CR, et al.: The problem of bacillus species infection with special emphasis on the virulence of bacillus cereus. Ophthalmology 88:833–838, 1981
7. Olson JC, Flynn HW Jr, Forster RK, et al.: Results in the treatment of postoperative endophthalmitis. Ophthalmology 90:692–699, 1983
8. Parke DW, Jones DB, Gentry LO: Endogenous endophthalmitis among patients with candidemia. Ophthalmology 89:789–796, 1982

# Index

Page numbers in *italics* indicate illustrations.
Page numbers followed by *t* indicate tables.

Acanthamoeba keratitis, corneal perforations in, 116–117
Actinic keratosis of eyelids, 18
Adenocarcinoma, mucinous, of eyelid, 22
Adenomas, sebaceous, of eyelid, 21
Adhesives, tissue, for noninfected corneal perforations, 89–93. *See also* Tissue adhesives for noninfected corneal perforations
Alkali-burned cornea, chronic corneal epithelial defects in, 61
Amphotericin B for endophthalmitis, 193*t*, 194
Antibiotics
  for endophthalmitis, 193–194
  for scleritis, 180
Aphakic corneal edema
  with hyaloid face intact, surgery for, 76
  with loose vitreous in anterior chamber, surgery for, 76
  penetrating keratoplasty for, 72–76
Ascorbic acid for chemical burns, 167
Avulsion of pterygium, 144–145

Bacterial keratitis, corneal perforations from, 107–110
Bacterial scleritis, corneal perforations from, 110
Bandage lenses, soft, for chemical burns, 167
Basal cell epitheliomas of eyelid, 19–20
Beta radiation after pterygium excision, 151
Bilateral acquired melanosis of conjunctiva and cornea, 130
Biopsy
  in eyelid lesion evaluation, 13, *14*
  in scleritis evaluation, 178–179
Bowen's disease of eyelid, 20–21
Bromhexine hydrochloride for keratoconjunctivitis sicca, 53
Burns
  alkali of cornea, chronic corneal epithelial defects from, 61
  chemical, 164–168. *See also* Chemical burns, mucous membrane abnormalities

Canthus
  lateral, defects of, repair of, *38–39,* 40
  medial, defects of, repair of, 27, *36–37,* 40
Carbonic anhydrase inhibitors for chemical burns, 166

Carcinoma
  meibomian gland, of eyelid, 21–22
  mucoepidermoid, of conjunctiva, 128–129
  spindle-cell, of conjunctiva, 129
  squamous cell
    of conjunctiva, 122–127, 128
    of cornea, 128
Cautery, thermal
  chronic corneal epithelial defects from, 61
  for superior limbic keratoconjunctivitis, 156, *158*
Cefazolin for endophthalmitis, 193
Chalazion, 14–15, *16*
Chemical burns, 164–168. *See also* Mucous membrane abnormalities
  clinical manifestations of, 164–165
  control of ulceration via chemical mediators for, 165–166
  intraocular pressure response to, 166
  treatment of, 166–168
Cicatricial pemphigoid, 159–161. *See also* Mucous membrane abnormalities
Clindamycin for endophthalmitis, 193*t*, 194
Collagenase inhibitors for chemical burns, 167
Comedo of eyelids, 23
Conjunctiva
  acquired melanosis of
    bilateral, 130
    primary, 130–132
  closure techniques for, for pterygium, 147
  grafts of
    for pterygium excision closure, 147–148, *149*
    for scleritis, 181–182
  intraepithelial neoplasia of, 121–127
    diagnosis of, 123
    treatment of, 123–127
  lymphoid hyperplasia of, 136
  malignant lymphomas of, 136–137
  malignant melanoma of, 133–136
  melanotic tumors of, 129–136
  mucoepidermoid carcinoma of, 128–129
  nevi of, 129–130
  papillomas of, 120–121, *122*
  recession and resection of, for superior limbic keratoconjunctivitis, 156, *157*
  resection of, for corneal perforations, 104–105
  shrinkage of, essential, 159–161. *See also* Mucous membrane abnormalities
  soft-tissue tumors of, 136–137
  spindle-cell carcinoma of, 129
  squamous cell carcinoma of, 122–127, 128

  transplantation of, for mucous membrane abnormalities, 169–171, *172*
  transplantation of, for recurrent/chronic corneal epithelial defects, 63
Conjunctival flaps
  for corneal edema, 81–84
  for exposure keratitis, 48–49
  for fungal keratitis, 115
  for noninfected corneal perforations, 102–103
  for recurrent/chronic corneal epithelial defects, 64–65
  for scleritis, 181–182
Contact lenses
  therapeutic
    for corneal edema, 71–72
    for exposure keratitis, 45
    in keratoconjunctivitis sicca, 53–54
    for noninfected corneal perforations, 88–89
    for recurrent/chronic corneal epithelial defects, 62
    for superior limbic keratoconjunctivitis, 156
Cornea
  acquired melanosis of, bilateral, 130
  alkali-burned, chronic corneal epithelial defects from, 61
  dystrophies of, recurrent corneal erosions from, 61
  edema of, 69–85. *See also* Edema, corneal
  epithelial defects of, recurrent and chronic, 59–66
    clinical conditions associated with, 60–61
    definition of, 59
    pathogenesis of, basic, 59–60
    therapy of
      medical, 61–63
      surgical, 63–66
  erosion of, recurrent, definition of, 59
  hydration of, regulation of, corneal edema and, 69, *70*
  infiltrates of, complicating, tissue adhesives, 93
  intraepithelial neoplasia of, 127–128
  lamellar graft of, for pterygium excision closure, 148, *150*
  perforations of, 87–118. *See also* Perforations, corneal
  squamous cell carcinoma of, 128
  transplantation of, for mucous membrane abnormalities, 172–173
  ulceration of, from chemical burns, control of, via chemical mediators, 165–166